Copyright statement

HEALTHY BUSINESS TRAVEL

*The essential guide to
Gatwick Airport's North Terminal*

Executive Travel Vitality

Acknowledgment of contributors and editors
Kathy Lewis
Patricia Collins
Julie Dennis
Brian Lynn
Jane O'Keeffe

Contents

Chapters

executive
travel
Vitality

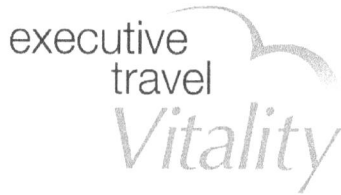

Executive Travel Vitality's team of travel health experts are all registered/chartered health professionals who travel regularly to advise on healthier travel practices. Their advice is underpinned by their professional registration with statutory and relevant governing bodies and based on scientific evidence in line with government and the World Health Organisation guidance. They have prudently tried and tested terminal facilities, products and services to provide business travellers with healthier options, techniques on how to improve their travel experience, and approaches to better health and wellbeing.

Visit us at www.executivetravelvitality.co.uk

Healthy Business Travel: Essential guide to Gatwick Airport's North Terminal

Welcome to Healthy Business Travel. The essential guide to reducing the stain of your business journey through Gatwick Airport's North Terminal and enhancing your wellbeing, long-term health and business performance en route.

London is renowned as the business capital of the world making Gatwick Airport a vital gateway for businesses, particularly those in the United Kingdom and Europe. It is situated only thirty miles away from the central London business districts, with excellent transport links, making it one of the easiest and quickest airports to access. Gatwick is ranked the second largest airport in the United Kingdom and the eighth busiest in Europe.

Each year, over 45 million business trips are made from the airports surrounding London. Gatwick Airport, being so close to London, handles nine million of theses journeys. In total, Gatwick serves over 220 destinations worldwide, comprising short and long-haul business trips.

Gatwick encompasses two terminals, the North and the South. The North Terminal being the younger of the two, having opened in 1988. While Gatwick is renowned for being the 'world's most efficient single runway', it isn't an ultra-modern airport and is currently being renovated. Despite, a billion-pound investment programme, the North Terminal still lacks the fundamental facilities and services which a modern airport needs, particularly when providing for frequent business travellers.

People who travel more than six times a year on business are more susceptible to poorer mental and physical wellbeing. On average, frequent business travellers have higher blood pressure, weight, blood cholesterol, lipids, sugar and stress levels. Consequently, they are not only at greater risk of cardiovascular disease, diabetes and cancer but also have higher levels of poor mental well-being.

Much of what a business traveller experiences regarding travel fatigue, strain and poor working conditions have a significant impact on their health and productivity.

Importantly, most of this can either be reduced by knowing what the choices are en route to the airport and what is available at the airport as you transit through.

This guide has been designed to provide an insight into how to become a more efficient and healthier business traveller by specifically pinpointing how to get the best possible use of the facilities and services when travelling through Gatwick Airport's North Terminal in your quest to be healthier and perform at your optimum level.

How to use this guide

The Healthy Business Travel guide aims to make business travel not just healthier but also easier. It does this by addressing the main constituents of poor business traveller health and subsequently providing practical solutions which can be easily mastered en route.

For expediency, the main elements of a healthy business travel life have been assigned to four sections, each with relevant chapters. The first section aims at reducing traveller fatigue, combating poor sleep, jetlag and revitalising the weary traveller. The second section provides an insight into how to lessen the strain while maximising any opportunity to meet work commitments. The third section deals mainly with lifestyle, including exercise and outdoor experiences to enhance relaxation, circulation, sleep, mental wellbeing and immune functions. The last part focuses on healthy eating and where to find healthier options within the airport.

Every chapter follows a similar format. The first portion explains the science and evidence behind the complications of a business travel lifestyle. It is followed by some practical advice on how to reduce the impact of the obstacle to achieve better travel wellbeing and lastly a 'where to find' segment, listing places and products within the airport and nearby which you can use to remove the strain of travelling.

To get the most out of this guide, you simply need to refer to the section or chapter which is most relevant to your travel lifestyle and difficulties you are likely to encounter, which will impact your wellbeing. Each chapter is self-contained, making it easy to skip an entire section or chapter so that you can read the most pertinent information first. So, if you are time-pressured, simply flick onto the contents page and use the hyperlink provided to go straight to the most appropriate chapter for your immediate needs and read the other sections at your leisure to plan for the next time.

If you are unsure of where to start, then read Chapter One on Travel Fatigue first. This chapter can be used as a board guide to which chapters within the book may be the most appropriate for you. It will quickly explain the benefits of changing one aspect of your travel lifestyle to enhance your overall wellbeing, which you can then follow up with practical suggestions in the relevant chapter.

Advancing to the appropriate chapter will also provide you with a greater understanding of the conditions you are experiencing during your business travels and what the benefits are for putting it right. Suggestions on 'how to' follow the chapter introduction and provide options for you to manage the problem more efficiently. Solutions have been provided for all sections, and all our suggestions have been tried and tested.

You will also find practical choices compiled by our Travel Wellbeing Consultants who have explored the Gatwick Airport's North Terminal to find alternatives for you. This guide is intended to take you a step beyond the usual general wellbeing advice, and subsequently, the additional advice ranges from the best places for Wi-Fi access to where to obtain healthy snacks items to take with you. Consequently, as a time pressured traveller, you can find what you need, and rely on us for information on where to obtain it quickly.

So, if it's work-life balance you are looking for, we have some practical suggestions for you. Alternatively, if you need to know which menu item is a healthy option to choose, then we've done the assessment and analysis for you.

Airport terminals, by their very nature, are dynamic places to pass through. Gatwick Airport's North Terminal is currently undergoing renovation and changes are expected to aspects of layout and facilities. Also, some restaurants and cafes modify their menus with changes to seasonal produce and tastes. While we aim to visit every six months to update the information within this guide and to reassess menu's, sometimes a restaurant may change their menu in between our visits. So, in addition to providing options for you on what to choose, we have also provided advice on how to choose.

All the food items we have listed as suitable for a healthy breakfast, lunch or snack have been assessed by a Registered Nutritionist or Dietitian and follow the government and current dietetic guidelines. In evaluating each item, we have relied on the information and analysis provided by the restaurant, café or food manufacturer. Hence, you will find foods listed which support a healthier business travel lifestyle along with their calorific and relevant nutritional information whenever possible. We've also provided suggestions on how to further reduce fat, sugar and salt intakes of some items.

We trust you will use the information in this guide to support your choices as much as possible and the provision of such will enable you to have a healthier business travel life, embracing stronger mental and enhancing longer-term physical wellbeing.

SECTION ONE: Rest and revitalise
Chapter 1: Travel fatigue

Business travel is fatiguing and isn't just caused by jet lag. Even if you are not travelling over time zones, you will still experience a sufficient amount of fatigue which will impact on your ability to function. Over time, the constant being on the move begins to add up. Frequent flyers (six times or more a year) have a higher level of stress than non-frequent business travellers.

Research shows a significant proportion of frequent business travellers are becoming 'burnt-out'. Over two-thirds of those feeling burnt-out report the wear and tear of business travel cause them to be less effective during and right after their trip. They also report feeling extra stress in the days before their trip and find it hard to lead a healthy lifestyle when travelling. Consequently, they are becoming less willing to travel, less satisfied with the outcome of their trips and less compliant to travel policies.

There are many factors which contribute to feeling fatigued when travelling on business. If you travel frequently, you will know these include aspects leading up to, during and post travel. Even before you leave, the additional strain in preparing to travel, attempting to get on a plane in good time and general disruption to your daily routine can be demanding. Coupled with the impact of spending time in a cramped space with little opportunity to move around, less oxygen in the environment, dehydration, limited food and drink choices, getting insufficient rest and the inability to relax en route. Finally, making your way from the plane to the relevant venue and keeping abreast of work demands once you arrive can be draining.

All these components ultimately add up, and if you are a frequent flyer, they start to wear you down, impacting on your psychological and physical health, your ability to concentrate and remain productive when on a business trip. The effect can become noticeable and of concern to work colleagues.

Travel fatigue has been found to significantly affect task performance, reduce the efficiency of processing information, inhibit memory recall, reduce alertness and psychometric coordination. The motivation to carry out a task has also been found to diminish, communication skills decrease, and interaction with the environment deteriorates, making the traveller more easily irritated and react more aggressively towards others.

The good news is that many of the contributing factors are within your control, and some can be managed easily en route to your destination without absorbing extra time when you are in the office or impacting on your commitments at home. When you get to Gatwick Airport's North Terminal, there are also plenty of resources to hand. It's just a case of knowing what to look out for and where to find what you need.

This chapter is aimed at helping you reduce fatigue when travelling through the North Terminal at Gatwick Airport. It will also guide you to relevant chapters in this book which will provide detailed information on how to improve your wellbeing and wherein Gatwick you can find resources to help.

How to reduce travel fatigue

1. Cast-off your cabin fever

Being packed into a cabin isn't very pleasant. While about a third of business travellers will travel business or first class on long-haul intercontinental flights, and 6% on short-haul international flights, the majority of us are left to the economy seating. Being crammed in, with insufficient room to move, limited space to work or restricted area to relax in is challenging enough, but there are many other factors which our bodies will react to which we also need to manage.

Various research suggests there is an analogy between flying and mountaineering, as both occur at altitude. When flying at 35,000 feet, the cabin is pressurised to altitudes of 6,000 to 8,000 feet to enable us to breathe easier. Because there is a corresponding increase in blood pressure, heart rate and respiration due to lower oxygen levels, the physiological efforts could explain the fatigue some passengers experience. The expansion of gas is also a consideration. It can make a somewhat uncomfortable journey!

When you're back on the ground, your body needs to readjust. If you are in transit or having a layover, then now is a good time to get those legs moving again to help your body readjust and improve your circulation. So even a single 15-minute walk will help by giving your body a chance to relax, unwind and reboot. Your heart rate will start to beat slower; blood pressure will reduce quicker, your respiration and gases will ease faster.

Some airports are difficult to navigate with people and obstacles everywhere. Finding a walking route of any substantial length could prove challenging if you don't know your way around. So, we've mapped out several walking routes in the North Terminal for those with only a short time before or between their flights. You will find a description, location and number of steps in Chapter 9 on Travelling Fit.

Another option is to take a quick shower. The warmth of the shower will help to ease muscle fatigue, increase circulation, stimulate creative thinking and problem-solving. Chapter 4 has more information on the benefits and where to find showers at Gatwick Airport or close by if you are on a stop-over.

2. Get plenty of rest!

Sounds obvious doesn't it, but just how easy is it to rest when travelling on business? We all believe in getting a good night's sleep and resting up, but we're travelling on business with work and travel deadline pressures.

Yet this is the time when we need sleep and rest the most. Otherwise, we fail to optimise our productivity which can affect the outcome of our business trip, not to mention the satisfaction that the journey was worth the cost and time away from other commitments.

When we travel on business, two-thirds of us report we sleep worse when away than at home, and it becomes poorer when we feel worn-out with nine in every ten business person reporting they sleep much worse when affected by the constant wear and tear of travelling.

Not getting sufficient sleep leads to reduced concentration, poor memory recall, impaired ability to make decisions, irritability and not to forget even more fatigue! In the long-term, regular poor sleep leads to weight problems, depression, diabetes and heart disease, all of which frequent business travellers have a higher incidence.

There are plenty of places to rest or even catch forty winks at Gatwick Airport's North Terminal. We have found the best quiet spots, where there is a low volume of people traffic, and listed them, along with hotels which have a half day or daytime rates, in Chapter 2 on Sleep and Productivity. If you have forgotten your sleep aids, then turn to Chapter 2 to find a list of stockers.

3. Reduce the strain

We are often our own worst enemies, frequently neglecting to schedule downtime, to relax or find a quiet space to catch up on demanding emails in the airport. Business travel often requires us to work en route or in the evening when we have reached our destination. Revitalising, relaxing and working efficiently to make more time for ourselves when we arrive can be problematic if not near impossible.

Not being able to work en route or connect to the internet are two of the biggest stressors for business travellers. If we improve our connectivity and are able to work more efficiently, we are effectively removing some of the strain which allows more time to relax once we have made it to our destination.

Gatwick Airport's North Terminal offers an abundance of places to work and connect – if you know where to find them. Section 2 of this book looks at ways to reduce travel strain in detail. We've also listed the best places to work productively, hold meetings, recharge your batteries and connect to the internet in Chapters 6, 7 & 8.

It can't be all work. Business travellers need the opportunity to take a break as well. Most importantly, you need time to relax your mind as well as your body, particularly if travel fatigue becomes a concern. When we are constantly focused on work, we are in our least problem solving and creative mode. By relaxing, we allow our mind to wander and give it some space to allow our ideas to surface. Being tense also means poor circulation, putting us at greater risk of injury and strain.

Taking time out en route isn't a luxury – it is a necessity to revitalise our battered wellbeing and arrive at our best. Which is why we've gone ahead and explored the North Terminal for you. We've found the quietest spots for you to relax and places where you can unwind in the Gatwick's North Terminal. These are listed in Chapter 5 along with some relaxation techniques and places to get a massage or spa before your flight.

4. Get some exercise!

Regular exercise makes us feel less tired in the long term, however travelling on business can interrupt normal fitness routines, making it harder to undertake each day. On the days when you are travelling, flexibility to your routine may be the key to keeping to your desired fitness target.

Ideally, we should aim for at least 150 minutes of exercise per week. Timing your exercise can also be advantageous. For example, some exercise in the late afternoon may help to reduce early evening fatigue and improve sleep. For those on long-haul, exercising outside to get sunlight is best timed to the appropriate sun exposure times to help reduce the effects of jetlag.

When you're travelling, you need to take the opportunities to incorporate different types of exercise into your schedule when you can. Some airports offer facilities on site such as exercise bikes, yoga rooms, gyms in connecting hotels, walking tracks and even ice-skating rinks!

If you have several hours before your flight, then you might be able to take advantage of nearby facilities. Immediately surrounding Gatwick Airport are some great running and cycle routes, along with picturesque golf courses, newly renovated tennis courts and fitness facilities.

Bearing in mind, you might be short of time and can't make a trip from the airport, we've listed some light exercises to undertake while on the go, places you can exercise at the terminal and connecting hotels with gym amenities in Chapter 9.

For those with several hours to spare or a layover, a list of nearby hotels with leisure facilities, golf courses and tennis courts is also provided in Chapter 9.

5. Get some sun

Sunlight is great reducer of tiredness for a variety of reasons. Typical symptoms reported during periods of low sun exposure include depression, fatigue, trouble concentrating, lack of interest in normal activities, social withdrawal and increased need for sleep.

Sunlight has a profound effect on our hormones which regulate our sleep-wake cycle and makes us feel more alert and active. It does this by stimulating the release of serotonin (happy hormone) and cortisol (alert hormone) and decreasing the level of melatonin (sleep hormone) during the day. By doing so, it resets our body clock every day, while also enhancing the quality and onset of our sleep in the evening, as well as improving our mood. Which is why it's important to get sunlight at the appropriate time when you reach your destination so it can also help to reduce any ill effects of jet-lag.

Another hormone that our body creates from direct sunlight is vitamin D. Not getting sufficient Vitamin D from the sun is one hazard of frequent travel. Research shows an association between low vitamin D status with low sun exposure, as well as seasonal disorders (SAD) and chronic fatigue syndrome.

Studies also show those suffering from SAD often have a lower vitamin D status than those that don't, although it remains unclear whether the depression is altering the diet or there was a lack of vitamin D to start with. While you can obtain vitamin D from your diet by including oily fish, eggs, meat, fortified cereals, soya milk and spreads, getting sufficient sunshine each day also has other health benefits.

If you have several hours before your flight or when in transit, then Gatwick Airport has some peaceful places where you can venture out and catch some sunlight. You only need about 10 – 15 minutes a day to synthesise vitamin D. When combined with a walk, it's an excellent way to remain alert and productive. You'll find these more tranquil places listed in Chapter 10. However, the UK is notorious for low sunlight levels during winter, so be prepared to get some sun at your destination as well.

If sunlight isn't readily available on the days you travel, then you can consider using light therapy which is also used as a treatment for mild SAD and to help regulate your sleep/wake cycle. You will find some light boxes listed available to purchase at Gatwick Airport's North Terminal in Chapter 3.

Another course of action is also to ensure you have sufficient Vitamin D in your diet. Seventy percent of Europeans and Americans are estimated to have insufficient vitamin D. So, the combination of getting more sunlight and a balanced diet will help raise your vitamin D status if it has dipped as a result of demanding business travel schedules.

Gatwick Airport's North Terminal has cafes and restaurants with menu items which offer good sources of vitamin D. We've listed menu items for you in Chapter 10.

6. Drink plenty of water

Fatigue is one of the main symptoms of dehydration. Even at 1% dehydration, you may start to feel tired. When you travel, your usual routine is interrupted, and you don't consume as many drinks throughout the day as you would when at your desk or home. On top of this, you may not eat the same foods which would typically contribute to your fluid intake. You may also find the air on the plane much drier than usual contributing to a small loss of water from your respiratory tract as you breathe and from your skin.

Health experts recommend aiming for a cup of water (200 ml) each hour to keep hydrated when travelling. If in doubt, check the colour of your urine. It should be a pale tint of yellow. Anything darker than a light lemon colour and you could probably do with a top-up of fluid. It does not include the alcoholic variety as alcohol is a diuretic and will serve to dehydrate you further. If you do have a glass of wine or spirits, then consider a low alcohol variety, diluting it with tonic water or taking a glass of water to match each time.

The price of bottled water varies in the North Terminal of Gatwick Airport. You won't be able to take bottles of water through security with you when you go into the Departure Lounge, which is a shame as water can be more expensive after you have passed through security than before. Hence, you will need to re-stock once through security. You are, however, usually allowed to take an empty bottle through and fill it on the other side.

To help you, we have listed where you can find free available water at Gatwick Airport's North Terminal in Chapter 11. We have also provided a list of all bottled water, together with the price so you can compare availability and cost. If water isn't something you enjoy drinking, then you might like to consider the other options we have listed in Chapter 11.

7. Eat at regular intervals

Eating at regular times is considered a factor in combating tiredness, as it keeps your blood sugar steady for more prolonged periods which reduces the onset of fatigue.

If it's been a while since your last meal, then your body will start to produce glucose to keep a constant amount of energy circulating to your vital organs and, in particular, your brain. As soon as your blood glucose drops below a certain level, it will trigger the body's response to produce more glucose to circulate. Eating a regular meal and a light snack (with fibre but low in sugar) every three to four hours is an excellent way to keep your energy levels constant, avoiding any peaks and troughs, rather than eating a large meal less often.

What's more, eating patterns affect your circadian rhythm by sending messages to your master biological clock. By eating at regular intervals, you are communicating with your metabolic processes the time of day, and your body knows from routine when your next meal is coming, controlling the feelings of hunger and sustaining your energy levels. It will also help regulate your awake/sleep cycle. So, if your fatigue is also added to by jet-lag then eating regularly may help to sync your body clock. You may need to readjust the time you eat if you travel long-haul to match the time when you reach your destination, therefore helping reduce the effects of jet-lag further. Chapter 3 has some great tips on how to synchronise your body clock.

It's wise to make sure you don't skip meals before boarding your flight if you want to maintain a state of alertness and be at your most productive during your journey. We've listed for you in Chapter 12 Healthy Eating where in the North Terminal you can find healthier light meals.

8. Eat slow burning carbohydrate snacks

Starchy foods which are high in fibre and low in sugar, such as whole grains, wholemeal bread, oatmeal bread, lentils and beans, make us feel full for longer by releasing energy gradually as they are broken down to be absorbed.

The fibre from the carbohydrates helps by further delaying the absorption of the food that has been broken down. Which means we are less likely to have peaks and troughs in our blood glucose as they supply a constant source of energy at a slower pace.

What's more, slow-burning carbohydrates contribute essential nutrients to the diet such as B vitamins which are used in energy production and the fibre helps to keep our bowels moving, along with lowering the risk of diabetes and heart disease which frequent business travellers have a higher incidence.

When complex carbohydrates are combined with a little protein, the collective snack offers an even greater variety of nutrients and keep us feeling fuller for even longer.

The key to a good snack is to avoid those which contain added sugar and high-fat contents, such as cereal bars, chocolate and pastries.

At Gatwick's North Terminal you'll find great snacks at the local shops and cafes. In Chapter 15, we've added a selection of healthier snacks and where to find them for you to buy to eat before you board (if you had a meal a few hours ago) or to take on board with you. We've also included a guide on when the best times to snack are and how to snack healthily.

9. Have a brilliant breakfast

Not having breakfast is a sure-fire way to start the day feeling tired. While you've been asleep, your body has been fasting. You've relied on the energy from the meal you had the evening before and then your liver's short-term storage of glycogen. But your liver's storage runs low after twelve hours and will gradually become entirely depleted, so unless you refuel it, it will need to take more drastic action to create glucose to feed your brain and vital organs.

Excellent breakfasts are those which combine complex/starchy carbohydrate, such as porridge, cereals, or wholemeal toast, with protein, such as dairy, fish, peanut butter or eggs, which enhances satiety. Complex, high fibre carbohydrates, such as porridge or baked beans on wholemeal bread, take a longer to break down than refined carbohydrates such as croissants or bagels. When complex carbohydrates are combined with protein, it takes even longer to digest breakfast, as the protein must be reduced to amino acids to be small enough for absorption across the intestinal wall. When those amino acids are finally absorbed into the bloodstream, they are either used for growth and maintenance or converted into energy for immediate use or storage. Overall, a combination breakfast will gradually break down and be absorbed over a longer period to provide fuel for the body's functions.

We've selected some great breakfast options for you in Chapter 12. These include breakfast meals which are light in calories for those either about to catch their flight and will eat again soon after boarding and those who want to lose weight, along with breakfast meals where the next meal might be at least 5 – 6 hours or not needing to reduce their daily calorific intake. All those listed are good sources of fibre and a combination of protein and carbohydrate.

10. Aim for five-a-day

Most fruits and vegetables have a high water content and subsequently contribute fluid to our daily diets. They also supply many other essential nutrients which are used in energy metabolism, along with being a good source of fibre which aids the movement of food and waste products. So, if you suffer from tiredness and are prone to traveller's constipation, then you still need to aim for, at the very least, five fruits and vegetables per day when travelling on business.

Fresh whole fruit is best, although dried fruit will offer valuable nutrients and fibre as well. Some of the restaurants, cafes and lounges now provide a basket of whole fruit at the counters, while other retail outlets sell dried fruit options along with sliced fresh fruit and vegetable pieces which are great for taking with you to the aeroplane. We have listed where you can purchase whole, dried fruit and sliced fruit and vegetables in Chapter 14.

While some restaurants and cafes only provide side vegetable dishes, soups and salads from their sit-down menu, others are now offering a takeaway service where you can purchase items to take on board with you. We have listed these in Chapter 14 as well but have excluded any dishes which are high in salt, fat and sugar.

Chapter 2: Sleep and where to get it

Sleep and Productivity: Sleeping really pays off

You're travelling for a reason; to enhance your business with better supplier arrangements, maintaining relationships with clients or increasing sales. Whatever the reason, you will want to ensure you maximise the return on the cost of your travel and add value to your company. So, by its very nature, business travel demands high performance. This performance will be affected by work relationships, the strains of travel, tight schedules, jet lag, personal health, family commitments, availability of food and late nights.

On top of this, the amount of sleep you have before, during and after your trip could seriously affect your work performance. Just a few hours of missed sleep before you travel, especially when combined with the stains of travel, will significantly reduce your performance during your trip and your long-term health if it becomes a regular occurrence.

Research has shown that losing as little as one and half hours for just one night will reduce daytime alertness by a third. With only six hours of sleep, your work performance is significantly diminished. Sleep deprivation will also cause slower reaction times, attention deficit, increased the risk of work-travel related accidents and mood alterations affecting your relationships with clients, suppliers, customers and colleagues.

Research also shows that on average, business travellers sleep only five hours the night before a business trip, the lowest duration in the seven days leading up to the journey. Business travellers who haven't slept well before they leave are at a decreased performance before they even start their journey. If travelling long-haul, the effects of jet-lag will also be more noticeable.

It is estimated that one in three adults suffer from poor sleep when at home. This abruptly rises when travelling on business due to the increased strain integral to any business trip. Yet the impact is greater than many of us initially imagine.

Over two-thirds (69%) of business travellers surveyed in recent research, for the Airliners Report Corporation, reported they sleep worse when travelling on business than at home. This rose to a staggering 86% for business travellers who said they felt nearly burnt out from business travel.

Poor sleep isn't just the domain of long-haul business travellers. Those who frequently travel (more than five times a year) but of short duration (1 - 5 days) are more likely to have a sleep deficit compared to non-travelling work colleagues in the same firm or those that travel for a longer duration. They are also more prone to report a greater lack of confidence in their continued ability to keep up with the pace of work and higher alcohol consumption, according to the recent survey of 13,000 multi-national company employees.

The impact of sleep deprivation on productivity and health is considerable. Immediate effects include impaired judgement, decreased mental and physical performance, reduced coordination and reaction times. Long-term sleep deprivation leads to chronic diseases such as diabetes, cardiovascular disease, obesity and mental ill health. Extensive research also repeatedly shows jet lag disrupts the body's internal clock and has a profound effect on cognitive function and health as well.

Not sleeping is depressing!

Poorer mental health caused by poor quality sleep, increased alcohol consumption and the inability to keep up with work is a specific concern for employers.

Alcohol consumption which rises with the frequency of travel, particularly when the trip is of short duration, is used by many business travellers to get to sleep, yet it reduces the quality of sleep and often results in daytime lethargy. Alcohol is also a diuretic which makes most travellers urinate more, often waking up during sleep time to do so. The symptoms of dehydration such as fatigue, lethargy and irritability may become exacerbated.

Both sleep deprivation and increased alcohol consumption when travelling are interrelated and linked with depression. When coupled with feelings of not being able to cope with workload there is an increased risk of mental health problems.

It can become a vicious cycle with the lack of sleep reportedly the biggest predictor of major depression. Work-related accidents increase, time off work rises and long-term mental health begin to affect work-related activities and family relationships.

The upshot is that travelling employees suffering from mental illness are likely to be absent from work up to seven and a half times longer than those with a physical disease.

If you think sleep medication might be an answer, then think again; if you take sleep medication, you are four times more likely to die earlier, as mortality rates increase four-fold with long-term sleep medication usage. Meanwhile, your physical health and wellbeing also suffer.

How sleeping impacts physical health and wellbeing

Physical illness remains one of the dominating effects of poor sleep. Poor sleep can disrupt the traveller's immune system, so they are more likely to suffer from viral ill health or traveller's tummy. Sleep deprivation or poor quality sleep (includes depth, the number of times waking up and duration) can also lead to metabolic conditions, including diabetes, heart disease and hypertension. Business travellers have a higher incidence of all these illnesses as well as a higher average weight when compared with non-business travellers.

For those who regularly sleep less than five hours, the risk of diabetes also increases. Studies show that missing out on sleep may lead to type 2 diabetes by changing the way the body processes glucose. Research suggests that sleep deprivation also affects the production of insulin, which regulates the uptake of carbohydrate and fat. More notably, is that the treatment of sleep disorders, i.e. getting a better quality of sleep which may improve glucose metabolism and energy balance.

Sleep is one of the essential components of a healthy business travel lifestyle; the others are proper nutrition and physical activity. So, sleeping can really pay dividends for the health and productivity of the business traveller.

The following chapter is aimed at helping you to maximise every opportunity to get some much-needed sleep when travelling on business.

Quick tips when planning for better performance

Planning for good performance means planning to be well rested and vitalised before, during and after your trip, and before you start to work. Here are some top tips for getting better performance by maximising your awake to sleep cycle.

Use your time wisely

If your business trip crosses several time zones, then schedule your meetings on your home time when you first arrive. Research shows that travellers performance is best during mid-day, not early morning which many consider the best time for productivity. So, choose mid-day hours on home time as your body will still need a chance to adjust.

Exercise when you can

Research has also shown that those who keep fit during their trip perform an astounding 61% better than non-exercisers. Regular exercisers have been linked with being in a better mood, and less stressed during the day. Research has also found that developing a regular exercise routine, even when travelling, helps to fight off sleep disorders. Developing your travel exercise routine might help you not only perform better, feel better but also ward off insomnia. To assist you, we have listed places where you can get some exercise in Chapter 9 on Fit Travel.

Accepting that not everything will go to plan lowers stress

Expect travel problems, such as delays, lost luggage, and slower than desirable WiFi (see Chapter 6 for the best WiFi reception). These are found to be the top three stress factors when travelling on a business trip. Travel stress will make you even more tired, so reframing your expectations can help to reduce the strain associated with travel. Inevitably, expectations which are too high can set us up for a fall. There's nothing worse than trying to control the uncontrollable, which is the nature of travel.

While problem-solving is a good coping strategy for business tasks that have gone wrong in the office, acceptance of possible eventualities is a far more effective coping strategy for reducing the strain when travelling on business. So, if your Wi-Fi is better than expected, your flight arrives on time, and your luggage hasn't been lost or stolen, then you've already exceeded expectations at the outset of your business trip! The rest is just 'as can be expected'.

Accepting that such events are inevitable at some point is an approach that will allow you some mental space to plan ahead. If you expect your flight to be delayed, then make sure your meetings are set to allow for a delay. Pack the necessary change of clothing (shirt and underwear) in hand luggage, in the event of baggage loss. Plan to do your emails where Wi-Fi is at its best and so on. You'll sleep much easier for it. Effectively, you are being proactive, rather than reactive to events around you.

Relax when you can

Stress and sleep go hand in hand. When attempting to reduce your stress level, you need to aim for a good sleep. Yet, when travelling, there is a tendency for most business travellers to become anxious about their plans for the next day. In fact, the recent survey conducted by the Airlines Reporting Corporation found that over half of business travellers feel extra stress in the days before a business trip and believe they are less effective during their work trips as a result.

When you become anxious at night about plans the next day, you inevitably disrupt your sleep and the quality of your sleep declines. Adopting some breathing exercises and relaxation techniques or just taking time out to relax on your trip is essential if you want to perform at your best. See Chapter 5 on Relaxation.

There is also a time and place when you simply need to switch your mind into 'default network mode'. This is when we are undertaking an undemanding preparatory task such as preparing breakfast, taking a shower or walking to the train station, and we are no longer consciously thinking about work or other cognitively demanding tasks. It is during these states of 'wakeful rest' when our brains can be at their most creative or problem-solving.

You'll find out more on default network modes and how to harness them to refresh and revitalise yourself in Chapter 4.

Prioritise getting a good amount of sleep before you set off

This might be easier said than done. However, the World Health Organisation recommend not being in a sleep deficit before you travel as a way of reducing the effects of jet-lag and enhancing performance. According to one study, business travellers often lose sleep the night before travel, and losing just one and a half hours for only one night reduces daytime alertness by a third.

How to nap comfortably when travelling

If you haven't had enough sleep before you set out to the airport, then here are some great tips on how and when to nap at Gatwick Airport's North Terminal.

Power nap sensibly

Contemplate having a short nap if feeling wiped out (10 - 20 minutes) before a short haul flight and save a longer nap (30 - 40 minutes) for the long-haul flight. A short nap is considered to help improve mood, alertness and performance without interfering with nighttime sleep if taken at a sensible time and in a tolerable environment.

We've found some quiet places in the North Terminal for you to rest your eyes momentarily. They are listed below these top tips. We've also added ways you can secure your possessions while you nap.

Consider taking an afternoon nap when travelling over several time zones

Taking an afternoon nap might be worth considering if you are travelling over several time zones westward. An afternoon naptime tends to coincide with a drop in our internal 'alerting system' which delays the body's increasing desire to fall asleep. After a nap, this drive to sleep lessens, making a person feel more alert and generally able to stay up for longer and need to sleep less. This is particularly useful if you are travelling and need to stay up to resync to a later destination time.

Don't snooze for too long

Sleep experts recommend not napping for more than 40 minutes to avoid going into a deep sleep. If you nap for longer and you start to go into a deep sleep, it will make it harder to wake up, leaving you feeling groggy and tired. So, if it is a nap – then make sure it is a short nap of fewer than forty minutes.

Be ready to nod off

Research shows that business travellers who rate their performance highly, over half will fall asleep unintentionally on the trip. So, have your sleep paraphernalia prepared and leave it with your toiletry bag. It might include eye masks, ear plugs, soft music, blankets, pillows, travel alarm clock and water.

If you haven't already packed these things, then we have listed where to find some of them at Gatwick Airport's North Terminal later in this chapter.

Plan your time in advance

Preparatory napping involves taking a nap before you get sleepy. It is a useful technique if you are to be up later than your usual bedtime. If you know that you have a five-hour gap at the airport, then plan what you can do with this time. To assist you in deciding on where you can nap, and in addition to the places we've listed for a quick snooze (20 minutes), we've also listed hotels onsite where you can have a longer rest depending on your schedule.

In Chapter 9 we've also listed places where you can exercise, to help improve the quality of your sleep, and where to find light meals in Chapter 13.

Choose your hotel room wisely

Gatwick Airport's hotels like to promote their sleep-friendly amenities. However, travellers should still ensure they request a room on a designated quiet floor or off the street with double-paned windows, room temperature control, black-out curtains and pillows to their preference, at the time of booking.

We have provided a description for hotels on the Gatwick Airport site along with a summary of guest reviews in the list below, noting that the experience of visitors differs in each hotel.

Get some sunshine

The key to easily getting to sleep when suffering from jet lag is to re-synchronise your body clock. This is best done by getting sunlight during the right time of day, avoiding bright lights at wrong times including laptops, mobile devices and television. There are apps which will work out the best time of day for you to seek sunlight when you arrive at your destination. We've listed some jet-lag apps for you to try in Chapter 3. We've also listed some quiet places outside the North Terminal where you can relax outside in Chapter 10.

Eat well

By this, we don't mean eating lots; we merely mean choosing foods that may reduce the time it takes to fall asleep. Foods high in melatonin promote sleep by helping to reduce the time taken to fall asleep, along with contributing to alleviating the feelings of jet-lag.

More information about foods which may help shorten the time taken to get to sleep and which are available at Gatwick International Airport's North Terminal is in Chapter 3 on Coping with Jetlag. We've checked out the snacks, breakfast and restaurants menus to help you to choose wisely. There's a comprehensive list of where to go and what is available.

Eat light

Large portions take some time to digest, and while you are digesting you may find it harder to fall asleep. High fat and high protein meals also take longer to digest, leaving you feeling fuller and uncomfortable in a cramped position. High-fat meals may make you feel sluggish, while high protein may keep you awake. In comparison, carbohydrate meals with fruit and vegetables and some protein are easier to digest and may make you feel sleepy.

Make sure you choose salads and fruit options whenever possible, as it is another approach to increasing your fluid intake while travelling so you will feel less thirsty and fatigued when you arrive. Complex carbohydrates, fruit and vegetables also provide fibre which will aid digestion and prevent traveller constipation, which may help to relieve any intestinal discomfort while on board.

Chapter 12 and 13 on healthy eating provides an extensive list of light menu items available while you are in Gatwick Airport's North Terminal, while Chapters 14 and 15 provide lists of healthy fruit, vegetables and snacks.

Preparing to nap in Gatwick's North Terminal

Although we don't recommend sleeping in an airport overnight, particularly when on a business trip, sometimes you just need to rest your eyes for a little while. So, if you are wiped out, suffering undue fatigue or severe jet-lag, encounter substantial delays, or find nearby hotels are all full, or transfer times between planes are short, then it's worthwhile to know the best places in the North Terminal where you can have a rest. Below are some suggestions on where you can catch some much-needed shut-eye.

First of all, make sure your possessions are secure to ensure a better chance of catching a few hours safely.

Securing your possessions

If you feel the need to catch forty winks while waiting for your flight, then make sure your belongings are safe first. Unfortunately, there aren't any luggage lockers at Gatwick Airport for security reasons. So, you'll need to make alternative arrangements.

Early Check-in

If you have luggage which can go in the hold, some airlines will allow you to check it in ahead of your flight check-in. The following airlines at Gatwick's North Terminal grant you check-in the day before you fly. Terms and conditions may vary with each airline, so you will need to check with your airline first. Generally speaking, you must be present at Check-in, and some require photo ID.

- **Easy-Jet**. You can check your bag in between 8.00 pm and 8.30 am if you are departing before 8.30 am the next day. No extra charge. Located on Check-in, Level One.
- **Virgin Atlantic** operates a twilight check-in service between 5.00 pm and 9.00 pm, with the exception of a dedicated Premium Economy desk. There is no additional charge, and all flights are eligible. Located in rows A in Check-in, Level Two.
- **Thomson Airways** Early check-in is available from 12.00 pm to 10.00 pm the day before for next-day departures before 12.00 pm. There is no additional charge. Located in rows C in Check-in, Level Two.

Luggage storage services

You can also put your luggage in storage for a few hours with Gatwick Airport's luggage services.

31

Excess Baggage Company's left luggage facilities are secure, and you can leave your luggage with them at your convenience. The facilities are manned with 24-hour CCTV and full security screening.

Location: Check-in Hall, Level One, right by the main entrance from the shuttle, just opposite London News Company, next to Costa Coffee.
Opening hours: 4.00 am to 10.30 pm
Telephone: +44 (0) 1293 734 888 **or email:** gatwick@left-baggage.co.uk
Website: www.left-baggage.co.uk

Cost: Up to three hours, the price is £6.00 per item. Between three and 24 hours it is £11.00 per item. Between 24 to 72 hours is £7.50 per item, and for 72 hours or more the charge is £5.00 per 24 hours. You can get a full quote on their online booking system if you wish to leave your luggage for more than 24 hours.

Wrapping your bag

If you're not able to check your bag in early and want to keep it with you rather than storage, then you could consider bag wrapping. This is also available from the **Excess Baggage Company,** located in the Check-in area on Level One, next to Costa Coffee and directly opposite London News Company. The cost starts at £12.50 per item for a Classic wrap and £13.50 for an Ultra wrap. This service trades under the name of Bag Wrap. You can find more about their services at http://www.bagwrap.com

There is also a small baggage wrap unit on Check-in, Level Two at the end of Row B & C.

Bag covers, brics, luggage skins and locks

Other alternatives are bag covers, brics and luggage skins. If you haven't brought a lock for your luggage, then you can pick one up from various stores at Gatwick's North Terminal. Prices indicated below are correct at time of review. Please use them as a guide.

Case Luggage & Accessories

Case is on the opposite side to the exit from security on the lower level of the Departure Lounge. They have several locks and luggage covers. You can pre-order via their website.

A reserve and collect service is available from Case Luggage. Simply reserve the items online and then collect as you pass through the airport's North Terminal. We've listed items available on their website below.

Opening hours: November to March 4.00 am to 8.30 pm; April to October 4.00 am to 10.00 pm
Telephone: 0129 356 9264
Email: gatwicknorth@caseluggage.co.uk
Website: www.caseluggage.com

Luggage skins include;

Small Cover AC0103 £20 Size 54(h) x 37(w) x 22(d) cm with a 1-year warranty.
Medium Cover AC0102 £22.00 68(h) x 45(w) x 26(d) cm with a 1-year warranty.
Large Cover AC0101 £25.00 78(h) x 50(w) x 29(d) cm with a 1-year warranty.

Brics include;

Covers for Bellagio BBG8303 £25.00 Clear Plastic with a 5-year warranty.
Covers for Bellagio BBG28304 £30.00 Clear Plastic with a 5-year warranty.
Covers for Bellagio BBG28305 £30.00 Clear Plastic with a 5-year warranty.
Cover for BLF15250 £23.00 Clear Plastic with a 5-year warranty.
Cover for BLF15251 £25.00 Clear Plastic with a 5-years warranty.
Cover for BLF15252 £28.00 Clear Plastic with a 5-year warranty.
Briggs & Riley Sympatico Covers £34.99 Medium Case Cover. Black Nylon 61 (h) x 45.5 (w) x 25.5 (d) Lifetime warranty that even covers airline damage.

Locks include;

Go Travel locks with two keys £8.99 TSA alert padlock. Assorted colours. Three dials solid brass padlock encased in nylon. TSA recognised.
Go Travel Large Brass Padlock £4.49 A solid brass padlock.
Tumi Alpha TSA Combination Padlock £21.00 Recognised by TSA, allowing TSA to open the lock should the need arise for a security search. TSA can relock it with no damage to bag or lock.

Boots the Chemist

Boots is located on the lower level of the Departure Lounge and in the Arrivals Hall. There are two Boots shops in the Departure Lounge. The one nearest to the security exit is the smallest. They stock padlocks with either combination lock or keys ranging from £5 to £8.00. The second, the larger of the two, is at the far end of the lower level and it also stocks padlocks with similar prices. You can pre-order via the Boots website, then collect the item from the airport if needed.

Opening in Arrivals: 24 hours
Opening in Departure Lounge: 4.00 am to 8.30 pm
Telephone: 01293 569606
Website: www.boots.com

Locks include;

Boots Travel Combination Lock £6.00 online Three digital combination lock. £6.50 airside and landside.

Boots Travel Key Luggage Locks £5.00 Two solid padlocks in assorted colours with three keys per lock. Encased in brass with sturdy steel shanks, they're suitable for securing your case while travelling. Available online, airside and landside.

Boots Travel TSA Recognised 3 Dial Lock £7.00 Designed to be quick and easy to use with a twist to set design. Ideal for USA travel. Allows your luggage to be unlocked and inspected by security authorities without damage. Available online and landside.

Go Travel Twist 'n' Set Lock £8.00 TSA accepted combination lock. Secure three dial design. No loose keys. Comes in three colours. Available airside and landside.

Go Travel My Date Lock £8.00 Calendar based lock with five dial design. Set using any memorable date, includes date, month and year. TSA accepted for travel in America. Available landside.

Go Travel Secure Lock £6.50 Combination brass padlock for luggage. Reliable three dial design. No need for keys. Easy to set code of choice. Available landside and airside.

Boots Travel Strap £5.00 Brightly coloured strap made from sturdy material and side release buckle. Available landside and airside.

Dixons Travel

Like Boots, it also has two stores on the lower level of the Departure Lounge. The first is smaller, opposite Weatherspoon Pub. The other is larger between Boots and Jo Malone on the right-hand side as you walk down towards the departure gates 101 – 113.

You can pre-order items from Dixon's Travel direct by phoning the Gatwick North Terminal store. They would be able to check and reserve your product for you. Unfortunately, you won't be able to order the item online.

If you stroll past the store, you will find some security items on the rack outside both stores, including a padlock at £4.92

Opening hours: 4.00 am – 8.300 pm daily
Telephone: 01293 569737

Locks include;
Go Travel Twist and Set lock £6.92 TSA approved. Error-free twist setting mechanism. No need for keys.
Go Travel Lock £5.99 Two solid brass padlocks with four keys. 20 mm to fit most zipped luggage.
Got Travel Combination Secure Lock £4.99. No need to worry about losing keys. Three–digit lock. Easy to set the code of your choice.

Excess Luggage Company
In addition to storing and wrapping your baggage, the Excess Luggage Company also stocks several locks. You'll find them on the rack near the doorway opposite their service counter.

Location: Check–in Hall, Level One, right by the main entrance from the shuttle, just opposite London News Company, next to Costa Coffee.
Opening hours: 5.00 am to 10.00 pm
Telephone: +44 (0) 1293 734 888 **or email:** gatwick@left-baggage.co.uk
Website: www.left-baggage.co.uk

Locks include;
Excess Baggage 1 lock and 2 keys £3.50 Solid single brass 25 mm lock with 2 keys.
Excess Baggage 2 brightly coloured locks and 4 keys £4.50
Excess Baggage 2 brass locks and 4 keys £5.99 Two small brass locks with 4 keys.
Excess Baggage Combination Lock and 2 keys £6.99 TSA approved.
Excess Baggage Combination Lock and 2 keys £7.50 Two plastic TSA approved locks and keys.
Go Travel Sentry Lock £5.99 Bright luggage lock with 2 keys. TSA approved for travel in the USA.

Go Travel Glo Locks £5.99 Lock locks with 6 keys. Available in 'hot' colours. Solid brass mechanism.

Go Travel My Date Lock £7.99 Calendar luggage lock which you set using a memorable date such as a special occasion. Secure five dial design. TSA accepted for travel in the USA.

Go Travel Big Dial Lock £9.99 3 large, easy to read dials with an error-free setting mechanism and set indicator. Sturdy zinc alloy, ABS plastic & steel construction. TSA accepted for travel in the USA.

Go Travel Dual Combi/key lock £9.99 Dual combination/key travel padlock. Opens via a three digit code or backup key. Fits most zipped luggage. TSA approved.

Go Travel Combi Cable TSA Lock £12.99 Ultra-strong steel cable system. Has flexible cable which feeds through small zipper holes. No keys required, easy-set three-dial combination lock. Made from robust zinc alloy and steel. TSA accepted for travel in the USA.

Straps include;

Go Travel Luggage Strap £4.99 Bold suitcase strap. Fully adjustable, durable and built to last. Fun, bright and easy to recognise.

Go Travel Stretchy Luggage Strap £12.99 Wide elasticated luggage strap which stretches to fit around your suitcase. Interlocking buckle.

Go Travel Glo Strap £6.99 Ultra bright luggage strap. Prevents luggage accidentally opening. Fully adjustable so to fit most cases.

The London News Company & WHSmith

It would be difficult to miss the many stores of WHSmith and the London News Company (owned by WHSmith). Both stock the same brand of products, so other than the name it is difficult to see any difference between the two. Which is rather fortunate if you are running late, as there is virtually a store on most levels of Gatwick Airport North Terminal. In fact, you will also find a mini WHSmith at Gates 101 – 113.

London News Company Locations: Opposite M&S Simply Food in the Arrival Hall; opposite Excess Baggage in the main entrance of Check-in, level one; upstairs of Check-in, level two just opposite Moneycorp Bureau de Change.

WHS Locations: Between The Bookshop and Fat Face, at the far end of the Departure Lounge next to Boots the Chemist; and Gates 101 – 113.

London News Company opening hours: Before and after security 4.00 am to 9.00 pm.

WHSmith opening hours: Before security 24 hours and post security 3.00 am to 10.00 pm
Website: www.whsmith.co.uk

Locks include;
Destination Travel TSA approved 1 lock and 2 keys. £9.99 Available airside and landside.
Destination Travel Combination Lock £8.49 Available airside and landside.
Destination Travel 2 Locks with 4 Keys £8.99 Available airside and landside.
Destination Travel 1 Lock 2 Keys £5.49 Available airside.
Gadget Shop 2 Locks and 2 Keys £12.99 Available landside.

Straps Include:
Destination Travel Strap £7.49 Strap with digit lock. Available airside and landside.
Destination Travel Combination Strap £12.99 Available airside and landside.

World Duty Free

There are four duty free shops in Gatwick's North Terminal. One is in arrivals as you exit into the Arrivals Hall past security. Another World Duty Free shop is located on the lower level of the Departure Lounge, as you pass through security and the departure gates 45 – 55 and 101 – 133.

Opening Hours in Departure Lounge: Open 24 hours
Opening Hours in Arrivals: Open 24 hours
Telephone: +44 (0)1293 502421 and +44 (0)1293 504260 **Email:** customerservices.uk@wdfg.com
Website: lgws.worlddutyfree.com

Locks include;
Go Travel Lock £6.00
Go Travel 2 Small Combination Locks £6.99
Go Travel Large Combination Locks £9.00

Money belts and body bags

Keeping your key documents and personal possession as close to your body as possible is crucial if you think you are going to doze off in the airport, particularly if travelling alone. Fortunately, there are a few retail shops which sell money belts and body bags.

Boots the Chemist

Boots is located on the lower level of the Departure Lounge and in the Arrivals Hall. There are two Boots shops in the Departure Lounge. The nearest one to the security exit is the smaller. They stock money belts which you can either purchased on the day or order online to collect.

Opening in Arrivals: 24 hours
Opening in Departure Lounge: 4.00 am to 8.300 pm
Telephone: 01293 569606
Website: www.boots.com

Money Belts

Boots Travel Money Belt £7.00 Lightweight fabric with two zipped pockets. The belt can be adjusted to fit a waist between 28 – 46 inch/75 – 115 cm. Available landside.
Go Travel Money belt £7.00 Unisex money belt. Soft and comfortable to wear. Can be worn to conceal passports, money and credit cards under clothing.
Boots Travel Waist bag £9.50 Black canvas.
Go Travel Stretchy Belt Pouch £13.00 Expands to carry keys and phones. Lightweight and ultra-stretchy. Discreet headphone cable port. Fully adjustable waistband.

Case Luggage & Accessories

Case is on the opposite side to the exit from the security exit on the lower level of the Departure Lounge. They have several money belts and pouches. You can pre-order via their website.
A reserve and collect service is available from Case Luggage. Simply reserve the items online and then collect as you pass through the airport's North Terminal.

Opening hours: November to March 4.00 am to 8.30 pm; April to October 4.00 am to 10.00 pm
Telephone: 0129 356 9264
Email: gatwicknorth@caseluggage.co.uk
Website: www.caseluggage.com

Money belts and pouches

Go Travel Stretchy Belt Pouch £14.99 Lightweight and stretchy, expands to carry phones, keys and more. Headphone cable port and reflective safety trim included.

Go Travel Money Security Belt £10.99 RFID money belt to block illegal scans of RFID chips embedded in modern-day passports and credit cards preventing personal data being stolen. Designed to be worn under clothing. Has two internal pockets for storage.

Go Travel Money Belt £9.16 Protects passports, credit cards and other valuables and blocks illegal RFID scanning equipment. Soft, padded & comfortable to wear.

Go Travel Body Wallet £9.16 Made from breathable, skin-soft fabrics. Comfortable and easy to wear concealed under clothing. One size fits all, fully adjustable.

Go Travel Passport Pouch £10.99 RFID neck pouch, soft and comfortable. Protects passports, credit cards and other valuables by blocking illegal RFID scanning equipment to safeguard against identity theft and digital crime. Comprises two secure zipped compartments.

Go Travel Shoulder Wallet £8.33 Soft & comfortable holster-style wallet. Conceals valuables such as passports, money & other valuables under clothing. Adjustable shoulder strap which goes across the body.

Bum-bags

Pack Society £20.00 Premium Cool prints bum bags 10(h) x 24(w) x 7(d) cm Made from polyester with water repellent treatment. Comprises one large compartment with zip closure and adjustable waist strap.

Eastpak Bum Bag £22.00 Authentic Casual Springer Bum-bag 16.5(h) x 23(w) x 8.5(d) cm The Main compartment has a zippered closure to keep your sunglasses, key and documents safe. The waist belt adjusts to fit. Secure back pocket to stash cards, passports and cash.

Cross Body bags

Eastpak £27.00 Authentic, The One – Across Body Bag. Comes in three colours 21(h) x 16(w) x 2.5(d) cm

Eastpak £40.00 Authentic, Casual flex across body bag 23(h) x 18(w) x 4.5(d) cm Comprises a main compartment with zipper closure, adjustable shoulder strap, zipped front pocket and inside pocket.

Eastpak £50.00 Leather 21(h) x 16(w) x 5.5(d) cm. Mini bag made from a waxy leather.

Kipling Small Across Body Bag £64.00 Basics Day bags, Small Across body bag. 24.5 (h) x 25.5(w) x 4(d) cm Small, slim shoulder bag. Roomy and light with zipped compartments. 24(h) x 23.5(w) x 5.5(d) cm A versatile, classic and compact cross-body bag or as a clutch. Fits an 8" inch tablet.

Kipling Basic Daybags £74.00 Ergonomically designed. Comfortable strap. Easy-going style with durable water repellent finish and plenty

Knomo £129.00 Mayfair 10 inch crossbody bag.

Converse Core Poly Cross Body £22.00 Core poly cross body 22(h) x 16.5(w) x 11.5(d) cm Comprises adjustable handles/straps, interior zipped pockets, zip closure on the main compartment and reinforced base of bag. Variety of colours to choose.

Dixons Travel

Like Boots, it also has two stores on the lower level of the Departure Lounge. The first is smaller, opposite the Weatherspoon's Pub. The other is larger between Boots and Jo Malone on the right-hand side as you walk down towards the departure gates 101 – 113.

If you stroll past the store, you will find some security items on the rack outside both stores.

Opening hours: 4.00 am – 8.30 pm daily
Telephone: 01293 569737

Money belts and pouches

Go Travel RFID Blocking Passport Pouch £12.99 Blocks illegal RFID scanning equipment to protect from identity theft and digital crime. Soft and comfortable neck pouch. This pouch has two secure zipped compartments.

Go Travel RFID Blocking Money Belt £12.99 Unisex money belt. Soft and comfortable to wear. Conceals passports, money and credit cards. Single zipped compartment.

Go Travel Body Pouch £5.92 Soft and comfortable neck pouch in unisex style. Designed to be worn under clothing.

Go Travel RFID Blocking Wallet £19.99 RFID blocking wallet. Real leather wallet which blocks illegal RFID scanning equipment. Also features eight credit card slots and two banknote compartments.

Got Travel RFID Blocking Organiser £19.99 Blocks illegal RFID scanning equipment to protect against identity theft & digit crime. Can carry up to 10 credit cards, passports and money all in one.

Go Travel Carry Clip It £6.92 Karabiner clip to carry clothing, attach bags etc. Strong, secure spring action. Pack contains three.

Where to rest your eyes at Gatwick's North Terminal

If needs must, then a short shut-eye can help when travelling. In the public areas, the best places are those that offer comfort, dim lights, no draughts, little noise and few interruptions.

Here are some places in Gatwick Airport's North Terminal which you might find conducive to resting.

Please note, that from time to time, Gatwick decides to relocate the rows of seating. These are correct at the time of review.

Arrivals, Ground Floor

Renovations are nearly complete in this part of Gatwick Airport's North Terminal. Subsequently, there are now several rows of seats just in front of International Arrivals, and UK and Republic of Ireland Arrivals exits. These are not very quiet places as people are coming and going constantly. However, there is one place which we found is much quieter than the public seating in the main Arrivals Hall area.

Costa Coffee

Here there is an alcove tucked away from the main thoroughfare, just behind the food service area on the right. When you enter the café, walk past the refrigerator, and just behind it is an alcove. It is lovely and quiet without many people passing. Here there are two large black soft leather couches.

If this is already full, then pop down to the back of the café which is also away from the main thoroughfare. It is much quieter here also, but unfortunately, there were no soft leather couches.

Check-in, Level one

There are few places to rest here if any.

Seated area next to Excess Baggage Company

The seated area is right by the main entrance to the airport shuttle, so it isn't very quiet, and there is a lot of natural light. However, one of the rows of seats does not have any armrests so that you can rest in a more relaxed position than the other seats. Naturally, the footfall is high, and the automatic doors keep opening, so we would recommend moving to Check-in, Level Two where there are some more peaceful places to rest.

Hampton by Hilton Hotel Business Centre and Public Bar.

You're less likely to be disturbed here than any of the other restaurants and cafes. There is a lounge bar which has a variety of seats and couches where you can relax. What's more, it's away from the main thoroughfare meaning less footfall and noise. This is probably the best place to rest in the airport before security.

Location: The entrance to this hotel is right near the Easy Jet Check-in on level one. You will see a sign above the entrance to the corridor for the Hampton by Hilton. Just follow the signs to the right of the check-in desk.
Directions: Turn right at the Easy Jet Check-in area and walk towards the end of the hall. Walk straight ahead through the entrance and follow the passage to the left. Walk through the automated double glass doors. The total distance is about 50 steps from the Easy Jet check-in to the hotel reception.

Check-in, Level Two

There is a greater opportunity here than level one to rest and achieve a few moments of drifting off.

Seating alcove behind Check-in rows B and C

Gatwick North Airport has just revamped their Check-in Area on Level Two, and in doing so, they have made a lovely rest area right out of the way of the main thoroughfare. Head towards the back of the check-in area, and you'll find several rows of seats at the end of Check-in aisles B&C. It's dimmer here during the daytime than the front entrance area and noise in low during a non-peak time, there are no draughts, and the foot fall is much lower than in other areas.

Next to Emirates Tickets and Customer Information

Next to the Emirates Tickets and Customer Information stand, near the far left-hand entrance to the airport from the shuttle, there is a seated area. Not the best place to relax, but there are so few before security.

Next to Jamie's Coffee Lounge

There are also a couple of rows of seats, on the other side of the entrance doors, next to Jamie's Coffee Lounge.

Departure Lounge, Lower Level

The quiet zone next to Boots the Chemist

Head down to the far end of the lower level in the departure hall, and to the right, you will find some seating just to the right of Boots the Chemist. This is one of the quietest spaces in Gatwick Airport North Terminal's Departure Lounge to rest. There is no thoroughfare here, so there is little footfall. The air conditioning unit works at a moderate temperature with little draught and a low noise level. Unfortunately, the chairs do have armrests, with the exception of the middle two seats in each row. So, sleeping horizontally would be difficult, but there is a little room to stretch out. Unfortunately, this area also has several large windows. Fortunately, you'll be right next to the stores which sell eye masks! Please see list provided below.

Quiet Zone, lower level, Departure Lounge.

If it's late in the day, then you might consider wandering down to the children's play zone when the children have already left for the evening. Some travellers have reported sleeping on the soft flooring in the play area when all have abandoned play for the day. It's apparently quiet, spongy, little noise and without draughts.

Corridor to Gates 45 - 55 and 101 – 113

Gatwick has recently moved some seating into the space at the beginning of the passage to the Gates. Walk through the entrance just between London News Company and the Children's play zone and turn to the left. There are several rows of chairs here. Unfortunately, they have armrests and sleeping horizontally would be challenging. However, the footfall just misses the area to the left of the entrance making it much quieter than the main Departure Lounge seating.

Departure Gates 45 – 55

There are several seats, usually four to a bench without armrests, along with the corridors to gates 45 – 55. There is low footfall making it generally quiet. However, there are large windows which provide ample light during the day, making it dazzling during summer hours. The seats are located at the following locations.

Opposite Gate 54 There are four benches of four seats without armrests.

Opposite Gate 53 There is a bench of four seats here without armrests.

Opposite Gate 51 and the toilets, there are three sets of four seats

The junction between Gate 50 and 49 – 46. There is a bench of four seats without armrests.

Soft seating in the restaurants

There is only one restaurant on the lower level. The other restaurants are located upstairs on the upper level.

Weatherspoon's Red Lion Bar has large sofa styled seats in an area outside the front of the restaurant. There is more noise here than other restaurants due to its location and high footfall. So, it is better to go upstairs to the upper level if your flight has been delayed and you are stuck in the airport in desperate need for some shut-eye.

Departure Lounge, Upper Level

Soft seating in the restaurants

Traveller reviews indicate that the restaurant benches on the higher level in the Departure Lounge are comfortable, there is a low noise level, no recorded announcements or buzzing noise from air ducts. While many of the restaurants do have cushioned benches, our researcher was not able to verify the suitability after hours. But it might be worth a visit if you're stuck overnight to check it out for yourself. Here are the restaurants and cafes that have soft or leather seats without armrests.

Armadillo has long brown leather sofas at the end of the restaurant dining area.

Comptoir Libanais has a quiet area at the far end to the right of the restaurant. There is a long leather bench.

EAT has a couple of brown leather benches at each end of their dining area inside the restaurant area.

Garfunkel's provided you can gain access, has some large round booths with comfortable seats.

Shake-a-hula has soft bench seats.

Starbucks has soft bench seats on the left-hand side as you walk towards Wagamama's restaurant. Also, there are two quiet areas away from the main thoroughfare. The first is the corner to the left of the long window looking towards the loading bay and runway. Here there is a long felt covered bench style seat. The second is behind the service area. When you walk towards the long window, turn right, and you find a long brown soft bench style seat.

Union Jacks Bar has soft green bench seats on the left. Here the footfall is lower. Unfortunately, Yo! Sushi can be quite noisy when operating.

Yo! Sushi, if you're really stuck, have small booths with bench styled seating for two people on either side of a table.

Not so public areas

Airport lounges

Aspire Lounge

The Aspire Lounge has two quiet areas away from the main buffet dining zone, suitable for reading, relaxation and catching up on emails. The first is located to the left of the main entrance. The second is at the end of the room on the right. The area on the left is a dedicated quiet zone and has been designed for comfortable working and resting. It contains many soft black leather chairs suitable for work as well as rest.

If you walk straight ahead when you enter, you will find another quiet area around the corner to the right. Although also secluded, the seats are comfortable soft leather.

Open: Open hours are from 4.00 am to 10.00 pm, with a slight seasonal variation.

Access: Welcomes anyone who is travelling, which means it may not be the quietest lounge to relax in.

Facilities: Large lounge chairs and quiet areas.

Cost: Lounge entry for adults is from £17.99 if you book in advance or £35 on the door without booking. If your flight is delayed and you want to stay longer, then you can buy additional hours.

Free access to: Diners Club, Dragon Pass, Aspire Platinum membership, Institute of Directors, Lounge Pass, Priority Pass and Vueling airline passengers.

Location: First floor of the Departure Lounge.

Directions: Head towards gate 103 – 113, as you pass London News Company, you will see a corridor on your right. Go through the double glass doors and take the lift to the first floor. The lounge is located on the right-hand side.

No. 1 Lounge

Probably the best of the lounges for resting your eyes. There are two quiet, low lighting locations in this lounge, both away from the hustle and bustle of the food and drink area.

The first is the darker TV corner in the main lounge. As you enter the room, you will see the buffet, bar and bistro on the left. Straight ahead are tables for diners, and to the right is a darker, quieter seating area. You might be lucky to find a spot here. There is a long leather bench facing the large screen television, and it is often full.

If you turn right when you enter the bar area and down some steps, you will move into the library. This is a quiet room, designated for work and relaxation. You will find lots comfortable seating conducive for a quick shut eye or two. Here there are large brown leather couches and large comfortable chairs with headrests which are suitable for resting your eyes. The lighting is dimmer in the corner areas, and there is plenty of power points so you can charge while you doze.

If you prefer to doze in front of the runway view, then you'll find swivel chairs with your back to the rest of the room in the main lounge area. Power points are located on the floor next to the chairs.

Open: 4.00 am to 10.00 pm.

Access: All travellers including groups and children.
Facilities: Soft seating with large leather couches in a quiet library zone.
Cost: Lounge entry for adults is £32.00 if you book in advance or £40.00 on the door without booking. If your flight is delayed and you want to stay longer, then you can buy additional hours.
Free access to: Dragonpass, Diners Club, Institute of Directors, Lounge Club, Priority Pass, Dining Club, Caxton FX.
Location: On the lower level of the Departure Lounge, after security, near gates 101 – 113.
Directions: Head towards gate 103 – 113, as you pass London News Company, turn right into the corridor, you will see another hallway on your right. Enter the hallway and walk through the double glass doors. No.1 Lounge is directly ahead.

My Lounge

A less formal lounge than the others, with a friendlier atmosphere for casual relaxation or catching up with emails. There are two private rooms at the far end. The first one is the 'den' with large leather bench styled seating with a television, and the second with a sofa, PS3 station and football table. Either room when less busy and within school term times could be conducive for a few minutes of resting your eyes.

Open: 5.00 am to 6.00 pm (4.30 am to 2.00 pm winter schedule)

Free access to: Institute of Directors, Lounge Club, Lounge Pass, Priority Pass, Diners Club

Facilities: Two private rooms for relaxation.

Cost: Lounge entry for adults is £20 if you book in advance or £25 on the door without booking. If your flight is delayed and you want to stay longer, then you can buy additional hours.

Location: Departure Lounge, lower level.

Directions: Head towards gate 103 – 113, as you pass London News Company, you will see a corridor on your right. Turn right and proceed through the double glass doors. The lounge is located on the left-hand side just before the lifts.

Airport hotels offering day rooms for resting

If you need a little more than a quick power nap and have more than 5 hours before your flight, then you could try the hotels which offer day rooms at reduced rates. The following hotels are on site. You can book either in advance or on the day. Day rooms can be booked direct (the website address is listed below) or via a day room booking website, such as the Between9and5 website (which reports being the world's first dedicated website for booking day rooms).

Sofitel London Gatwick

This four-star hotel is directly connected to the North Terminal and offers a day room for those that need to rest before their next scheduled flight or meeting. There are 518 rooms with Mybed mattress for a good rest. Rooms have easy to control air-conditioning and dark curtains.

Reviews from previous guests comment on how much they appreciate being able to pre-book a day room so they can manage their travel wellbeing in advance when travelling through the North Terminal.

Guests have also raved about the soft, comfortable mattresses and pillows, which are now also available to purchase. Foam pillows are also an option.

While the hotel is silent to external noise with excellent soundproofing reported, there does appear to be an odd issue with noisy air conditioning in some rooms. Make sure you ask for a designated quiet floor or room away from families and functions.

You can book this day room either directly with the hotel or via www.between9and5.com

Telephone: +44 (0) 1293 567070 **or email** reservations3@sofitelgatwick.com
Website address: www.sofitelgatwick.com

Day Room time availability: 10.00 am to 5.00 pm
Room Rate: £79.00 inclusive of VAT per day
Location: The Sofitel hotel is connected to Gatwick Airport through a covered walkway on the right-hand-side of the shuttle on the North Terminal, Level two.
Directions: From the terminal exit on level one, walk straight ahead to the right of the shuttle to a covered walkway sign posted Sofitel Hotel. Walk down the corridor, and you're at the entrance within 2 minutes. If you are arriving by car, you will find the entrance to the hotel on the ground floor next to the Hotel's car park. Alternatively, you can park in the Airport car park with easy access to both the hotel and airport terminal on level one.

Hampton by Hilton

Connected to the Hotel and only two minutes from the Check-in desks on level one of the Departure Lounge, this highly rated hotel by guests offers rooms at a reduced rate during the day. It also provides fully air-conditioned rooms with blackout curtains and a choice of comfortable pillows.

Reviews from previous guests comment on the many pillows available as well as the type of pillows ranging from foam to feather. If a soft pillow is your preference, then these have been a definite favourite amongst past guests.

Although there appears to be excellent sound proofing from the noise of the runway, some guest commented they found the internal noise too loud on occasions. The rooms on the top floor are reportedly the quietest, so make sure you request this if you are a light sleeper or find getting to sleep difficult.

Telephone: +44 (0) 1293 579999 **or email** russel@hbhgatwick.com
Website address: www.hbhgatwick.com

Day Room time availability: 9.00 am to 18.00 pm
Room Rate: £69 which is a flexible rate with payment taken upon arrival and free cancellation policy up until midnight day before arrival. The price includes complimentary breakfast available from 4.00 am to 10.00 am.
Location: The entrance to this hotel is near the Easy Jet Check-in on level one. Just follow the signs to the right of the check-in desk. You will see a sign above the entrance to the corridor for the Hampton by Hilton.
Directions: Turn right at the Easy Jet Check-in area and walk towards the end of the hall. Walk straight ahead through the entrance and follow the passage to the left. Walk through the automatic double glass doors. The total distance is about 50 steps from the Easy Jet check-in to the hotel reception.

YOTEL, South Terminal

Located on level one of the Arrivals Hall in the South Terminal, Yotel is ideal if you want a quick nap before your flight or when continuing your journey. Business travellers often enjoy this conveniently located hotel as an option for a short stay between flights.

Past day guests comment positively on the suitability for a day room. The cabins are snug, but more than useful for a quick nap. Each cabin has an en-suite bathroom with a monsoon rain shower, shower accessories, towels, workstation and TV.

Reviewers have compared the Yotel facilities to other hotels in the area for a day stay, commenting that the sleep quality at Yotel is better than dayrooms at other hotels, as you won't hear all the normal workings of a hotel. They also report the rooms are adequately sound-proofed, the beds are comfortable, and the shower facilities are excellent.

Dayroom rates start at the minimum four-hour stay for £39; then you pay for any additional hours on top.

Telephone: +44(0) 207 100 1100 **or email** customer@yotel.com
Website address: https://www.yotel.com/en

Includes: Complimentary tea/coffee, Luxury towels and all-natural body wash/shampoo

Dayroom time availability: Short stay of up to four hours is £39. You can pay for additional hours after the minimum charge for four hours. Payment via debit or credit card. No cash accepted.

Location: South Terminal Arrivals on the ground floor.

Directions: Catch the airport shuttle to the South Terminal, head towards the Arrival Hall turn right at Marks and Spencer, and you'll see the lift located on the right-hand side of the Arrivals Hall. The lifts are between Costa Coffee and Moneycorp Bureau de Change. Simply take the elevator down to the entrance on the ground level and turn left.

BLOC Hotel, South Terminal

Situated in the South Terminal, the entrance is right next to security control on the upper level in Departures. Guests comment on how exceptionally convenient it is to the restaurants and other shops being within the South Terminal and how modern the facilities are. Despite being so close to the airport runway, guests also report on how quiet it is, with no external noise. You can also request a view over the runway upon check-in at the hotel reception and not worry as the soundproofing is superb.

Despite the small sized bedrooms, the amenities are positively reviewed as a good option for a day room. The beds are seemingly comfortable, the electric black-out curtains work well, and the monsoon shower facilities offer the opportunity to revitalise just prior to or recovering from a long-haul journey. One guest summed their day room stay as "would definitely stay here again".

The BLOC hotel offers a day-time rate at the half price of the night rate for use between 7.00 am in the morning until 4.00 p.m. The cost is from £29.00 for a standard room.

Telephone: +44(0) 020 3051 0101 **or email** bookingslgw@blochotels.com

Website address: https://www.blochotels.com/

Day Room time availability: 7.00 am to 4.00 pm

Rate: Minimum day room rate of £29.00.

Includes: Day room facility includes Zenology shower products and "soft fluffy" towels.

Location: The hotel is in Gatwick South Terminal. The reception is located on the upper level of Departures right next to the security entrance.

Directions: You can also get to the hotel from level two in the Arrivals, via the stairwell next to the toilets just opposite Boots the Pharmacy.

Hilton London Gatwick Airport, South Terminal

The Hilton is a four-star hotel with over 800 bedrooms. There is direct access to Gatwick's South Terminal via a covered walkway. It offers dayrooms which are spacious, clean and comfortable at a lower cost than the night rate. The soundproofing is reportedly excellent with past guests commenting they couldn't hear any aeroplane noise.

High recommended by past business travellers for an excellent sleep and shower. Past guests report full black-out curtains, however, have provided mixed reviews about the air conditioning working and some have commented the mattress was somewhat 'worn-out'. The good news is the Hilton is about to undergo a significant refurbishment (2018 – 2018).

Telephone: +44 (0) 1293 610 828 **email:** london.gatwick@hilton.com
Website address: http://www3.hilton.com

Dayroom availability: 9.00 am to 6.00 pm
Dayroom rate: From £75.00 per day.
Location: South Terminal Gatwick Airport, Gatwick RH6 0LL
In the corridor which connects the hotel with the terminal right opposite the Costa Coffee.
Directions: Simply take the shuttle to the South Terminal from the North Terminal. Walk from the shuttle to the Hotel.

Airport hotel offering overnight rooms

In addition to those hotels mentioned above, there are other hotels right next to the North Terminal which you might like to consider for a good night's sleep.

Premier Inn

This hotel guarantees a good night sleep. They are so confident you'll have a great night's sleep that if you don't, they will give you your money back! To assist in this quest, they have reportedly very comfortable mattresses and offer a pillow menu so you can request a pillow to suit your individual preference.

Blackout curtains and soundproofing are also standard in rooms. Many reviewers have commented on how quiet their rooms were despite being so close to the Gatwick Airport's North Terminal.

While the air-conditioning can be controlled in the room, some reviews by previous guests indicate they found the room too warm and stuffy. The main reason provided was the inability to open a window for fresh air, and the lowest temperature was reportedly only 19°C. However, the majority of reviewers indicated the room was just right, and only a few felt the room was too cold.

So, if you need fresh air and prefer to sleep with a window open, it would be best to enquire when booking on the feasibility of such, bearing in mind that it will then also be very noisy. The alternative would be to choose a hotel not so close to the airport.

Telephone: 0333 003 8101 or 0871 527 9354
Website address: www.premierinn.com

Room Rates: average price from £67.50 with no refunds or £79 on a flexible booking with the cancellation policy. Early booking might secure discount rates, according to some reviewer comments.
Locations: Directly opposite the North Terminal drop-off point.
Directions: Simply walk outside the main entrance of the terminal on level 1, down the escalator on the left of the shuttle and cross the road. You can't miss it!

Must have sleeping aids

Forgotten your sleep accessories? You can get various items to aid getting to sleep at the following outlets. Some of these stores allow you to purchase or order online, and they will have the item reserved for you to collect once you reach the airport.

Boots the Chemist

There are several Boots the Chemist at Gatwick's North Terminal, including one before security (in the Arrivals Hall) and two within the Departure Lounge. You can pre-order online and collect either from Boots the Chemist within the North Terminal Departure Lounge or before security at Unit 2 near M&S Simply Food, opposite Costa Coffee on the ground floor, post-exit from Customs and Excise.

Opening in Arrivals: 24 hours
Opening in Departure Lounge: 4.00 am to 8.300 pm
Telephone: 01293 569606
Website: www.boots.com

Items to aid sleep

Earplugs

Boots Earplugs and Eyeshade Travel Set £5.50 Two memory foam ear and a fully adjustable sleep mask. Available airside and landside.

Boots Travel Reusable Earplugs £4.00 Contains three pairs of reusable earplugs in super soft memory foam. Carried in a hygienic carry case. Available in store airside and landside.

Auritech Sleep Hearing Protectors £19.95 Advertised as superior to traditional foam, wax or silicone earplugs, reducing annoying noises, e.g. snoring, but allows you to hear normal conversations or alert sounds. Order online.

BioEars Soft Silicone Earplugs with active aloe, three pairs, £4.99 Soft Silicone earplugs that are hygienic and effective to reduce noise. Order online.

Boots Pharmaceuticals Soft Disposable Earplugs £6.99 Contains 20 pairs of earplugs and a carry case. Designed to reduce harmful or irritating noise and are comfortable to wear. Order online.

Boots Foam Earplugs £7.19 Contains twenty pairs of earplugs. Designed to reduce harmful or irritating noise. Comfortable to wear. Ideal to use when sleeping, working, travelling or swimming. Order online.

Boots Pharmaceuticals Soft Disposable Foam Earplugs Three Pairs with carrying Case £2.69 Designed to fit most ear canals. Contains three earplugs and a carry case. Order online.

Boots Pharmaceuticals Muffle Wax Earplugs (5 pairs) £2.69 Effectively reduce harmful or irritating noise and moulds to fit the shape of the ear. Ideal for travelling. Order online.

EarPlanes Two earplugs (one pair) £9.99 Reusable, extra soft earplugs, tested by US Navy Pilots.

Pluggerz-Sleep-Earplugs £8.29 Reusable earplugs that offer full protection when worn continuously. Can be used over 100 times. Order online.

Boots Flight Earplugs (One pair with a carry case) £4.69 Relieves in-flight ear discomfort associated with air pressure changes during flights. They also help to reduce noise. Available landside and online.

Sleep Masks

Prices from £4.99 for a sustainable sleep mask to £7.00 for a silky travel mask.

EcoTools Sustainable Sleep Mask £3.33 Made with rayon from bamboo to create a product that is both durable and allows the skin to breathe. Available in store airside and landside.

Boots Eyeshade & Earplug Set £5.50 A deluxe sleeping mask designed to shut out any light and unsightly travel partners together with earplugs to provide an uninterrupted sleep for a long journey. Available airside and landside.

Boots Silky Sleep Mask £7.00 Available airside.

Go Travel Nightshade Sleep Mask £6.50 Extra comfortable sleep mask to block out any unwanted light. Soft, silky fabric on inside and out. Suitable for both genders and features a wide elasticated headband for comfort. Available airside and landside.

Go Travel Silky Eye Mask £7.00. Luxury silky eye mask. Blocks out unwanted light to promote sleep during travel. Gently padded with a fleecy lining and features a wide elasticated headband for comfort. Available airside and landside.

Alarms with special effects.

Lumie Bodyclock Starter 30 £56.99 Provides an initial 30 minutes of sunrise to help walk you up. 760 g. Order online.

Lumie Bodyclock Go 75 £74.95 Wakes you up with a 20, 30 or 45-minute sunrise. It reportedly contributes to reset your sleep/wake cycle to help you feel refreshed. 760 g. Order online.

Lumie Bodyclock Active 250 £99.95 Wakes you with the sunrise to help reset your sleep/wake cycle. Heavier than the first two body clocks at 1.02 kg. Order online.

Travel pillows

Boots Travel Holiday Beach Pack £10.00 Design and go super snoozer neck pillow with eyeshades and earplugs.

Boots Comfy Travel Sleep Pillow £10.00 Available airside and landside.

Boots Inflatable Travel Pillow £6.50 Suitable for packing in hand luggage. Available airside and landside. Can also order online. Available airside and landside.

Boots Memory Foam Travel Neck Pillow Delux £15.00 Made from memory foam with a soft cover to enable greater comfort while travelling. It provides head and neck support for long flights or car journeys. Available airside and landside.

Go Travel Sleep Set £10.00 Neck pillow and mask. Available airside and landside.

Go Travel 2 in 1 Travel Pillow £14.00 Bean pillow which has two configurations. It can be worn as a U-shaped neck pillow or as a rectangular travel cushion. For maximum comfort, it has a soft velour exterior. Available airside.

Go Travel Super Snoozer Pillow £10.00 Inflatable travel pillow. Flat-back design fits snuggly around your neck and head to reduce neck strain on long journeys. Ergonomically designed for correct anatomical support. Available landside and airside.

Go Travel Memory Foam £15.00 Super deluxe memory foam travel pillow. Moulds to the head, neck and shoulders. Flat-back design for upright sleeping comfort. Removable, washable cover. Button & loop fasting to attach to wheeled luggage. Available landside and airside.

Go Travel Supreme Snoozer £14.99 Inflatable travel neck pillow. Air and foam hybrid design. Soft removable jacket. Folds small for easy packing. Flat back shape to support the head. Available airside and landside.

Go Travel Ultimate Memory Pillow £24.99 Structured travel pillow. Snug 360 fit which instantly moulds to the chin and neck. Adjustable close to prevent head tipping forward. Rear grip to secure pillow to a headrest. Includes a carry pouch. Available landside.

Case Luggage

Case Luggage is situated on the lower level of the Departure Lounge between Harrods and Accessorize offers various travel essential items, including sleep aids. A reserve and collect service is available from Case Luggage. Simply reserve the items online and then collect as you pass through the airport's North Terminal.

Opening hours: November to March 4.00 am to 8.30 pm; April to October 4.00 am to 10.00 pm
Telephone: 0129 356 9264 Email: gatwicknorth@caseluggage.co.uk
Website http://www.caseluggage.com

Items to aid sleep

Microbead Pillow Two for £18.00 In the bargain bin at the front of the store.

Go Travel Super Snoozer £9.16 (£10.99 on high street or online) Inflatable neck pillow. Ergonomic design for correct anatomical support. Flat-back to fit snuggly around the head. Available airside.

Go Travel Double Decker Pillow £16.49 Bean pillow which can be worn in two ways. The flat-back mode provides more support around the neck. The head-rest mode offers additional support at the back of the head. Available online.

Go Travel Ultimate Memory Pillow £27.49 for upright sleeping comfort. This pillow has been designed to mould instantly to the circumference of the neck to provide a 360° fit. Soft velour cover with a rear gip to secure the pillow.

Go Travel Silky Eye Mask £6.66 Luxury silky eye mask, blocks out unwanted light. Gently padded with a fleecy lining with an elasticated headband for comfort. (£7.99 online or high street).

Dixons Travel

Like Boots, it also has two stores on the lower level of the Departure Lounge. The first is smaller, opposite the security exit. The other is larger between Boots and Jo Malone on the right-hand side as you walk down to the departure gates 101 – 113.

You can pre-order items from Dixon's Travel direct by phoning the Gatwick North Terminal store. They would be able to check and reserve your product for you. Unfortunately, you won't be able to order any items online.

If you stroll past the store, you will find some travel essential items on the rack outside both stores.

Opening hours: 4.00 am – 9.00 pm daily
Telephone: 01293 569737

Items to aid sleep

Go Travel Super Snoozer Pillow £7.92 Inflatable travel pillow with a flat-design to fit comfortably around the head and neck to reduce neck strain on long journeys. Ergonomically designed for correct anatomical support.

Go Travel Memory Pillow £12.99 Super deluxe memory foam designed to mould to the head, neck & shoulders. Flat-back design for upright sleeping comfort. Removable, washable cover.

Go Travel Ultimate Memory Pillow £19.99 for upright sleeping comfort. This pillow has been designed to mould instantly to the circumference of the neck to provide 360º fit. Soft velour cover with a rear gip to secure pillow.

Travel Pillow £12.99 or 2 for £20 You'll find these in the large bin near the front of the store.

Travel Blanket £12.92 or 2 for £20 Look out for the giant bin near the front of the store.

Sleep Masks

Go Travel Nightshade Eye Masks £5.92 Comfortable sleep mask, blocks out any unwanted bright light. Soft and silky fabrics in and outside. Unisex design with a wide elasticated headband for comfort.

Go Travel Quiet Zone Earplugs £7.99 Sound filtering earplugs. Yellow filter blocks out low-frequency sound and the white filter blocks out the high-frequency sounds. Earplugs soften to the shape of the ear. Comes with a hygienic travel carry case.

Excess Baggage Company and Bag Wrap

You can pick up travel accessories from Excess Baggage Company as you walk from the shuttle to the Check-in area. When you pass through the main entrance, you will see Excess Baggage on your left opposite London News Company and next to Costa Coffee.

Opening hours: 5.00 am to 10.00 pm
Telephone: +44 (0) 1293 734 888 **or email:** gatwick@left-baggage.co.uk
Website: www.left-baggage.co.uk

Items to aid sleep

Go Travel Ear Plugs £3.99 Reusable foam earplugs. Three pairs per pack. Hygienic travel carry case. Moulds to fit the ear canal. Made from soft memory foam. Available landside.

Go Travel Super Snoozer Pillow £9.99 Inflatable travel pillow. Ergonomically designed for correct anatomical support. Flat-back design fits snuggly around your neck and head to reduce neck strain on long journeys. Available airside.

Go Travel Plush Pillow £9.99 Soft travel neck pillow. Supports head and neck for sound sleep. Fits snug around the neck. The fleecy jacket can be machine washed. Button & loop fastening attaches pillow to wheeled luggage.

Go Travel Bean Snoozer £12.99 Flat-back bean travel pillow. Supports the head without pushing it forward to reduce neck strain on long journeys. Comines soft padded foam with air-light poly-bean filling. Fits snug around head and neck.

Go Travel Memory Foam £14.99 Super deluxe memory foam travel pillow. Moulds to the head, neck and shoulders. Flat-back design for upright sleeping comfort. Removable, washable cover. Button and loop fasting to attach to wheeled luggage.

Go Travel Nightshade Sleep Mask £5.99 Extra comfortable sleep mask to block out any unwanted light. Soft, silky fabric on inside and out. Suitable for both genders and features a wide elasticated headband for comfort. Available airside and landside.

WHSmith and London News Company

It would be difficult to miss the many stores of WHSmith and the London News Company (owned by WHSmith). Both stock the same brand of products, so other than the name it is difficult to see any difference between the two. Which is rather fortunate if you are running late, as there is virtually a store on most levels of Gatwick Airport's North Terminal. In fact, you will also find a mini WHSmith at Gates 101 - 113.

London News Company Locations: Opposite M&S Simply Food in the Arrival Hal; opposite Excess Baggage in the main entrance of Check-in, level one; upstairs of Check-in, level two just opposite Moneycorp Bureau de Change.

WHS Locations: Between The Bookshop and Fat Face; and Gates 101 – 113.

London News Company opening hours: Before and after security 4.00 am to 9.00 pm.

WHSmith opening hours: Before security 24 hours and post security 3.00 am to 10.00 pm

Website: www.whsmith.co.uk

Sleep Masks

Destination Travel Eye Mask and Earplugs £6.99 Eye mask is adjustable, elasticated with velcro strap and super soft for extra comfort. The earplugs are made from soft foam which seals without pressure within the ear. They are reusable and come in a protective carry box. Available airside and landside.

Cabeau Sleepmask £14.99 Midnight magic Sleep. Comfortable, adjustable sleep mask, made from memory foam. Guaranteed black-out. Side pockets for earplugs and an adjustable nose bridge.

BioEars earplugs £4.99 Soft silicone earplugs. Sound reducing with a 22-decibel noise reduction rating.

EarPlanes £8.99 Made of soft hypoallergenic silicone. Safe, soft and disposable. Relieves air pressure discomfort. Tested by US Navy Pilots. Noise reduction 20 decibels.

Pillows and blankets

Cabeau Fold and Go Blankets£19.99 Pillow, blanket, cushion and seat lumbar support.

Cabeau Micro Lightweight Comfort Pillow £29.99 Raised side support, superior quality microbead, 360 side-head chin & comfort, breathable micro-pocket for phone or music player with adjustable support. Available airside and landside.

Destination Travel Blow-up Pillow £5.00

Cabeau Evolution Pillow £19.99 Available landside and airside.

World Duty Free shop

There are four duty free shops in Gatwick's North Terminal. One is in arrivals as you exit into the arrivals hall past security. Another World Duty Free shop is located on the lower level of the Departure Lounge, as you pass through security and the departure gates 45 – 55 and 101 – 133.

You can now reserve and collect online or by phone. You won't need to pay for the items until you receive your order so if travel plans change or you change your mind you won't need to worry about refunds. In the event of travel delays, the World Duty Free shop will keep your order for collection up to 48 hours after your scheduled departure time.

If the items listed below aren't yet available online to pre-order, then you can call or email the customer services. If you don't wish to take the items away with you, then you can tell the sales assistant when you pay for your items that you want to collect on return.

Opening Hours in Departure Lounge: Open 24 hours
Opening Hours in Arrivals: Open 24 hours
Telephone: +44 (0)1293 502421 and +44 (0)1293 504260 **Email:** customerservices.uk@wdfg.com
Website: lgws.worlddutyfree.com

Items to aid sleep

Travel Blue Sleep Rest £8.50
Travel Blue Eye Mask, £3.00 Soft sleeping mask, designed for comfort and rest.
Travel Blue Flight Mate Earplugs £9.99 Pressure reducing ear plugs. Reduces pressure in your ears during flight while not blocking normal voices.
Travel Blue Travel Set £12.49 Mask and neck pillow.
Travel Blue Inflatable Pillow £10.00 Classic inflatable neck pillow for rest. Made of soft, anti-allergenic fabric. Comes with a travelling pouch.
Travel Blue Ultimate Pillow £10.00 Designed to support the neck. Combination of the inflatable pillow with an additional layer of luxury soft synthetic down. Outside is microfibre for additional comfort. Hand washable.
Travel Blue Comfy Pillow £9.99 Supports the neck during rest on long journeys. Made of luxuriously soft, thick fleece material. Hand washable.
Travel Blue Neck Pillow £10.80 with micro pearls. The micro pearls make the neck pillow exceptionally soft and comfortable. Ideal for sleep or relaxation during a business trip. Outside is high-quality velveteen material. Inside is filled with micro-beads.
Travel Blue Memory Foam Pillow £19.99 Exceptionally soft and comfortable pillow. Ideal for sleep during travel. Made of velveteen material filled with memory foam. Good neck support. Variety of colours.
Travel Blue Infinity Travel Pillow Tranquility £23.33 Memory foam material for soft support, specially designed for travellers. Ergonomically designed to mould softly to

your shoulders and neck. Comes with a built-in pocket to keep it clean and save space.

Chapter 3: Coping with Jet Lag

Most of us experience travel fatigue and sleep disruption when travelling, but jet lag takes fatigue and poor quality sleep to a whole new level when travelling on business. Studies on international business travellers have found that jet lag is one of the most common health problems, with one recent study reporting three-quarters (74%) of all business travellers cite jet lag as their primary health concern.

According to the World Health Organisation, jet lag will leave the passenger with reduced physical and mental performance, indigestion and disturbance of the bowel function, general malaise, daytime sleepiness and difficulty in sleeping at night. Even if you usually sleep well, you are susceptible to the effects of jet lag.

Jet lag is simply a term used to describe the symptoms caused by the disruption of the body's internal clock and the circadian rhythms it controls. The circadian rhythm normally controls our hormone regulation, eating times, body temperature variation, thyroid function, metabolic process, and various other functions. Disruption of the body clock occurs when travelling across multiple time zones, e.g. when going east towards west or west towards east on a high-speed aircraft.

When flying over several time zones, the body clock becomes out of synchronisation with the destination time, i.e. the traveller experiences day and night time contrary to the body's current rhythms. If the natural pattern of releasing hormones, controlling temperature, eating and sleeping are upset and out of time, then travellers may notice the effect and feel out of sorts with their normal functions.

The symptoms are quite varied, depending on the time of day, the amount of time zone alteration and individual differences. The body will attempt to synchronise itself, but it can take days to get one's natural timings back again. It will depend on how many time zones the traveller has crossed.

How long will it take to adjust?

It is estimated that to re-adjust fully to the new destination's time zone, recovery of one day per time zone should be used as a guideline. Which doesn't seem very helpful if you're on a short duration business trip!

The rate at which people adjust to a new destination time zone really depends on the individual, as well as the direction of travel. Some sleep experts state that one in three adults will experience severe jet lag, one in three mild jet lag and one in three hardly noticeable at all. Older business travellers may also experience jet lag more than younger business travellers.

If the journey is trans-meridian, then the symptoms travelling eastwards may be worse than going westwards. This is because when you are travelling east, your body clock has to be advanced which is harder than delaying sleep when you go west. Most people have a circadian rhythm which is slightly longer than the 24-hour clock, so lengthening the day becomes more problematic than shortening it.

Jet lag is less likely to happen, if at all, if you travel from north to south over the same time zone. For example, a trip between the Pacific and Atlantic may well result in jet lag, but a journey from Europe to South Africa would not cause jet lag as there isn't any time difference.

How does your body clock re-sync?

Essentially, there are two separate processes which are related to your biological timing. The first being the circadian rhythm, which is the regulation of the body's internal processes which influence the level of alertness, and the second is homoeostasis. Homoeostasis sleep propensity (inclination to sleep) is simply the result of the combination of the amount of time elapsed since the last sleep and the biochemical substances which drive sleepiness.

Circadian rhythms are controlled by a master clock, the suprachiasmatic nucleus (SCN), located in the hypothalamus of the brain. There are also periphery body clocks located in other tissues. It is the role of the master clock (SCN) to send signals to the peripheral oscillators in the tissues, and this helps to synchronise them for their physiological functions. The peripheral clocks also respond to internal signals such as food intake and nervous stimuli. Tissues such as muscles, liver, lungs and other organs all synchronise at different rates.

The master clock (SCN) is regulated by light hitting the retina, which causes a hormonal reaction that regulates our sleep-wake cycle. At night time, when the sun goes down, the pineal gland becomes active and releases a substance called melatonin which makes us less alert. In the morning, when the light hits our retina, the pineal gland becomes inactive, and there is a rise in the level of cortisol, our wake-up and alert hormone. Senior executives travelling on business may notice jet lag more, as levels of melatonin in our blood have been found to decrease with age.

As light is a powerful catalyst, it is essential to get sunlight and darkness at the relevant times of day to help trigger a release of hormones from the SCN at the correct times. It is also the role of peripheral clocks to send signals to the master clock. So, sticking to your usual routine at the destination time may help realign the master clock.

This second synchronisation of the independent clocks may explain some of the other symptoms. Travellers adapt their sleep-wake cycles with light from the environment. However, as other tissues adapt at different rates, this could explain some implications for health and mood.

The effects of jet lag

Jet lag & productivity

If you feel after years of long-haul travel and jet lag that you're processing information slower and don't recall facts as well, then you might just be right! And here's why. Studies are showing frequent transmeridian business trips are associated with cognitive deficits over the long-term. Cognitive defects include poorer performance on mental tasks, impaired concentration, the inability to complete a task, impaired working memory and poorer coordination.

Business travellers who frequently fly long-haul across several time zones, experiencing jet lag over several years, also tend to have a higher cortisol level. Cortisol is a 'get up and go' hormone and plays a significant role in making us more alert in the morning. There is good evidence that long-term exposure to raised stress hormones can impair mental skills and memory.

Chronic disruption of circadian rhythms reportedly raises cortisol levels during the working day, and the levels are found to be significantly higher in those with a history of repeated jet lag than those working on the ground. Research has also shown a significant difference in cognitive functions between those experiencing frequent jet lag and those not undertaking transmeridian flights.

Jet lag and travel fatigue

Being tired before you fly on long-haul really isn't much fun either! When jet lag is combined with the tiredness caused by the preparation for and the journey itself, the effects can be quite devastating for the traveller.

Travel fatigue symptoms include general fatigue, diminished ability to process information, impaired memory recall, disorientation and headaches. These symptoms are independent of time zone travelled and are caused by a cramped space, little chance to move around, low-oxygen levels, disruption of sleep and other routines, and dehydration due to limited fluid and restricted food intake. Travel fatigue will make your recovery from jet lag even more challenging and possibly prolonged.

If this sounds familiar, then avoiding a sleep deficit and reducing fatigue before boarding the plane may help to manage some of the symptoms of jet lag. Chapter 4 provides information which can assist in reducing travel fatigue as you pass through Gatwick's North Terminal.

Jet lag, mood and mental health

Long-haul travel can really take it out of you. Being able to manage all the demands, deadlines and incidentals that only pop up en route can make any traveller irritable or anxious. Unfortunately, business travellers experience higher levels of work-related stress on top of their travel. Anxiety and depressed mood are also symptoms of frequent long-haul travel when experiencing reoccurring jet lag. Other common jet lag symptoms include increased fatigue, headaches and irritability.

Research shows that frequent sleep disturbance is the single most significant predictor of major depression, suggesting sleep plays a major role in preventing depression. Travel and work-related stress can exacerbate the inability to get good quality sleep.

Research has also shown the shift of body temperature, melatonin production, quality of sleep and changes in other rhythms increases the incidence of suicide, affects individuals with bipolar diseases more, and major affective and psychotic disorders occur more frequently when more time zones are crossed.

Jet lag and digestion

If that's not enough, then there are the problems with digestion, including indigestion, changes in the frequency of defecation, the consistency of stools, along with reduced appetite and enjoyment of food. Research shows the majority (60%) of business travellers on transmeridian flight report gastrointestinal problems, including nausea, constipation and diarrhoea.

It's simple when you put into the context of the discussion above on synchronisation. Jet lag disrupts the circadian rhythm which influences the production and secretion of digestive enzymes and insulin.

Jet lag and weight maintenance

If you're wondering why you've been gaining weight over the last few years or finding it difficult to lose weight while travelling long-haul on business, then the first point to mention is that you're not alone. Frequent business travellers report a higher BMI than non-frequent travellers.

The second point to confirm is there are many variables as to why business travellers may put on weight, and yes you've guessed it - one of them is linked to jet lag and the regular disruption of the circadian rhythm. Others, as you probably already know, include healthy food availability, business entertainment, reduced activity and changes to your usual food intake.

Sleep researchers have deduced from their studies how the master clock (SCN) regulates our energy balance. The master clock (SCN) sends signals to our peripheral tissues by hormonal, nervous and behavioural pathways to regulate the peripheral clock's control of fuel use. There is also regulation of food intake and activity to maintain an energy homoeostasis (balance of energy intake and energy expenditure). It is through regulation of food intake, physical activity and metabolic processes that both the brain and peripheral clocks contribute to long-term weight stability.

It is the disruption of the precise balance of energy intake and energy expenditure which may explain to some degree why some travellers have a higher BMI than non-travellers. As researchers continue to explore this issue, there is growing evidence that the timing of meals has an impact on weight as well as the secretion of certain hormones. The composition of a meal may also affect weight gain. In a comparison of two diets of the same energy value, the proportionally higher fat diet consumed at the wrong time is more likely to result in weight gain.

Jet lag and long-term health

Research is now linking circadian disruptions with cardiovascular disease, diabetes and cancer, which explains why employees with long-term circadian rhythm disturbances, such as shift workers, have a higher incidence of these diseases. So, it isn't surprising that frequent travellers, particularly business people travelling long-haul, are also reporting higher blood pressure, raised cholesterol, triglycerides and sugar in clinical blood results than non-frequent travellers.

While the precise metabolic changes are still being explored, sleep experts have found a circadian misalignment will elevate blood pressure. One explanation is that the rise in cortisol (alert hormone) later in the day and reduction in melatonin production (sleep hormone) will cause blood pressure to rise. Over time, a regular increase in blood pressure may increase the risk of cardiovascular disease.

Research is also finding a change in the way we metabolise fatty acids when there is a phase shift in our body clock. The circadian system regulates fat absorption, storage and fat transportation. So, our metabolism will be affected by any change in our sleep-wake cycle. Not just the amount but also the type of fat in your diet is important as saturated fat appears to cause more lipid storage than polyunsaturated when faced with a circadian phase shift. This may help to explain why there is a reported rise in blood cholesterol and triglycerides in frequent long-haul business travellers.

Frequent long-haul flyers are also more at risk of developing diabetes. Previous research evidence suggested blood sugar levels increased with circadian rhythms shifts, placing individuals into a pre-diabetic state. Sleep experts are now finding circadian misalignment decreases glucose tolerance and insulin secretion. Similar results are found with studies reporting on short sleep, sleep deprivation and poor quality sleep.

While the precise mechanism for the increased incidence of certain cancers isn't known, we do know that shift workers who experience a regular shift in their body clock have a higher incidence of cancer. We are yet to find out why.

What can you do to reduce jet lag?

Consider the length of your trip

If it is a short trip, less than four days, you may be better off just living in the home time zone, and waiting until you can actively reduce the effects of jet lag. Taking into account that your body may not have the opportunity to synchronise fully to the new time zone; it may make it harder to re-synchronise when you reach home again.

Sleep deficit

Get as much rest as possible before departure. If you fly when you're tired, it will make the jet lag feel worse. Try to get some sleep on the flight if you are flying overnight so you can stay up until night-time when you reach the destination.

The World Health Organisation recommends using any opportunity to rest before and during medium to long-haul flights. They suggest that even short naps (less than 40 minutes) can be helpful.

If you need to find a place to sleep in Gatwick Airport's North Terminal, then refer to Chapter 2. We've listed the most restful areas, along with on-site hotels for short naps, day rooms, and overnight stays.

Reset your watch at the beginning

Routine is an important mechanism to re-aligning your body clock. If your trip is several days, then you might be better off adjusting your watch at the beginning of your flight to the destination time. Once changed, keep to the schedule at destination time, amending your food intake and sleep routine to the new time.

Adjust your bedtime gradually before leaving

If you are travelling over several time zones, you might find it useful to change your sleep pattern to match the schedule at your destination before you go. Some sleep experts recommend travellers adjust their sleep and awakening times by an hour per day for several days before travel to coincide with the destination time.

If you're going east, try going to bed an hour earlier than your usual time, and if you're travelling west, try to go to bed an hour later. For westward travel, it is preferable to delay sleeping until bedtime at the destination. For eastward with more than nine hours' time difference, it might be easier to delay the internal body clock than to advance it. During the flight, try to sleep in accordance with your destination's time zone.

Anchor your sleep

A minimum block of four hours sleep during the local night is referred to as 'anchor sleep'. It is believed this is the minimum amount of time to allow the body's internal clock to adapt to the new time zone. The World Health Organisation recommends when you reach your destination try to make sure you have a minimum of four hours sleep every 24 hours, even if it means having naps throughout the day.

Stop-over on long-haul flights

If you find it difficult to sleep on a plane when travelling long-haul, then try including a stop-over to make the adjustment to a new time zone easier. It will also help reduce fatigue once you arrive. Many airports are now offering onsite accommodation or hotels joined to the departure lounge. Some hotels even do short stay (up to 4 hours) or day room availability (9.00 am to 5.00 p.m.) at a reduced rate. We've listed those on site at Gatwick Airport's North Terminal in Chapter 2 on Sleep.

Go west!

Losing time is harder to adjust to than gaining time. When we travel east, we lose time, and west we gain time. It can be difficult to fall asleep at an earlier bedtime, keeping you up during the first part of the night. When going west, it is easier to fall asleep, but harder to wake up. Studies show that performance is generally better when travelling westward.

Research also reveals that you need to adjust for half the number of time zones crossed when going west compared to two-thirds the number of time zones crossed when travelling east. In fact, travelling east by six to nine times zones is reportedly the worst as the exposure to light to realign the body clock doesn't match the day/night cycle at the destination.

This is where a jet lag app can help by estimating the best time of day for you to seek light and when to avoid it. We discuss these later, and detail where you can download them for free.

Switch off the blue-lights

Avoid looking at your electronic devices and in-flight videos at least half an hour before bedtime. Blue lights are the lights emitted by electronics and in-flight video screens. During the day, blue lights may be beneficial as they boost attention, reaction times and mood. Blue-light also suppresses melatonin secretion, our 'go to sleep' hormone, making it harder and take longer to fall asleep.

If you don't already have sunglasses which filter blue light, you'll find the outlets at Gatwick Airport's North Terminal listed below.

Keep hydrated

Make sure you have plenty to drink, preferably water. Dehydration makes it more difficult for the body to adjust to a new rhythm. What's more, symptoms of dehydration include fatigue and lethargy, and may contribute the feelings of jet lag.

Travel health professionals recommend aiming for at least one cup of fluid per hour (200 ml). Tea and instant coffee count, neither are now considered to have a significant diuretic effect but do not consume within 4 - 6 hours of an anticipated period of sleep time as the caffeine is a stimulant. The World Health Organisation also suggest that if coffee is drunk during the day, small amounts every two hours is preferable to one large cup. Keep consumption to your destination time zone.

Alcohol is best avoided as it increases urine output and disrupts the sleep cycle. While it may help to fall asleep, the effect is short-lived, with disruptions to get up during the night, as well as impairing the quality of sleep. A hang-over, no matter how mild, will exacerbate the effects of jet lag and travel fatigue.

So, when they come around with the trolley – opt for water, milk, juice, and maybe tea or coffee. Stay away from drinks that are aerated as they cause a sensation of bloating.

Not sure where to get bottles of water to take with you on the flight? We've listed all the outlets in Chapter 11.

Exercise

Keeping up your fitness routine is also recommended as a good way to help manage the effects of jet lag. For some individuals, vigorous exercise after arrival has been reported to be helpful, and some research on animals has found exercise can help adjust the internal clock.

The effects of exercise are being researched further, and it is now thought that activity-based routines can have an essential role to play in the synchronisation of the body clock. It is considered that exercise may help to force a state of alertness, promote more restful sleep and induce arousal in the central nervous system which impacts on the internal clock.

The World Health Organisation had also looked at the research so far and recommended exercise during the day may help to promote a good night's sleep when jet-lagged, but cautions to avoid strenuous exercise within 2 hours of trying to sleep.

Want to exercise before boarding your flight? Then turn to Chapter 9 to find the best places at Gatwick Airport's North Terminal, along with nearby fitness facilities.

Diet

Simply being aware of re-adjusting your watch to the time of your destination can play a prominent role. It influences both the peripheral and master body clocks to realign to the new time zone.

Extreme food regimes have been tried out, but research on intense regimes lack evidence and data to support any recommendation. We can only recommend proven strategies where any nutritional or health claims have been approved. For example, the feast/fasting diet is a diet based on the idea that a high-protein meal in the morning will increase alertness, whereas high carbohydrate meals in the evening will raise the amount of tryptophan available from protein foods and will increase levels of serotonin, a precursor of melatonin which makes you sleepy.

However, research on this regime is limited, and the design of the methodology for fasting/feasting has been questionable. The effect of these types of foods have also not been confirmed sufficiently by research, consequently the European Food Safety Authority (EFSA), upon reviewing the research to date, has not approved the use of tryptophan or tyrosine as nutrients which promotes sleep and alertness.

We can, however, advise on foods which are light, healthy and contribute nutrients approved by the EFSA for nutritional properties and health claims. This includes our healthy meals and snacks in Chapters 12, 13, 14 and 15 respectively, along with the consumption of melatonin-containing foods listed below.

Melatonin

Timed administration of melatonin is another way of adjusting the sleep/wake cycle. However, in most countries, this is a prescription based drug, and the World Health

Organisation warns against over the counter remedies in other countries. Some sleep experts recommend the use of foods which have a high content of melatonin such as Montmorency cherries or tart cherry juice. Research on this has been quite promising, and the EFSA has approved nutrition and health claims regarding the effect of melatonin.

More information on the use of melatonin is provided later in this chapter, along with advice on where you can purchase foods which can contribute melatonin to your evening diet while at Gatwick Airport.

Get some sun

The cycle of light and dark is one of the most critical factors in resetting your body clock. When light hits the retina, it triggers the master clock to send signals to the pineal gland. The pineal gland becomes inactive, and our 'wake-up' hormone, cortisol, levels rise. The timing of the exposure of bright sunlight at the destination will help you to adapt to a new time zone quicker.

The deliberate exposure to light at the right time is essential in helping people to synchronise their sleep/wake cycle having reached their destination. Bright light in the morning will cause a phase advance and bright light in the evening will cause a phase delay. The World Health Organisation recommends when flying west to have exposure to daylight in the evening and avoidance in the morning. Conversely, when travelling east, one should have exposure to the light in the morning and avoidance in the evening.

Health professionals might also use light therapy which requires timed exposures. Some health professionals recommend special glasses which provide light to eyes at certain times: others simply recommend dark glasses or blue-light glasses to inhibit light and encourage the secretion of melatonin at certain times. The WHO also suggest wearing dark glasses to help avoid undesired periods of light exposure.

We have provided more information on where to get products at Gatwick Airport's North Terminal below.

Use an app

Some sleep experts have been involved in designing applications for estimating the relevant times to sleep and seek sunlight. These are beneficial if you wish to reset your body clock based on light and sleep patterns. They are listed below.

Apps for jet lag

Over the last couple of years, several apps have been released for mobile devices which can be used to advise on how to reduce the effects of jet lag. These generally focus on the key components which have a significant influence on readjusting your body clocks, such as destination time, sunlight and daily routines.

We have mentioned some of the more popular apps below and, although we neither endorse nor recommend any specific app, we have provided some information on each. Whichever app you decide to use is entirely up to you. We suggest you try a few out and let us know how you have found them. They are all free of charge.

British Airways Jet Lag Advisor

British Airways has worked in conjunction with a leading UK sleep expert, Dr Chris Idzikowski. The app works by asking you simple questions, such as what time you normally wake up, whether or not you sleep well, what the time will be at your destination and what time it is at home.

The aim is to advise you on the best things to do to minimise your jet lag. You will receive advice on when to seek sunlight, when to avoid light and why you need to adjust your meals and exercise.

There are no gimmicks with this app. It's simple to use and provides expert advice in a nutshell. Like all the other apps we have listed, it is free to access.

Website: www.britishairways.com/travel/drsleep

Jet Lag Rooster (iOS)

Jet Lag Rooster was developed by Jay Olson, when working for Swan Medical Group, to assist frequent travellers and airlines training their pilots and flight crew. It is free to use and offers the user three categories of advice.

A little more detailed than the British Airways Jet Lag Advisor above. You put in where you are flying from and the destination, along with the date, time of departure and arrival. The app will also ask you for your normal sleep routine and if you are taking melatonin. There is an assumption you are flying from the United States, but this is a simple operation to change.

In addition, it will ask you when you want to start shifting your sleep pattern. Choices within this question, include after arriving, after departing or up to 3 days before leaving. This will determine the nature of the advice given.

Website: www.jetlagrooster.com

Entrain

Entrain is a free app for iPhone. It was developed at the University of Michigan and works by recommending light schedules that adjust your body's clock as fast as possible to a new time zone. As with other apps, this starts by asking questions about your current and destination time zone.

You can adjust your schedule by choosing a brightness setting and moving the time of arrival to an earlier slot if you want to shift your body clock before you depart. Once you have scheduled your travel, a graph is used to represent your circadian rhythms (current and target rhythm) over several days.

Itunes webpage: https://itunes.apple.com/us/app/entrain/id844197986?mt=8&ign-mpt=uo%3D4

Where to buy products that may reduce jet lag

There are a few simple products on the market which may help you minimise the effects of jet lag. Some of these work on the basis that if you restrict the amount of light stimulating your suprachiasmatic nucleus (master body clock) at appropriate times, you can control the release and levels of melatonin in your body and thereby reset your body clock. Others work by simply enabling a better sleep, whereas others have a direct effect on the levels of melatonin in your blood. Mostly, they are based on scientific theory and often recommended by sleep experts to either help sleep at the right time or to help regulate your body clock.

Why not try a few out and see how you get on. The majority are relatively inexpensive and lightweight. We've searched Gatwick Airport's North Terminal on their availability and listed the various retail stockists and prices where appropriate.

Sleep Masks

Shutting out the light when it is time to sleep, particularly if you are a sensitive sleeper, can be problematic when travelling on an aeroplane or the room is too light when trying to adjust to the time at your destination. According to research conducted, sleep masks can help to reduce the time it takes to get to sleep, increase the amount of rapid eye movement sleep and improve the quality of sleep. Researchers have also found that those who wear a sleep mask have higher levels of circulating melatonin in their blood.

When choosing a sleep mask, choose one that sits comfortably and is snug, but not too tight. Look at the quality of the fabric and the fit rather than the external look. A good design will allow you to open your eyes comfortably. Some people don't like the sensation of eyelashes touching the material so look carefully at the type of design.

There is a choice of stores in Gatwick's North Terminal which stock sleep masks. These are listed below.

Boots the Chemist

There are several Boots the Chemist at Gatwick's North Terminal, including one before security near M&S Simply Food, opposite Costa Coffee on the ground floor, post-exit from Customs and Excise and two within the Departure Lounge.

Opening in Arrivals: 24 hours
Opening in Departure Lounge: 4.00 am to 8.300 pm
Telephone: 01293 569606
Website: www.boots.com

Travel Masks

EcoTools Sustainable Sleep Mask £3.33 Made with rayon from bamboo to create a product that is both durable and allows the skin to breathe. Available in store airside and landside.
Boots Eyeshade & Earplug Set £5.50 A deluxe sleeping mask designed to shut out any light and unsightly travel partners together with earplugs to provide an uninterrupted sleep for a long journey. Available airside and landside.
Boots Silky Sleep Mask £7.00 Available airside.
Go Travel Nightshade Sleep Mask £6.50 Extra comfortable sleep mask to block out any unwanted light. Soft, silky fabric on inside and out. Suitable for both genders and features a wide elasticated headband for comfort. Available airside and landside.

Go Travel Silky Eye Mask £7.00. Luxury silky eye mask. Blocks out unwanted light to promote sleep during travel. Gently padded with a fleecy lining and features a wide elasticated headband for comfort. Available airside and landside.

Case Luggage & Accessories

Case is on the opposite side to the exit from passport control & World Duty Free on the lower level of the Departure Lounge. They have a range of travel accessories, including sleep masks.

Opening hours: November to March 4.00 am to 8.30 pm; April to October 4.00 am to 10.00 pm
Telephone: 0129 356 9264 Email: gatwicknorth@caseluggage.co.uk
Website: http://www.caseluggage.com

Go Travel Silky Eye Mask £6.66 Luxury silky eye mask, blocks out unwanted light. Gently padded with a fleecy lining with an elasticated headband for comfort. (£7.99 online or high street).

Dixons Travel

Dixons Travel also has two stores on the lower level of the Departure Lounge. The first is smaller, opposite the Weatherspoon's Pub. The other is larger and located between Boots and Jo Malone on the right-hand side as you walk down to the departure gates 101 – 113. You'll find a sleep accessory stand usually located outside the front entrance of the store.

Opening hours: 4.00 am – 9.00 pm daily
Telephone: 01293 569737

Sleep Masks
Go Travel Nightshade Eye Masks £5.92 Comfortable sleep mask, blocks out any unwanted bright light. Soft and silky fabrics in and outside. Unisex design with a wide elasticated headband for comfort.

Excess Baggage Company and Bag Wrap

Excess Baggage Company is located at the front entrance to the Check-in, level one, opposite the London News Company and next to Costa Coffee. You'll find the following items on the accessories stand at the entrance of the stores.

Opening: 4.00 am – 8.30 pm

Telephone: 0129356900

Go Travel Nightshade Sleep Mask £5.99 Extra comfortable sleep mask to block out any unwanted light. Soft, silky fabric on inside and out. Suitable for both genders and features a wide elasticated headband for comfort. Available airside and landside.

London News Company & WHSmith

There are six stores of WHSmith and the London News Company (which is owned by WHSmith). They both stock the same brand of products, so other than the name it is difficult to see any difference between the two. Which is rather fortunate if you are running late, as there is virtually a store on most levels of Gatwick Airport North Terminal. You will also find a mini WHSmith at Gates 101 - 113

London News Company Locations: Opposite M&S Simply Food in the Arrival Hall; opposite Excess Baggage in the main entrance of Check-in, level one; upstairs of Check-in, level two just opposite Moneycorp Bureau de Change.
WHS Locations: Between The Bookshop and Fat Face, at the far end of the Departure Lounge next to Boots the Chemist; and Gates 101 – 113.
London News Company opening hours: Before and after security 4.00 am to 9.00 pm.
WHSmith opening hours: Before security 24 hours and post security 3.00 am to 10.00 pm
Website: www.whsmith.co.uk

Sleep Masks

Destination Travel Eye Mask and Earplugs £6.99 Eye mask is adjustable, elasticated with velcro strap and super soft for extra comfort. The earplugs are made from soft foam which seals without pressure within the ear. They are reusable and come in a protective carry box. Available airside and landside.
Cabeau Sleepmask £14.99 Midnight magic Sleep. Comfortable, adjustable sleep mask, made from memory foam. Guaranteed black-out. Side pockets for earplugs and an adjustable nose bridge.

World Duty Free

There are four duty free shops in Gatwick's North Terminal. One is in arrivals as you exit into the Arrivals Hall past security. Another larger World Duty Free shop is located on the lower level of the Departure Lounge, as you pass through security and there are two smaller ones at the departure gates 45 – 55 and 101 – 133.

Opening Hours in Departure Lounge: Open 24 hours
Opening Hours in Arrivals: Open 24 hours
Telephone: +44 (0)1293 502421 and +44 (0)1293 504260 **Email:** customerservices.uk@wdfg.com
Website: lgws.worldddutyfree.com

Sleep Masks
Travel Blue Sleep Rest £8.50
Travel Blue Eye Mask £3.00 Soft sleeping mask, designed for comfort and rest.
Travel Blue Travel Set £12.49 Mask and neck pillow.

Lightboxes

Sunlight is a very effective way to readjust your body clock once you have reached your destination or just before you depart. However, the timing of light stimulating your suprachiasmatic nucleus (master clock) is vital. Get it wrong, and you may end up with feeling more exhausted and less able to concentrate.

So, if you need to source light when it is dark outside, then turning on a bright bathroom light or using a light box may help. There are several light boxes on the market now. It is suggested that one should choose a light box which is very bright (10,000 or more lux) to be effective at stimulating the release of cortisol and inhibiting the release of melatonin. A bathroom light is usually somewhere between 200 to 400 lux so less effective, but often brighter than other domestic lights.

You can either purchase a light box at Gatwick Airport North Terminal or take one you have purchased in advance. Choose one which is lightweight and above 10,000 lux. We've also listed several items on our website which are highly rated.

Boots the Chemist

There are several Boots the Chemist at Gatwick's North Terminal, including one before security and two within the Departure Lounge. You can pre-order online and collect either from Boots the Chemist within the North Terminal Departure Lounge or before security at Unit 2 near M&S Simply Food, opposite Costa Coffee on the ground floor, post-exit from Customs and Excise.

Opening in Arrivals: 24 hours
Opening in Departure Lounge: 4.00 am to 8.300 pm
Telephone: 01293 569606
Website: www.boots.com

Lumie Zest Combination SAD Light and Wake-up £149.99 This portable, lightweight SAD light provides bright light therapy and includes a wake-up light option to start the day with a gradual sunrise. The blue-enriched light provides 2,000 lux at 50 cm. Weight 260 g

Lumie Arabica SAD Light £119.95 Lumie Arabica SAD light provides a bright light (10,000 lux). It weighs 1.7 kg and is 38 x 22 x 17 cm in size.

Lumie Brightspark SAD and Energy Light £138.00 Slim SAD light for use at home or work. Provides 10,000 lux at 20 cm. Weight 1.9 kg A little bulky for hand luggage!

Lumie Brazil SAD Light £178.80 Lumie Brazil SAD light also provides a bright light (10,000 lux).   It weighs 3.1 kg and is 50 x 32 x 15 cm in weight. Not so travel-friendly for hand luggage!

Alarm clocks with light

It is equally important that you wake up at the right time. If you find it difficult to wake when it is very dark, then a combination light clock might be the answer when you are travelling. Combination light and alarm clocks gently adjust the light in the room. The aim is to reduce the production of melatonin and to stimulate cortisol, which is your alert hormone.

Boots the Chemist

Boots the Chemist offers three combination alarm clocks which you can order online in advance and collect upon arrival either from the Departure Lounge, lower level or after customs in the Arrival Hall, ground floor at Unit 2 near M&S Simply Food, opposite Costa Coffee on the ground floor, post-exit from Customs and Excise.

Opening in Arrivals: 24 hours
Opening in Departure Lounge: 4.00 am to 8.300 pm
Telephone: 01293 569606
Website: www.boots.com

Alarms with special effects.

Lumie Bodyclock Starter 30 £56.99 Provides an initial 30 minutes of sunrise to help walk you up. 760 g. Order online.

Lumie Bodyclock Go 75 £74.95 Wakes you up with a 20, 30 or 45-minute sunrise. It reportedly contributes to reset your sleep/wake cycle to help you feel refreshed. 760 g. Order online.

Lumie Bodyclock Active 250 £99.95 Wakes you with the sunrise to help reset your sleep/wake cycle. Heavier than the first two body clocks at 1.02 kg. Order online.

Blue light-wave blockers

Blue light waves have a stronger effect on the body clock than other light rays. While during the day, it can help boost attention, reaction times and mood, they can have the most disruptive effect during sleep. Research indicates that blue light suppresses melatonin secretion more than other light waves. Electronic devices omit blue-light, hence why it is essential to cease working on your device at least half an hour before bedtime.

Specialist glasses which block blue wave light have been designed to aid sleep and reduce jet lag if worn at predicted times. They are relatively inexpensive and can be purchased through Amazon. You can also have an anti-blue light tint added to your prescription glasses.

Designer sunglasses which block blue light are also available at the following outlets. Although they tend to be more expensive than others selected, they may also offer other features such as photochromic lenses which lighten or darken depending on the time of day.

Boots the Chemist

Boots the Chemist also offers designer sunglasses which block blue light waves. You can order online in advance and collect upon arrival either from the Departure Lounge, lower level or after customs in the Arrival Hall, ground floor at Unit 2 near M&S Simply Food, opposite Costa Coffee on the ground floor, post-exit security.

Opening in Arrivals: 24 hours
Opening in Departure Lounge: 4.00 am to 8.300 pm
Telephone: 01293 569606
Website: www.boots.com

Oakley Holbrook £99 One of the best-selling Oakley glasses. The lenses block 100 percent of UVA/UVB/UVC rays and blue light up to 400 nm.
Oakley Silver £132 Made from a lightweight O-Matter, these glasses can be worn all day. They block 100 percent of UVA/UVB/UVC rays and blue light up to 400 mm.

Oakley Half Jacket 2.0 XLSports Sunglasses £100 Polished black, with black iridium polarised lenses. They block 100 percent of UVA/UVB/UVC rays and blue light up to 400 mm.

Serengeti Granada £179 Driver lenses with a Classic style frame. Granada frame is constructed from lightweight Monel metal for comfort and durability. Block most blue light and are also photochromic.

Serengeti Nuvino £133 Rimless frame, so it doesn't box in your view. It's also lightweight and durable. The CPG lens protects against glare, fines tunes light transmission and blocks most blue light, along with being photochromic (lighten and darken with the conditions).

Ray-Ban

Ray-Ban is located in the middle of the lower level of the Departure Lounge. All their lens apparently block harmful light up to 400 nanometers. You can also choose some styles which offer blue-light blocking properties. Select from the following models and choose Green Lenses G-15 which blocks most of the blue light.

Aviator Classic £172 Originally designed for US aviators in 1937, now one of the most iconic models in the world.

Original Wayfarer Classic £127 Choose G-15 polarised lenses to block out the blue light.

Erika Classic £136 Frames come with a choice of lenses. Choose the Green Classic G-15 for blue light blocking.

Clubmaster Folding £200 Combines retro style with a new functional design. Can be easily folded and stored for convenience. Offered in a variety of frame colours and lens treatments, including the Green Classic G-15 for blue light blocking.

New Wayfarer Classic £118 An updated version of the classic Wayfarer style, which includes a smaller frame and slightly softer eye shape. There are a variety of lens treatments, including Green Classic G-15 and G-15 polarised.

Dark sunglasses

Dark Sunglasses may help to keep the bright or sunlight out at less desirable times, and by doing so, it is believed they may help readjust your body clock by not inhibiting the release of melatonin at inappropriate times.

There are several shops at Gatwick Airport's North Terminal where you can purchase a new pair of sunglasses. We found the following stores have a good stock of sunglasses to choose from.

Accessorize

Accessorize is situated in the Departure Lounge on the Lower Level, next to Case Luggage Company. They stock women's sunglasses.

Opening hours: 4.00 am to 9.00 pm
Location: Departure Lounge, lower level next to Case Luggage Company.
Telephone: +44 (0) 1293 579817
Website: http://uk.accessorize.com

Boots

There are several Boots the Chemist at Gatwick's North Terminal, including one before security and two within the Departure Lounge. Boots stock a range of sunglasses for men, women and children. You can order in advance online and collect from the store, both before security and in the Departure Lounge. You simply nominate the relevant store when you select store delivery the website.

Opening in Arrivals: 24 hours
Opening in Departure Lounge: 3.00 am to 9.00 pm
Telephone: 01293 567625 and 01293 569606
Website: www.boots.com

JD Sports

JD Sports are situated in the Departure Lounge, upper level, in between Pret A Manger and Sunglass Hut. They have a range of sunglasses for both men and women.

Opening hours: 4.00 am to 9.00 pm
Location: Departure Lounge, upper level, between Pret A Manger and Sunglass Hut.
Telephone: +44 (0) 1293 223016 **email:** customercare@jdsports.co.uk
Website: www.jdsports.co.uk

Ray-Ban

Ray-Ban is situated in the middle of the lower level of the Departure Lounge. They only stock Ray-Ban sunglasses.

Opening hours: 4.00 am to 9.00 pm
Location: In the Departure Lounge, lower level.

Telephone: +44 (0) 1293 579404
Website: www.ray-ban.com/uk

Sunglass Hut

There are two Sunglass Huts in the Departure Lounge. The first is on the lower level, on the left-hand side, between Ted Baker and Dune as you pass out from World Duty Free, and the second is upstairs on the upper level next to JD Sports and Wagamama's. They have an excellent range of sunglasses for men and women.

Opening hours: 4.00 am to 9.00 pm
Location: In the Departure Lounge, lower, next to World Duty Free and upper level between JD sports and Wagamama's.
Telephone: +44 (0) 1293 507610
Website: www.sunglasshut.com/uk

World Duty Free

There are four duty free shops in Gatwick's North Terminal. One is in arrivals as you exit into the arrivals hall past security. Another World Duty Free shop is situated in the lower level of the Departure lounge as you exit from security and head towards the lounge pavilion. Lastly, there is also a World Duty Free at the departure gates 45 – 55 and 101 – 133.

They stock over 25 brands including Ray-Ban, Ted Baker, Jimmy Choo, Gucci, Prada and Oakley.

Opening Hours in Departure Lounge: Open 24 hours
Opening Hours in Arrivals: Open 24 hours
Telephone: +44 (0)1293 502421 and +44 (0)1293 504260 **Email:** customerservices.uk@wdfg.com
Website: lgws.worlddutyfree.com

Melatonin

Melatonin is a natural hormone made by your body to help induce sleep. During the day, when it is light, the gland producing melatonin is inactive. When the sun goes down, or it is dark, the pineal gland is activated by the master body clock (Suprachiasmatic Nucleus) and releases melatonin. When melatonin rises sharply in your blood, you begin to feel less alert. This usually occurs about 9.00 p.m., and melatonin stays elevated in the blood for about 12 hours. So, if your body clock is six hours out, you will begin to feel less alert about 3.00 p.m. or 3.00 a.m., depending on the direction of travel. Either way, you will need melatonin to be released into the blood at a more relevant time.

Unfortunately, as we age, we produce less melatonin, thereby making us more susceptible to jet lag. This may be a contributing factor as to why senior management travelling on business suffer more with frequent long-haul travel.

Melatonin by consumption

You can also either obtain melatonin by prescription (UK & Australia) or purchase it over the counter in other countries (such as the USA). If you are flying from Gatwick Airport's North Terminal, you won't be able to obtain melatonin over the counter at the airport without a prescription.

The WHO also warns travellers about taking over the counter melatonin, for example in the USA it is considered a food supplement and is not a regulated medicine. The WHO doesn't recommend the purchase of over-counter tablets on the basis that the effects from such tablets are not fully evaluated, and the side effects are not entirely known. This is mainly due to the non-standardised manufacturing methods meaning the dosage per pill varies considerably, and some harmful compounds have been found present in unregulated tablets.

Another option is to eat or drink foods which contain melatonin or precursors of melatonin. The European Food Safety Authority has approved claims on melatonin relating to the regulation of the sleep-wake cycle and jet lag. Foods which are good sources of melatonin are advocated to be consumed on the first day of travel and the following few days after arrival at the destination. To help alleviate the feeling of jet lag, you will need to consume at least 0.5 mg close to bedtime.

Food sources of melatonin

Foods high in melatonin include tart cherry juice, whole tart cherries, and to a lesser extent, walnuts and raspberries. Other food sources are corn, rice, peanuts, barley, oats, asparagus, tomatoes, broccoli, strawberries, olives and sunflower seeds. However, the level of melatonin in these following sources is low, and large quantities would need to be eaten to supply an adequate dose of melatonin.

Sleep experts have researched the consumption of tart Montmorency cherry juice about 30 minutes to 1 hour before sleep and now recommend this to be effective in reducing the time for the onset of sleep and improving sleep quality. Montmorency cherry juice concentrate has at least ten times whole tart cherries and at least fifty times more melatonin than other foods, including sweet cherries. This is probably your best bet for increasing melatonin levels naturally just before bedtime as the juice is easy to consume and quickly digested.

Some airlines provide meals items which contain melatonin or one of its precursors (tryptophan) to help induce sleep on long-haul flights. You may have noticed the odd dessert or snacks with walnuts or cherries as part of the ingredients on the menu. To claim a reduction in the time taken to fall asleep, the European Foods Standards Authority (EFSA) state foods which contain 1 mg of melatonin per portion need to be consumed close to bedtime. This is hard to achieve, but some melatonin present in some restaurant or snack items may contribute small supplementary amounts.

Some research suggests that pineapple, bananas, oranges and kiwifruit may also help to raise the level of melatonin within 2 hours of consumption. Likewise, some research suggests foods high in tryptophan (an amino acid which is eventually converted to melatonin) might help to induce sleep when combined with carbohydrate. Consequently, you may also have noticed a combination meal made of carbohydrate and protein containing tryptophan such as rice and salmon as part of your evening airline meal. However, neither of these two examples are approved EFSA approved health and nutrition claims, and some research defies scientific evidence regarding basic biochemical pathways.

Where to find food items which contribute melatonin

You can pick up foods which are natural sources of melatonin to take on board with you from the following outlets at the Gatwick Airport's North Terminal.

The best two foods, as they have the highest contents, are Montmorency cherries (juice contains a higher concentration) and walnuts. Unfortunately, we couldn't find any Montmorency cherry juice available post-security. Other food sources are available, although the quantities needed to reach 1 mg to shorten the onset of sleep or 0.5 mg to reduce the effects of jet lag might be difficult to consume! Certainly, no single portion of food will provide sufficient to meet the EFSA guidance.

However, selecting a mix of food items might have a cumulative effect by contributing supplementary melatonin in addition to your body's production. Consequently, any of the portions we mention below contribute melatonin, but may not have a sufficient quantity of melatonin on their own to meet the EFSA's required amount to have a single significant effect.

Arrivals, Ground Floor

Marks & Spencer

Marks & Spencer's Simply Food store is located before security. Provided you are purchasing solid food items you will be able to take them through security. However, liquid items and gels over 100 ml are prohibited.

Opening Hours: 24 hours
Location: You will find Marks & Spencer in the Arrivals Hall, ground floor, next door to Boots.

Items include:

Walnuts 85 g Walnut halves. Walnuts are one of the richest sources of melatonin. However, they are also high in calories owing to the fat content, making an energy dense snack. Those who wish to lose weight might feel inclined to restrict their portion. The good news is the fat is mainly monounsaturated, and walnuts are also a good source of vitamin E.

Lightly Salted Giant Corn 140 g Giant corn kernels, lightly salted. Corn contains some melatonin. Despite the label stating lightly salted, this product is moderate to high in salt at 0.9g per 100g. So, if you eat the whole packet and not the portion size which is indicated at 30g, you will be adding a lot of salt to your daily diet.

Jalapeno Corn 140 g Contains corn (80%), sunflower oil, salt and spices. Corn contains some melatonin. These are higher in salt than the lightly salted, but not by much given the amount is 1.08 g salt per 100g. Similar to the lightly salt giant corn above, if you eat the whole packet, it will contribute a lot of salt to your diet.

Fruity Mix 70 g Mixture of sweetened dried cherries, raisins, sultanas, dried cranberries and dried apricots. Due to the high added sugar content, it would be healthier to combine some of this mixture with some other items such as nuts, such as walnuts or cheese.

London News Company and WHSmith

London News provides a couple of snack packets containing cherries. Tart or sour cherries are the variety which contains the most melatonin.

There are several London News Company and WHSmith stores at Gatwick's North Terminal, of which three are before security. WHSmith is on the right-hand side as you walk from the shuttle, car parks and Sofitel Hotel into the North Terminal, level 1. There is also a smaller London News Company on the ground floor in the Arrivals Hall next to the Bureaux of Change, and a smaller one in Check-in on Level 2 at the end of Zone E opposite the Moneycorp Bureau de Change. There are another three stores in the Departure Lounge on the Lower Level and some small units near the departure gates.

Opening Hours: Arrivals 24 hours
Opening Hours: After security in the Departure Lounge 4.00 am to 8.30 pm

Items include

Urban Fruit – Cheeky Cherry 90 g Just cherries (and the occasional pip) gently baked. 240 kcal (1006 kJ) per packet

Graze All Day Energiser 34 g Contain sour cherries, pears and walnuts. Both the walnuts and sour cherries provide the melatonin in this snack. A small packet contains 150 kcal (631 kJ).

Graze Dark Chocolate Cherry Tart 40g Contains dried sour cherries (20%) which provide a source of melatonin, along with pecans, chocolate buttons and raisins. High in fibre but also contains added sugar content from chocolate. A small punnet (40g) contains 184 kcal (767 kJ).

Boots the Chemist

Boots the Chemist has various snack items which you can choose. You can either shop for snack items in the Boots before security or from the two within the Departure Lounge. The one in the arrival hall is located on the ground floor at Unit 2 near M&S Simply Food. The larger store in the Departure Lounge is down the far end and is the better store for snack items.

Opening in Arrivals: 24 hours
Opening in Departure Lounge: 4.00 am to 8.30 pm

Items include:

Walnuts 40 g or 200g Walnuts are one of the best sources of melatonin. They are also high in monounsaturated and polyunsaturated fats. The packet of 200 g is very in high fat and calories.

Mixed nuts and raisins 40 g, 200 g or 400 g Includes walnuts and peanuts which are both a source of melatonin, and other nuts which are high in tryptophan a precursor to melatonin. Comprises raisins, peanuts, hazelnuts, walnuts, almonds and brazil nuts. A small portion (40 g) is 206 kcal (856 kJ)

Nairn's Gluten Free Oats & Fruit Biscuit Breaks Comprises over 70% wholegrain oats which are a source of melatonin and tryptophan (precursor to melatonin). Also, high in fibre to support digestive function and low in sodium. These biscuits come in a handy pouch so are easy to pop in your hand luggage for a snack on the go.

Nairn Gluten Free Biscuit Breaks Oats & Stem Ginger Approximately 65% whole grain oats and only 46 calories per biscuit. Oats aren't just a source of melatonin but also tryptophan (precursor to melatonin). High in fibre to aid digestion and traveller's constipation. These biscuits come in a handy pouch so are easy to pop in your hand luggage for a snack on the go.

Check-in, Level One

Costa Coffee

Costa Coffee doesn't offer a lot in the way of tart cherry food items, but it does provide a small snack bag with walnuts. There are a couple of Costa Coffee. Both are located before security, in Check-In hall on level 1, next to the excess baggage, on the left-hand side of the lobby as you enter from the train station and a larger one in the Arrivals Hall at the far end, near M&S Simply Food store.

Locations: Arrivals Hall, right next to the International Arrivals exit, and Check-in Level 1.
Opening in Arrivals: 24 hours
Opening in Check-in: 4.00 am and 8.00 pm

These dishes contain foods with a melatonin content.

Fruit and nuts 40 g £1.10 contains walnuts (15%) which are a good source of melatonin, mixed with almonds (good source of tryptophan) and raisins.

Departure Lounge, Upper Level

The upper level of the departure lounge comprises restaurants and cafés. Many of these sell meals containing ingredients which supply some melatonin and precursors of melatonin. We've listed some of the menu items below, although noting that many contain some melatonin but not sufficient to meet the EFSA approved guidance on specified quantities.

Armadillo

Mexican food often includes rice and corn within dishes or as side dishes. Both rice and corn contain a little melatonin. You would need to eat a rather lot to reach a 1 mg dose to aid sleep, making it rather impossible in the time-frame! Even though not sufficient by themselves to have a noticeable effect, they all contribute some melatonin.

Open: 4.00 am to 8.30 pm
Location: In the middle of the upper level of the Departure Lounge, overlooking the lower level below.

These dishes contain foods with a melatonin content.

Grilled Corn on the Cob cayenne aioli & Grana Padano. Corn is one of the top ten foods containing contain melatonin.
Jambalaya Comprises of spiced rice, black beans, sliced chorizo, chicken prawns, roasted rainbow veggies, spinach and sweetcorn. Both rice and sweetcorn contain melatonin.
Pan Roast Salmon Fillet pickled beetroot, mouli, carrot, charred corn, Served with green rice.
Green Rice A side dish of rice with herbs. Rice contributes a small amount of melatonin.

Comptoir Libanais

Comptoir Libanais is a Lebanese canteen. Middle Eastern Cuisine comprises many ingredients which contain some melatonin. Perhaps this is one good excuse to enjoy a Mediterranean diet.

Open: 4.00 am to 8.30 pm
Location: First restaurant on the upper level, next to the stairs and directly opposite the security entrance.

These dishes contain foods with a melatonin content.

Olives A mix of green and black olives, both containing some melatonin.
Halloumi & Olive Wrap. Marinated halloumi cheese, black olives, cucumber and tomato. All contain melatonin or tryptophan, a precursor of melatonin.

Halloumi Cheese Flatbread Oven baked flatbread with halloumi cheese, thyme, sesame seeds and fresh mint. Served with fattoush salad and pickles.

Pan Roasted Salmon Pan roasted salmon fillet served with vermicelli rice, harissa sauce, pickles and fattoush salad.

Halloumi Salad Grilled Halloumi cheese, romaine lettuce, tomatoes, cucumber, spring onion, olives, radish, olive oil & lemon juice. Halloumi is a good source of tryptophan, a precursor of melatonin, while tomatoes, cucumber and olives all contain some melatonin.

Sirine Salad Lebanese spiced chicken breast, feta cheese, romaine lettuce, spring onion, mint, vine tomato, topped with pomegranate seeds and pumpkin seeds.

EAT

EAT offers a small snack packet of dried fruits, nuts and seeds. They also now offer some healthier alternatives to their current bakery range, which contain some ingredients that offer a little melatonin. One items which might be worth trying is the Cherry Berry Almond Smoothie due to cherries having a higher melatonin content than other foods.

Open: 4.00 am to 20.30 pm
Location: Halfway along the upper level, just opposite Shake-A-Hula.

These dishes contain foods with a melatonin content:

Cherry Berry Almond Smoothie Cherries, blueberries and oats blended with almond milk. 162 kcal (678 kJ)

Fruits, Nuts & Seeds 40 g, contains pumpkin seeds, almonds, sunflower seeds, cashews, golden raisins. Almonds and sunflower seeds contain a small amount of melatonin, and as well as the other nuts and seeds are a good source of tryptophan, a precursor to melatonin. However, the quantities of seeds are small within this packet.

Texan Chilli Beef, beans, tomatoes, red peppers and wild rice. Served with Crème Fraiche.

Super Nutty Fit Box Quinoa, black rice with beetroot, houmous, chargrilled broccoli, cashew nuts and pistachio nuts. Black rice, broccoli and pistachio nuts contain melatonin.

Pret A Manger

Pret A Manger range of snacks has grown considerably over the past few years. We found one snack item with walnuts and fortunately, Pret A Manger has added some new items since our last visit which offer some melatonin content.

Open: 3.00 am to 8.30 pm
Location: Far left-hand corner on the upper level, overlooking the World Duty Free and main departure board.

These dishes contain foods with a melatonin content.

Greens, Grains & Chicken Salad Avocado, edamame beans, British chicken breast, broccoli florets, spinach, peas, mint, parsley, brown rice & red quinoa and seed mix. The brown rice and broccoli both contribute some melatonin. Seeds can also add melatonin.

Chicken, Broccoli & Brown Rice Soup Chunky broth made with vegetables, baby broccoli florets and brown rice.

Coconut Chicken Curry Side Soup Ground curry spices gently stewed in coconut milk with butternut squash, onion and tomatoes. Cooked with new potatoes, gungo peas, brown rice, red pepper, turmeric, mustard, ginger puree, lime juice and diced chicken thigh.

Veggie Chilli Soup Combination of three beans (black turtle beans, red kidney beans and black-eyed beans), pepper, sweetcorn, brown rice and quinoa, with a hint of lime.

Avocado & Chipotle Chickpeas Salad Wrap Avocado, chipotle chickpeas and charred corn & black bean salsa topped with fresh coriander and mixed salad leaves.

Mexican Avocado Flat Bread Refried black beans, avocado, charred corn & black bean salsa, tomatoes and fresh coriander.

Sweet Potato Falafel & Smashed Beets Veggie Box Turmeric and sweet potato falafel, smashed beets humous, avocado and broccoli on a bed of brown rice and red quinoa.

Roast Beets, Squash & Feta Veggie Box Roasted baby beets, butternut squash, diced feta, spinach and mixed seeds. Served with brown rice & red quinoa, and a pot of French dressing.

Starbucks

Starbucks is offering more healthy options now than previously. However, only a few items contain ingredients with any notable content of melatonin and tryptophan. Both are healthy meal options.

Open: 24 hours a day
Location: Situated at the far end of the upper level of the Departure Lounge, between Wagamamas and the Flying Horse.

These dishes contain foods with a melatonin content.

Grilled Veg and Grain Salad Bowl A vegan salad with a chimichurri dressing, complete with shredded carrots, pea shoots, sugar snaps, char-grilled broccoli, corn, chargrilled red peppers, roasted pumpkin seeds and wild rice. Brown and black rice, broccoli, peppers, pumpkin seeds and corn all offer some melatonin.

Courgetti, Broccoli & Halloumi Cous Cous. Cous Cous, quinoa & barley with a smoky tomato sauce, courgetti, halloumi, red pepper & tender stem broccoli.

WHSmith and the London News Company

Renowned for its books, stationery and snacks, WHSmith and London News Company offers some snack items which contain melatonin. Ideal if you want something to take on board to add to your other foods contributing melatonin.

London News Company Locations: Opposite M&S Simply Food in the Arrival Hal; opposite Excess Baggage in the main entrance of Check-in, level one; upstairs of Check-in, level two just opposite Moneycorp Bureau de Change.

WHS Locations: Between The Bookshop and Fat Face; and Gates 101 – 113.

London News Company opening hours: Before and after security 4.00 am to 9.00 pm.

WHSmith opening hours: Before security 24 hours and post security 3.00 am to 10.00 pm

These dishes contain foods with a melatonin content.

Urban Fruit – Cheeky Cherry 90 g Just cherries (and the occasional pip) gently baked. 240 kcal (1006 kJ) per packet

Graze All Day Energiser 34 g Contain sour cherries, pears and walnuts. Both the walnuts and sour cherries provide the melatonin in this snack. A small packet contains 150 kcal (631 kJ).

Graze Dark Chocolate Cherry Tart 40g Contains dried sour cherries (20%) which provide a source of melatonin, along with pecans, chocolate buttons and raisins. High in fibre but also contains added sugar content from chocolate. A small punnet (40g) contains 184 kcal (767 kJ).

Chapter 4: Revitalise and refresh

Freshen up for the day ahead

Arriving at your destination looking and feeling revitalised and ready for business can certainly reduce the impact of travel strain and aid productivity. Simple approaches can work wonders and can include anything from a good nap, using a hydrating moisturiser to a quick shower. If you travel short or long haul, then a refreshing shower is one of the most effective approaches to feeling revitalised.

Taking a shower when travelling has many physical and psychological benefits. Most of us associate the feeling of being revitalised following a shower with being cleaner and better groomed, but this is not all that a shower does for us.

Showers help our muscles to relax. The warmth from the water promotes better blood flow and circulation while loosening joints, tendons, tissues and muscles. If you can't get a massage, then a shower may be the next best thing for a stiff neck or hunched shoulders, particularly after working on your mobile device or being crammed into a seat for an extended period.   So, if you are feeling tense just before or after a flight, then a shower might be worth the small investment in time before travelling to your venue or business appointment.

Showers also give us some private time when we are alone with our thoughts. In brief, showers help to put our minds into a semi-meditative state. Our established routine in the shower is undemanding, providing some time to let our minds wander while we go through the motions of washing.   You become less aware of your travel environment and more aware of your internal thoughts. When you consider that we have all been crammed into a small space on board a flight, continually conscious of those around us, focused on the business ahead and acutely aware of work constraints, then the benefits of some private time are clear; it allows us an opportunity to collect our thoughts and relax. Our brains are no longer focused on the outside world and are now in a 'wakeful rest' state.   Neurologists call the processing of information during undemanding preparatory tasks the 'default mode network', and it is activated when the processing of cognitively demanding tasks is no longer taking place.

Distraction is also an excellent reason to take a shower. The running water provides a 'white noise' which helps clears your mind. Being distracted from travelling and business problems for a short time while you attend to your personal needs, may just provide a sufficient break from being entirely focused on the business travel that lies ahead. And yes, that is often a good thing. Here's why: this is what psychologists call the 'incubation period' for your ideas. While you've been working hard on business, you are now giving your mind the chance to wander, and your ideas can surface into your conscious mind.

Ultimately, the combination of relaxing, being in a semi-meditative state and being distracted helps create a feel-good factor, and it is during this time that dopamine is released into our brains. As a consequence, research has found that this more relaxed state where our thoughts are unconstrained while undertaking a preparatory task can lead to a more creative and problem-solving mental state. We are no longer hounded by the hustle and bustle of the terminal, we can't check our emails, and we can no longer hear our fellow passengers. So, we are left with the unconstrained 'voices' in the back of our head telling us something. This is why so many people claim their best thinking or problem-solving is done while in the shower! The answer to our work problems may have been there all along during the trip. We just need to take a little time, switch our processing to the default network mode (from cognitive thinking to preparatory tasks) and gain some private space to listen to our thoughts as they spontaneously surface.

So, when you are heading out on your business travels, or just after landing, taking a quick shower might just be more worthwhile and revitalising than you previously imagined.

Most airports offer showers for weary travellers, and while these tend to have the reputation of being for the 'smelly' traveller, business lounges and hotels are now beginning to provide similar facilities for their business travellers as they recognise the benefits for their clients and the market's changing needs.

We have searched Gatwick International Airport's North Terminal for you, and here are some options to consider.

Where you can shower

Public showers at the North Terminal

Unfortunately, there are no public showers in the North Terminal where you can freshen up after your flight or before boarding unless you have access to the Emirates Lounge.

If you are not flying with Emirates, then your best bet is to either hire a day room to freshen up and shower or to hop on the free shuttle service to the South Terminal where there are public and private showers (lounges or hotel facilities). The shuttle service only takes three minutes.

Public showers at the South Terminal

There is only one set of public showers at the South Terminal now, as Gatwick have recently closed the others down. If you are arriving from the North Terminal, then you'll only find the showers in the Departure Lounge just after security. It is only of any use if you intend to travel out from the South Terminal. Otherwise, you will need to either rely on business and private lounges or hotels for a shower.

Directions: Catch the shuttle from the North Terminal. Walk through security. Turn left as you exit security. There are showers both within the Men's and Women's toilet areas.

Lounges with showers at the North Terminal

The Emirates lounge is the only private lounge which now offers showers at the North Terminal. Reviewers have, however, rated the facilities highly, in fact, higher than other lounges.

Emirates Lounge

This lounge is restricted to business and first-class travellers or members. Reviewers have highly rated it for the facilities and service.

Access: Emirates First Class and Business Class travellers or as an Emirates Skywards Platinum or Gold member departing on an Emirates flight. One guest is allowed if travelling on the same flight.

Opening hours: First departure to the last departure
Location: First floor of the Departure Lounge.
Directions: Head towards gate 103 – 113, as you pass London News Company, you will see a corridor on your right. Go through the double glass doors and take the lift to the first floor. The lounge is located on the left-hand side.

Lounges with showers at the South Terminal

Regress Express Business Centre

The new Regus Express business lounge at the South Terminal is one of many Regus Business Centres worldwide. It's the perfect place to freshen up. There are five shower suites to choose from, and they supply towels, so you needn't worry about bringing your own.

Telephone 0870 880 8484
Access: Accessible to all travellers regardless of ticket class. Regress operates a drop-in entry policy. Complimentary access to Institute of Directors members
Open: 6.00 am to 6.00 pm Monday to Friday.
Cost: Showers are £20.00 and include an hour in the lounge, along with supply you a towel.
Location: South Terminal Arrivals on the ground floor.
Directions: To get to the lounge from the arrivals area, simply take the lift between Costa Coffee and Moneycorp, down to the entrance on the ground level and turn right. If you are coming from the train station, then turn right at Marks and Spencer, and you'll see the lift located on the right-hand side. Take the elevator to the lower floor and turn right.

Showers at hotels at the North Terminal

Hampton by Hilton

Connected to the Hotel and only minutes from the check-in desks on level one of the Check-in areas, this hotel is highly rated by guests and offers rooms at a reduced rate during the day. As part of the day room rate, you have access to all the facilities. Much more than just a shower!

Telephone: +44 (0) 1293 579999 **or email** russel@hbhgatwick.com
Day Room time availability: 9.00 am to 6.00 pm

Rate: £69, flexible rate with payment taken upon arrival and free cancellation by 11.59 pm the day before arrival.

Includes: Fluffy towels, bathroom amenities, breakfast, WiFi, business centre, fitness room, snack shop, lounge.

Location: The entrance to this hotel is near the Easy Jet Check-in on level one. Just follow the signs to the right of the check-in desk. You will see a sign above the entrance to the corridor for the Hampton by Hilton.

Directions: Turn right at the Easy Jet Check-in area and walk towards the end of the hall. Walk straight ahead through the entrance and follow the passage to the left. Walk through the automatic double glass doors. The total distance is about 50 steps from the Easy Jet check-in to the hotel reception.

Sofitel London Gatwick

Sofitel London Gatwick Hotel is close to the check-in at the North Terminal and offers a day room if you would like to shower. Although Sofitel has been praised as a five-star hotel, the price for a shower might be somewhat more than you need to pay; however, they offer far more than just a shower in their day room rate.

Telephone: +44 (0) 1293 567070 **or email** slg@sofitelgatwick.com

Day Room time availability: 8.00 am to 5.00 pm

Day Rate: £79.00 inclusive of VAT per day.

Includes: Towels, ESPA skincare and bathroom amenities, use of the gym, complimentary internet, business centre.

Location: The Sofitel hotel is connected to Gatwick Airport through a covered walkway on the right-hand-side of the shuttle on the North Terminal, level one.

Directions: From the terminal exit on level one, walk straight ahead to the right of the shuttle to a covered walkway sign posted Sofitel Hotel. Walk down the corridor, and you're at the entrance within 2 minutes. If you are arriving by car, you will find the entrance to the hotel on the ground floor next to the Hotel's car park. Alternatively, you can park in the Airport car park with easy access to both the hotel and airport terminal on level one.

Showers at hotels at the South Terminal

YOTEL Hotel

Located in the South Terminal, Yotel is ideal if you want a shower before your flight (or even a quick nap). The on-site airport entrance is located within the public area of the arrivals hall which is just around the corner from the shuttle. Each room has an en-suite bathroom with Monsoon rain shower. Yotel doesn't take advanced bookings for their shower cabins. Just show up, and the shower cabin will be allocated on a first come, first serve basis.

Telephone: +44(0) 207 100 1100 **or email** customer@yotel.com
Shower Rate: A minimum of a 4-hour stay for this Yotel. Payment via debit or credit card. No cash accepted.
Includes: Complimentary tea/coffee, Luxury towels and all-natural body wash/shampoo
Day Room time availability: Short stay of up to 4 hours is £39.00. You can pay for additional hours after the minimum charge for 4 hours.
Location: South Terminal Arrivals on the ground floor.
Directions: If you are coming from North Terminal, via the shuttle, walk from the shuttle to the South Terminal arrivals hall, turn right at Marks and Spencer, and you'll see the lift located on the right-hand side. The lifts are between Costa Coffee and WHSmith. Simply take the elevator down to the entrance on the ground level and turn left.

BLOC Hotel

BLOC hotel is located in the heart of Gatwick Airport's South Terminal, just steps from the Departure Lounge. They offer a day-time rate at half price of the night rate which you can have the use of between 7.00 am in the morning until 4.00 p.m. After which time, if you need a shower, you will need to pay the full night rate. Past guests have rated the Italian tiled wet-room style, monsoon-drench showers highly.

Telephone: +44(0) 020 3051 0101 **or email** bookingslgw@blochotels.com
Day Room time availability: 7.00 am to 4.00 pm
Rate: Minimum day room rate of £29.00.
Includes: Day room facility includes Zenology shower products and "soft fluffy" towels.
Location: The hotel is in Gatwick South Terminal. The reception is located on level 3 of the Departures Lounge right next to the security entrance.
Directions: You can also get to this from level 2 in the Arrivals, via the stairwell next to the toilets just opposite Boots the Pharmacy.

Other ways to revitalise

There are several alternatives which can also help you feel rejuvenated when you travel through Gatwick Airport's North Terminal. One is to take care of your skin, nasal passages and eyes which can become dried out when flying.

The atmosphere in the plane is rather arid. According to the World Health Organisation, the humidity is usually less than 20%, which is lower than when you are at home (typically over 30%), so there can be a noticeable discomfort to the eyes, mouth and nose. Advice is to use a skin moisturiser and to protect the eyes by wearing glasses rather than contact lenses.

Here are some relevant ways to help revitalise your skin and eyes.

World Duty Free

The World Duty Free offers free skin consultations and can recommend moisturisers to match your skin type. Different product ranges also offer various consultations to help freshen and hydrate the skin. All consultations are free and are designed to take between two and ten minutes. All you need to do is pick the right counter for your needs.

Counters and their products include;
Clarins – Fragrance Consultation: Application of daytime moisturiser plus one drop of double serum and foundation of choice.
Clinique – a moisture makeover to quench thirsty skin with a burst of refreshing hydration, while infusing the skin with deep and lasting hydration.
Estee Lauder – for products to revive fatigued eyes.
Lancome – for a skin diagnosis and moisture application.
Sisley – for eye contour relaxing treatment.

Jo Malone

No complimentary treatments here, alas! But there are plenty of hand and body lotions to help hydrate and condition your skin while you are on board, along with vitamin E hand treatments and body balms to soothe dryness. You can view these items on their website. Although click and collect is an option, there wasn't an option to collect from Gatwick Airport's North Terminal store. Alternatively, you could telephone ahead to check availability.

Telephone: 01293 502 029

Website: www.jomalone.co.uk
Opening hours: 04.00 am to 10.00 pm
Location: After security in the main Departure Lounge, lower level, on the right-hand side as you walk towards the departure gates, between Dixon's Travel and Hour Passion stores.

Some items include:

Lip Conditioner £23.00 for 15 ml. Incorporates Vitamin E. Prepared to help soften, smooth and care for vulnerable skin.

Eye Crème £38.00 15 ml. Formulated with vitamin E, reportedly designed to moisturise the delicate skin around the eyes while helping to reduce the look of fine lines and dark circles.

Lime Basil & Mandarin Body and hand lotions £20.00 for 100 ml. Formulated to hydrate and condition the skin. Other fragrances are available in larger bottles.

Geranium & Walnut Hand Cream £22.00 50 ml Soothe and soften your hands. Lightweight, softly scented with apricot kernel oil which absorbs quickly, leaving the hand feeling moisturised.

Vitamin E Gel £65.00 30 ml Moisturises dry, dehydrated or weathered skin. Vitamin E is high in anti-oxidants.

Vitamin E Hand Treatment £42.00 100 ml. Conditions the skin while protecting from harsh environmental conditions.

Boots the Chemist

Boots the Chemist offers a variety of moisturisers, nasal sprays and refresh products for you to choose from. You can order online in advance and collect upon arrival either from the Departure Lounge, lower level or after customs in the Arrival Hall, ground floor next to M&S Simply Food, opposite Costa Coffee on the ground floor, post-exit from Customs and Excise.

Opening in Arrivals: 24 hours
Opening in Departure Lounge: 4.00 am to 8.30 pm
Telephone: 01293 569606
Website: www.boots.com

Some items include:

Nasal Sprays

NeilMed Sinus Rinse £17.99 Provides natural relief from the symptoms of allergy and various nasal conditions.

Travel Kits

Nivea Travel Essentials £7.50. Nivea items include shower cream, refreshing cleansing wipes, deodorant, moisturiser and lip care.

Bull Dog Travel Kit £10.00 Items are 30 g and include; moisturiser, face wash and shave gel.

Elizabeth Arden Ceramide Travel Kit £25.00 Contains 5 ml Superstart Skin Renewal Booster, seven pieces Advanced Ceramide Capsules and 15 ml Ceramide Lift & Firm Day Cream SPF30.

No. 7 Protect & Perfect Intense ADVANCED Travel Kit £26.00 Contains the essentials for your skin care. Includes: 15 ml Serum, 25 ml Day Cream and 25 ml Night Cream.

Simple Kind to Skin Hydrating Light Moisturiser £1.50 50 ml For all skin types, this moisturiser keeps it replenished and nourished. Quickly absorbed and contains Vitamin E.

Clinique Turnaround Overnight Revitalising Moisturiser 50 ml £38 Revitalising moisturiser.

Quick Bargain Shopping Basket Items

Cocoa Butter Formula with Vitamin E £1.35 50 ml Softens and smooths rough and dry skin, twenty-four-hour moisture.

Nivea Hand Cream £1.59 30 ml Smooth and nourishing hand cream to combat dryness.

Sanctuary Spa Illuminating Moisture Lotion SPF15. £2.99 15 ml Evens tone and refines texture for skin that glows from first use. Twenty-four-hour hydration.

Boots Expert Dry Skin Concentrated Hand & Nail Cream £2.75 Hypoallergenic, fragrance-free. Purified lanolin, to immediately increase skin's natural moisture content by one-third and continues to soften smooth and protect up to 8 hours.

Nivea Hydro Care £1.65 4.8 g Caring lip balm. It provides long-lasting moisturisation and rehydrates.

London News Company & WHSmith

London News Company and WHSmith have a bargain bin of small travel items which include moisturisers and lip balms.

There are several London News Company and WHSmith stores at Gatwick's North Terminal, of which three are before security. London News Company is on the right-hand side as you walk from the shuttle, car parks and Sofitel Hotel into the North Terminal, level 1. There is also a smaller London News Company on the ground floor in the Arrivals Hall next to the Bureaux of Change, and a smaller one in

Check-in on Level Two at the end of Zone E opposite the Moneycorp Bureau de Change. There are also three

Opening Hours: Arrivals 24 hours
Opening Hours: After security 4.00 am to 10.00 pm

Essential Bargain Shopping Basket Items
To protect lips;
Vaseline Petroleum Jelly 20 g £2.99
Grab It Lip Balm 4 g £1.49
Chapstick Original £2.99
Lipsal £2.99
Carmex Moisturising Lip Balm 10 g £2.99 Helps to moisture and relieve dry, cracked lips.

A quick cleanse;
Nivea Cleansing Wipes £1.99. 3 in 1 refreshing cleansing wipes. Cleansing lotion with vitamin E. Seven wipes.

To moisturise;
Grab It Hand Cream £1.49 25 ml
Nivea Cream £2.49 50 ml White tube
Nivea Smooth Nourishing Hand Cream £2.49 30 ml Smooth and nourishing hand cream to combat dryness.
Simple Light Moisturiser £2.49
Atrixo Enriched Moisturising Cream 50 ml £1.50 For soft, smooth hands. Contains chamomile.

SECTION TWO: Working Productively
Chapter 5: Relaxation

Business travels in the fast lane.

It's hard to relax when travelling. There is so much to deal with, schedules to keep and extra work to undertake. So, it's hardly surprising frequent business travellers report poorer psychological health than non-travellers. Studies have repeatedly shown that employees with low mental wellbeing scores are likely to perform below the norm. While businesses generally choose employees who are high performers to travel and represent the company, studies show over time that high performers' productivity will suffer as a result of declining psychological health due to frequent business trips.

One study commissioned by the Institute of Travel and Meetings (ITM) found frequent travellers had psychological well-being scores typical of the bottom 40% of performers at work. Scores for work-life balance and overall health were also reportedly very low. The key issues affecting work-life balance for frequent business travellers were cited as excessive travel time, insufficient spare time, transit through airports, jet-lag, long hours and 'work' interfering with personal time.

Not having sufficient spare time to relax exacerbates travel stress. A recent study by Booking.com which surveyed more than 4,500 business travellers aged between 18 and 65 from eight countries, reported 93 % of us feel stress at some point during our business journey. Nearly half of all business travellers (47%) report being anxious over delays and cancellations, a third (32%) felt anxious over missing a flight, while chronic fatigue, including jet lag, accounted for more than 42% feeling stressed.

Another study undertaken by Carlton Wagon Travel showed the strain was greatest in the airport just before take-off for managerial workers, which traditionally is when there is less time to relax. Does the extra stress affect performance? The recent study conducted on behalf of the Airlines Reporting Corporation (ARC) reports half of all business travellers feel extra strain in the days before business trips and believe they will be less effective during their journey as a result. Frequent travellers are feeling the impact.

Notably, travellers experience more strain when they travel than they do when in the office, so it is essential to find time to relax during a business trip, particularly just before boarding. The more strain travellers experience, the more difficult it becomes to work productively and effectively when away on business. This makes it essential to find an approach which enables you to unwind and refocus when travelling.

A suitable approach might be to find a quieter spot in Gatwick Airport's North Terminal where you can chill out and relax. Alternatively, you might seek out a spa with a masseur before arriving at the airport to relieve pre-flight muscle tension. Sometimes, just finding a room with a view where you can watch the aeroplanes take off or taking time out for reflection and meditation can work wonders, particularly if you're short of time. For others, maximising the efficiency of their journey time works best, so when they reach their destination, they can then relax without the need to catch up on emails.

Whichever approach you decide will depend entirely on what's available at the airport, your work to flight schedule and your personal preferences.

In this chapter, we look at how to shed anxieties, tips on how to make time to relax, suitable relaxation techniques when travelling, and most importantly where you can relax in Gatwick Airport's North's Terminal. We have explored Gatwick Airport's North Terminal from end to end. You'll find appropriate places to relax listed below our top tips.

Why relaxation is vital for business travellers

There are many reasons why relaxation is vital when travelling on business. Here are just a few reasons why frequent business travellers should consider prioritising relaxation if they wish to be in good health when regularly conducting business away from the office.

Reduces blood pressure

Relaxation helps to slow down your heart rate as well as reduce your blood pressure, and it slows your breathing down, relieves muscular tension, improves concentration, mood, and cardiovascular systems. All of these are important if you've been travelling at altitude in a confined space. Flying at altitude can raise blood pressure as it is a way of increasing the supply of oxygen around your body. If high blood pressure is not addressed, it can cause some health issues including headaches, digestive problems, anxiety and inability to focus. However, symptoms of sustained high blood pressure are not always obvious. Over the long term, frequent flyers reportedly have higher blood pressure than non-flyers. In time, higher blood pressure can lead to more chronic cardiovascular disease.

Improves your immunity

Flying in a confined space also means you're subjected to more germs and travelling with strangers means some of these will be germs your body hasn't encountered before. Research suggests that relaxation may lower your risk of catching a cold. In fact, some research has found that chronic stress, i.e. lasting more than 40 days, doubles a person's risk of catching a cold. Stress can hamper the body's ability to fight inflammation over the long term due to raised levels of cortisol in the blood. Cortisol helps to reduce inflammation, but over time, the body's efforts to reduce the inflammation also suppresses the immune system. So, constant stress induced by frequent travel and work pressures cause increase havoc to the immune system, making the traveller more susceptible to viruses.

Boost your memory

Constant travel stress over the long term may also trigger changes to your mental ability and behaviour by affecting the part of your brain which controls the high-level executive functions, such as working memory, recognition, suppression of distraction, novelty seeking and decision making. Research is also beginning to show that shorter bursts of stress impair the centres of the brain involved in memory and learning. So, if you are frequently flying, i.e. more than six times a year, then relaxing en route may be a powerful factor in helping to maintain a desirable level of cognitive performance.

Relaxing helps you to make better decisions

Being tense and tired means that you might not always think so clearly. Research has shown that stress can change how we calculate risk, adverse outcomes and reward. When we are tense and tired, our decision-making process becomes cloudy, and we tend to focus more on the positive outcomes or rewards and avoid the negative possibilities. As a result, when people are making a difficult decision under stress, they may pay more attention to the upsides of the alternatives they're considering and less to the downsides. Subsequently, riskier decisions are best made when you are more relaxed and more likely to weigh up the negative and positive outcomes equally.

Improves mood, reduces anger and frustration

Relaxation and meditation, when practised regularly not only relieve anxiety but can also improve mood. Travelling is tiring and being stressed, tired or jetlagged can increase the level of irritability, frustration and anger that a frequent traveller may typically experience. In particular, long trips, frequent changes in travel dates and the high number of stressors encountered during a journey will all increase stress levels and, consequently, mood.

When you become stressed or angry, your breathing rate and heart rate increase. Methods to reduce the impact of the stressor, such as breathing techniques can reverse some of the anger building up as deliberately slowing down breathing and systematically relaxing your tense muscles.

While removing the stress factor is a more effective stress management technique, relaxing can help you to maintain control over some of the unavoidable travel stressors you may be experiencing.

Remove stress factors and create more relaxation time

There's little chance of escaping negative work carry over, the spillover of work into your personal time when you're travelling on business. So, it's little wonder the strain of a business trip can become all-pervading, and for a significant number of business travellers, it can lead to burn-out where they are no longer able to cope with the demands of travelling on business effectively. The combination of extended working hours, taking your work with you to your hotel room, business meetings planned over dinner to avert the effects of jet-lag, interrupting family commitments and not having sufficient personal time to relax or pursue leisure activities can all add up.

Even though the pressures of business travel might be unavoidable, there are ways to relieve some of the strain and reduce the overall impact. Finding time to relax is vital in helping to manage stress, and travel stress is no different, if not even more important. By putting your body and mind back to a state of rest, you will lower your heart rate, decrease blood pressure, increase blood flow to major muscles, reduce muscle tension, reduce fatigue, be less irritable or frustrated and improve concentration and mood. All the benefits we talked about above.

So here are our top tips on how to reduce anxiety and travel strain and create more time for relaxation.

Plan your schedule wisely: create buffer time

Nearly half of business travellers are anxious over delays and cancellations, and the second top stress factor is poor or no internet connections to catch up on work emails. So, make sure your schedule allows for 'buffer time' to cope with delays in travel, longer meetings than expected, and poor internet connections to meet deadlines. This way you'll have a chance to cope without feeling you are under undue strain. It might also create some unscheduled time for a quick break in between planned activities to relax or to catch up on emails before you head to your next aeroplane or appointment. If connectivity has become an issue before you board, then turn to Chapter 6 where we have itemised all the best places to connect to the internet at Gatwick Airport's North Terminal.

Plan for downtime

Plan to relax and unwind. While it is tempting to pack in as much business or as many working dinner meetings as possible, the consequence of trying to do too much without time to relax will make it less rewarding and effective. Work-life balance is key to combating travel stress and fatigue. Strain intensifies from the lack of relaxation time, negative work carryover and poor sleep, leaving you feeling less productive when you travel, or when you eventually return to the office. So, plan to take time out.

We've listed below some quiet places you'll find in the North Terminal where you can relax. We've even included the best views of the runways, and where you can find the most comfortable seats. You'll find these listed below in the next section.

Build in rest days

When business travellers were recently asked to rank potential improvements to travel policies, they cited the ability to work from home the day before or the day after a trip in their top five changes. If having a rest day means you're not 'hitting the wall' around two in the afternoon in the office after a return flight the day before, then you're doing the right thing by taking a rest day. Presenteeism, attending work in body but not in mind, increases for frequent business travellers, particularly when suffering from jet lag and travel fatigue. At the very least, ask your employer to adapt their travel policies to include the option of working from home the day after you return or book return flights on a Friday when your rest day is at the weekend.

Build in flexibility for flight connections

Make sure you allow sufficient time for any connecting flights, particularly if you are boarding at Gatwick Airport's North Terminal having arrived at the South Terminal. You may need to walk through arrivals, airport security, catch the shuttle to the North Terminal and back through security if your connection is to the other terminal. Allow at least two hours, so you have time to grab a drink or a snack, toilet breaks, relax or take a chance to catch up on a few emails before your next connection.

Know your terminal and departure areas

Knowing what facilities are at your terminal in advance is a good approach to reducing the strain when travelling. Finding out before you leave for the airport where to find a quiet place, connection points for electronic devices, water fountains for water bottle refills, showers and massage chairs is essential for reducing strain when in an airport for the first time. Don't panic! You'll find the answers to all these questions in this book.

Utilise speedy boarding options

Travel options such as speedy boarding, premium security and passport control, where you pay a little extra might also be advantageous when flying on business. It will enable you to get seated and organised before everyone else has boarded. There is less waiting, so you can spend more time relaxing, or if need be, checking your emails before switching over to flight mode.

Gatwick offers both Premium Security, where you can 'breeze through with ease', and Premium Gatwick Passport Control to reduce the time through passport control. Both particularly useful late at night when those queues can appear endless and add at least another half an hour to your landing time.

Premium Security is located to the left of the security area and provides a dedicated route, greater efficiency and a 'tranquil environment'. It is open from 4.00 am to 8.45 pm.

Premium Gatwick Passport Control reduces the time through checking your passport. You will need to book it at least 24 hours in advance. It is open from 06.00 am to 12.00 am. Both services can be booked via the Gatwick Airport website, along with access to the No.1 Traveller Lounge, My Lounge and Aspire Lounge facilities.

Relaxation techniques to use when travelling

Health professionals are increasingly encouraging business executives to undertake techniques to reduce work-related strain, such as mental relaxation and visualisation. They recognise the importance of finding a way to reduce the heart rate, blood pressure and reducing muscular tension in an attempt to decrease long-term ill health for employees.

Relaxation techniques can work well when you are travelling on business. They are free, easy to use and can be done almost anywhere, anytime. Typically, they simply involve refocusing your attention off the trip ahead onto something more pacifying. They function by increasing your awareness of your body which helps you to relax any of your tight muscles.

There are several different types of relaxation techniques. They include the top four techniques mentioned below, along with other more common approaches found in some airports which we have also listed below this section.

Autogenic relaxation

It is where you use visual imagery and body awareness to reduce stress. Fundamentally, the relaxation comes from within you. For example, you might imagine a peaceful setting and then focus on controlled breathing to slow your heart rate down, then use different physical sensations, for example relaxing your feet, arm or leg, each one at a time.

Patricia Collins, a relaxation consultant, has written a quick description on how to do this later in this section.

Progressive muscle relaxation.

It is when you focus on slowly tensing and then relaxing each muscle, in a leisurely manner, from head to toe (or toes to head). You can do this sitting, lying down or standing up and it's a technique worth practising before your trip. It can take some time to go from head to toe, so it is better suited to when you have fifteen to thirty minutes before making your way to the departure gate.

Further down in this section we've provided a link to a podcast produced by the National Health Service in the UK for you to try.

Visualisation

It is where you create a mental image to take a visual journey to a peaceful, calming place or situation. People often use a beach, a holiday or a 'happy place' from when they were a child. It's ideal for the boarding gate when other techniques might be too time-consuming, and you're beginning to feel a little anxious. It may require some professional guidance during the first couple of times.

Later in this section, we've provided a link further down to a podcast produced by the National Health Service in the UK for you to try.

Deep breathing exercises

These are controlled slow breathing techniques. They may be best suited to a tranquil environment. We have made some suggestions about where you can go to practice this technique later in the chapter.

Choose any relaxation technique that you feel is most suitable for you, as it doesn't matter which relaxation one you choose as long as you find it effective. Do try to practice any relaxation techniques regularly to gain the benefits. As you practice, you will become more aware of what tense muscles and sensations of travel strain feel like. When you start to feel stiff, a few moments of using relaxation techniques can make the business trip more enjoyable and productive.

To get the full benefits, you should also look at reducing stress factors which might be causing strain. We talk about the main stressors which business travellers report in our next three chapters. These include simple issues such as connectivity, phone charging and being able to work productively when travelling. We've already discussed how to get some rest, cope with jet-lag, reduce fatigue and how to revitalise in the first four chapters. You will also find chapters on exercising and healthy eating at Gatwick North Terminal in Section 3 and 4.

Simple breathing exercises

Here are two passive activities you can do to reduce stress and anxiety when travelling. One focusses on breathing, the other muscle relaxation. These have been specifically designed for business travellers by Patricia Collins, a relaxation consultant from Australia. They are quick and easy to master and can be undertaken at the rest places we recommend in Gatwick Airport's North Terminal in the section below.

Firstly, secure all your belongings in bags which are close to you. Sit in a quiet spot if possible but if there is a crowd just let it be part of the scene.

Place your feet evenly on the floor and, hands on your lap. You can now test for muscle tension by:-
* Making tight fists then, letting go, feel the difference.
* Repeat a few times and do the same with your toes. This will help with your circulation.

Now; to turn off the pressure.
* Close your eyes if you feel safe if not; look down at the ground.
* Take a deep breath and slowly let go, out, out, out. Repeat until you feel the tension ease.

To loosen muscles, visualise your toes, let them uncurl, think of your lower legs and loosen them, moving up do similar to your knees, thighs and hips.
This is where sitting will lock up energy. Move on your seat, tighten the buttock muscles then let go.

Repeat a few times to feel the tension go and your circulation return.
Return to the breathing exercises and enjoy feeling in control of your stress and anxieties.

Here is another fun activity. Make a mental picture of all your anxieties about flying for business. Put them in a box tied with a red ribbon, attach a red balloon and see it rise away into the universe.

Relaxation podcasts

If relaxation exercises are new to you, then you might prefer to listen to a couple of podcasts which take you slowly through each stage of relaxation and visualisation. We have listed some options for you to try out and practice while at the airport. These have been recorded by the National Health Service in the United Kingdom. They aren't as quick to go through as the ones above which Patricia Collins has written for you. However, they will take you through a step by step relaxation and visualisation process.

If you haven't got any earphones handy to listen to this privately, then you can purchase earphones at Boots, WHSmith and Dixon Travel.

Progressive muscular relaxation exercise

http://www.moodjuice.scot.nhs.uk/downloads/progressivemuscularrelaxation.mp3

Muscular tension can be quick to build up en route to the airport and during your flight, causing pain and even more anxiety. Undertaking some muscular relaxation exercises can help control some of the unpleasant symptoms of muscular tension. By reducing physical tension, you will become more relaxed overall. This podcast takes you slowly through exercises which tense, then relax your individual muscles. It is only 30 minutes long, and you can do these at any of the quiet locations in the airport we have compiled below.

With practice, you will be able to recognise and respond to the onset of tension.

Visualisation podcast

www.moodjuice.scot.nhs.uk/downloads/visualisation.mp3

Another technique which you can use to help you relax is visualisation. This podcast takes you through a visualisation process. Its objective is to improve your mood and reduce your anxiety or stress level by calming your mind, which is particularly worthwhile if time permits before your flight. It is twenty-four minutes long, so you will need to find a quiet place in Gatwick's North Terminal where you can plug in your earphones, and you won't be disturbed. We have listed all the best quiet locations in the airport down below.

Other relaxation methods

Massage

Massage is often employed to relax tense muscles by pressing, rubbing or manipulating muscles and soft tissues. There are reportedly over 80 massage therapies to choose. We've listed some places near Gatwick Airport's North Terminal where you can have a massage in the section below this. Unfortunately, there are no massage facilities within Gatwick Airport's North Terminal itself.

Yoga

Some airports are now offering a yoga room for busy travellers. The main benefits of using yoga when travelling include lessening anxiety, increased muscle strength and tone, along with cardio and circulatory health. Unfortunately, Gatwick North Terminal does not have a yoga room.

Meditation

Gatwick Airport North Terminal has a Chapel where you can meditate. You'll find more details under 'Where you can rest at Gatwick Airport's North Terminal below'. Also, suitable for visualisation exercises.

Music

Some Airports are now having music therapy as part of the customer experience. Gatwick Airport occasionally offers music recitals, however not very often.

Art Therapy

Similarly, some airports have art pieces in a circuit to encourage wandering. Gatwick's North Terminal has art in memory of the Queen's Jubilee en route to passport control after you land. Unfortunately, Gatwick Airport North Terminal doesn't have permanent art pieces in the Departure Lounge areas.

Where you can relax

Relaxing the mind

Quieter public spaces within the terminal

If the hustle and bustle of the airport terminal get to you, then stepping away and finding a quiet area is well worth the effort. Here are a couple of places we've discovered in the North Terminal of Gatwick Airport which are more peaceful than the main thoroughfare and have a lower footfall.

Arrival, Ground Floor

By its very nature, this very busy hall does not lead itself well to relaxation, as it is fast moving and has a high footfall. The best option if you need a few moments to yourself before meeting someone, is to head straight to Costa Coffee.

Costa Coffee

An unlikely quiet spot, however, if you head straight down to the back of the café on the right-hand side, this is the most peaceful spot in the arrival's hall. Alternatively, if you turn right at the service counter, you'll find a little alcove tucked away behind the refrigerator. There are even some nice soft leather couches to relax on.

Check-in, Lower Level

This bustling part of the terminal doesn't lend itself well to relaxation. There are a couple of rows of chairs just in front of the main entrance on either side. One is next to the London News Company, and the other is next Excess Baggage. The footfall is high here, so if you desire a more tranquil environment, we suggest you head to either the Chapel/Prayer room or the Hampton by Hilton Business Centre and Bar.

Chapel/Prayer Room

Head straight towards the Easy Jet check-in counters and turn right just past the reserved seating for special assistance. Head straight to the corridor marked Hampton by Hilton, and just before you reach the walkway, you will find the Chapel/Prayer Room on the right-hand side.

Starbucks in the Hampton by Hilton

Starbucks has recently been absorbed into the Hampton by Hilton Bar and Business Centre. It remains hidden away from the rest of the bustle of the airport. Consequently, not many travellers know it is there, and it is less frequented than the other eateries in the terminal. There are some nice couches to relax in on the left-hand-side of the room.

Check-in, Level Two

There are several seating areas on level two. This is where you enter security for departure.

Seating near Emirates check-in counter.

Just as you come up from level one on the escalator, turn right and walk towards the far right-hand corner. As you pass, Emirates ticket and information desk, there is a row of seats here.

Seating next to Jamie's Coffee Lounge.

There are a couple of rows of seats next to Jamie's Coffee Lounge and the entrance from the carpark.

Seating at the back of level two.

Behind the Check-in counter rows A& B there is a new alcove area with several rows of seats. The footfall is lower than the front of the Check-in hall, and consequently, it is much quieter.

Departure Lounge, Lower Level

Quiet zone between Boots and Dixon's Travel

One of the most peaceful public seating areas is at the far-right end of the North Terminal between Boots the Chemist and Dixon's Travel on the right-hand side. The foot fall here is much lower than the other public seating areas within the North Terminal. There is also plenty of natural light and power sockets for recharging your electronic devices while you relax. The air conditioning works at a moderate temperature with a little draft and low noise level.

Just opposite the departure gate exit

If you walk towards Gates 45 – 55 and 101 – 113, as you turn down the corridor just past London News Company and the children's play zone, you'll find several rows of seats. It is away from the main thoroughfare and bustle within the Departure Lounge. The bonus being several power points on the columns for charging your mobile devices.

Gates 45 – 55 Along the corridor for gates 45 – 55, it is often very quiet, and there are several seats.

Opposite Gate 50 Our researchers found four seats at the very end of the corridor, opposite from Gates 50, were quiet, and away from the main footfall. Here some calm reflection is possible until your flight departure gate is called. There are also power points on the nearby columns and a vending machine.

Other seats along this corridor included;

Gate 51. just opposite the toilets are three sets of chairs with four seats on each.

Gate 53. There are four seats here.

Gate 54. There are four benches with four seats here.

Gates 557 – 574

The corridor to Gates 557 – 574 may get busy at certain departure times, but there is ample time in between flight departures for some peace, particularly in the afternoon when the airport is at its slowest. Our researchers found gates 574 to be the quieter end of the corridor. We recently discovered the airport had relocated spare seating to this corridor, which makes it an excellent place to sit and relax, especially when the sun shines through the large windows.

Weatherspoon's Red Lion Pub

There are not many places to eat on the lower level. The Red Lion Pub at the end closest to the entrance from security is bustling with people during busy times, but if you head down the inside to the far left of the pub, you'll find a spot by the window. The view isn't great, but this is the quietest place in the pub.

Departure Lounge, Upper Level

The upper level of the Departure Lounge plays host to many restaurants, but not all of them are quiet enough for some time out. Here is a couple which you could try if you long for a drink and something to eat in a more peaceful environment.

Comptoir Libanais

Comptoir Libanais has a quiet space inside to the right at the back. There is a table for four people and a large window. The view isn't great, but at least it is quiet, and there is natural light.

Pret-A-Manger

Pret-A-Manger at the far end near the escalator is busy during peak times but has a quieter area down the back of the café where there is little footfall.

Starbucks

Starbucks has a couple of quiet spots near the window. If you turn right after collecting your food and drink and walk towards the window, then you'll find a quiet spot to the left and the right. The right, behind the service counter, is the more peaceful of the two places. There are four tables and a long soft couch bench, along with some power points. The sun shines in on a warm day, and although the view of the runway is obscured by the roof of the terminal gates below, it is the best spot on the upper level of the Departure Lounge.

Private Lounges

Not all lounges are quiet! There may be a lot of business chatter and general chit chat as people relax socially. However, some lounges do have dedicated quiet zones where you can sit and relax. Here is a couple we've found in the North Terminal.

Aspire Lounge

The Aspire Lounge has a quiet area away from the main buffet dining zone for reading, relaxation and catching up on emails. It is located to the left of the main entrance and is a dedicated quiet area. There are several large comfortable black leather lounge chairs. If you walk straight ahead when you enter, you will find another quiet area around the corner to the right.

Open: Open hours are from 4.00 a.m. to 10.00 p.m., with a slight seasonal variation
Facilities: Large lounge chairs and quiet areas.
Access: Welcomes anyone who is travelling, which means it may not be the quietest lounge to relax in.
Cost: Lounge entry for adults is £17.99 if you book in advance or £35 on the door without booking. If your flight is delayed and you want to stay longer, then you can buy additional hours.
Free access to: Institute of Directors, Lounge Pass, Priority Pass, Diners Club, Dragon Pass, Aspire Platinum membership and Vueling Airline Passengers.
Location: First floor of the Departure Lounge.

Directions: Head towards gate 101 – 113, as you pass London News, you will see a corridor on your right. Go through the double glass doors and take the lift to the first floor. The lounge in located on the right-hand side.

No. 1 Lounge

There are two quiet, dimly lit locations in this lounge, both away from the hustle and bustle of the food and drink area. The first is the dimly lit TV corner in the main room. As you enter the lounge, you will see the buffet, bar and bistro on the left. Straight ahead are tables for diners, and to the right is a dimmer, quieter seating area. You might be lucky to find a spot here.

If you turn right and go down the steps, you'll enter the library. It is a dedicated quiet room, designated for work and relaxation. Here, you will find soft, comfortable seating conducive for relaxing. There are several large black leather couches and some lounge chairs to chill out on.

Open: 4.00 am to 10.00 pm
Access: All travellers including groups and children.
Facilities: A designated quiet area for relaxation.
Cost: Lounge entry for adults is £30 if you book in advance or £37.50 on the door without booking. If your flight is delayed and you want to stay longer, then you can buy additional hours.
Free access to: Dragon Pass, Diners Club, Institute of Directors, Lounge Club, Priority Pass, Dining Club, Caxton FX.
Location: On the lower level of the Departure Lounge, after security, near gates 101 - 113.
Directions: Head towards gate 101 – 113, as you pass London News, you will see a corridor on your right. Go through the glass double doors. No.1 Lounge is directly ahead.

My Lounge

A less formal lounge than the others, with a friendlier atmosphere for casual relaxation or catching up with emails. There are two private rooms at the far end. The first is the 'den' with large sofa type seating, and the second has a sofa, TV, PS3 station and football table.
Open: 6.00 am to 8.00 pm

Facilities: Two private rooms for relaxation.

Cost: Lounge entry for adults is £18 if you book in advance or £24 on the door without booking. If your flight is delayed and you want to stay longer, then you can buy additional hours.

Free access to: Institute of Directors, Lounge Club, Lounge Pass, Priority Pass, Diners Club

Location: Departure Lounge, lower level.

Directions: Head towards gate 101 – 113, as you pass London News, you will see a corridor on your right. Go through the glass double doors. The lounge is located on the left-hand side just before the lifts.

Meditation

Putting your body in a state of semi or full meditation will help to reduce the impact of your body's reaction to travel strain. Most airports have a prayer room or Chapel for passengers to have a quiet reflection. At Gatwick Airport's North Terminal, there is a Chapel and prayer room just before security.

Prayer/Chapel

The chapel and prayer rooms are open 24 hours a day for people of all faiths to have quiet reflection, prayer and meditation. Users are requested to turn off their mobile phone and to leave the chapel tidy after use. There are services which support several denominations through the day.

Location: The Chapel and prayer room is situated in Check-In on level One, next to EasyJet customer services, just before the entrance of the corridor to Hampton by Hilton

Directions: As you enter the Airport through the main entrance from the shuttle station, turn right, after the phone charge area and the reserved seating for special assistance. You'll find the Chapel/prayer room on the right at the end of the Easy Jet Check-in area, just before the corridor to Hampton by Hilton Hotel.

Open Spaces outside the terminal

Riverside Gardens

Riverside Gardens is a mixture of woodland and grassy glades with a stream which runs through it and a sizeable human-made lake. It offers well-used public open spaces and is a local favourite for dog-walking and fishing. There is also a cycle path to get to and from Gatwick Airport. The walk is delightful during the warmer months.

Location: On the southwestern edge of Horley, Surrey, adjacent to the A23, London Road.

Directions from Gatwick Airport: Riverside Gardens are easily accessible from the South Terminal.

North Terminal: Hop on the shuttle to the South Terminal. It takes approximately three minutes. The exit to the path to the gardens is in the shuttle terminal. When you come out of the shuttle, walk towards the station, before you go through the entrance to the terminal, turn right and come back along the shuttle to the far end. At the end, there are stairs to the ground level and an exit; this will lead you to the footpath. The path runs adjacent to the London road (A23) leading up to Gatwick Airport, alongside Gatwick Stream and under the Airport Way.

South Terminal: Take the stairs down to ground level, turn right and cross over Caledonian Way. Keep walking for approximately 50 steps until you come to two underpasses. Take the underpass on the right; signposted "Sussex border path 1989 #21" and "Car Park B". Keep walking on the path until you come to a second underpass. Go through the second underpass which proceeds under the Airway and the shuttle, until you reach the lake. You'll find some benches to sit at just before the lake. It is approximately 600 steps in total.

Rooms with a view

Watching the world go by can be quite a challenge when you are travelling in haste. Yet, a few minutes out to watch the planes taxi or people watching can be quite relaxing, and there are plenty of opportunities to do just that at Gatwick Airport's North Terminal.

No. 1 Lounge

We found the No. 1 Lounge had the best view out of all three airport lounges. It looks directly across the runway. When you walk into the room, just head towards the far right of the lounge. In front of the window, there are swivel chairs, and power points are located on the floor next to the chairs. Alternatively, enter the library which also has large windows facing the runway. In the first section of the library, there is a bench along with window, with power points, for you to read.

Open: 4.00 am to 10.00 pm.
Access: All travellers including groups and children.

Cost: Lounge entry for adults is £30 if you book in advance or £37.50 on the door without booking. If your flight is delayed and you want to stay longer, then you can buy additional hours.

Free access to: Dragon Pass, Diners Club, Institute of Directors, Lounge Club, Priority Pass, Dining Club, Caxton FX.

Location: On the lower level of the Departure Lounge, after security, near gates 101 – 113.

Direction: Head towards gate 101 – 113, as you pass London News, you will see a corridor on your right. Go through the glass double doors. No.1 Lounge is directly ahead.

Restaurants with a view

Check-in, Level Two

Jamie's Coffee Lounge

If you need some brightness to your day and enjoy watching the crowds, then Jamie's Coffee Lounge has seating along with front entrance of the airport. Directly in front of the window is a work style bench which has a prime view of passers-by.

Nicholas Culpeper

Head straight upstairs in the Nicholas Culpeper restaurants for a table by the window if you want some natural light. The view isn't great, but it's good enough to let your thoughts wander while soaking up some daylight.

Departure Lounge, Upper-Level, view of the runway

Only a couple of the restaurants on the upper level offer an excellent view of the runway. So if you are looking for somewhere to watch planes while drinking a cup of tea/coffee or having a meal and need to time out of your work schedule or emails for a few minutes, to help yourself to relax, then head to the following restaurants.

Jamie's Bakery

Jamie's Bakery has a limited view of the runway, but only because of the size of the bakery.

Jamie's Italian

Jamie's Italian restaurant has the next best view of the runway on the Upper Level. From the large window, nearest to the far end of the airport, you can get a reasonable view. The restaurant itself can be quite popular during peak times, so the noise level may not be as desirable as other quiet areas.

Wagamama

Wagamama's has the best view of all the restaurants on the upper level of the runway. Although partially obstructed by the roof of an airport building, still well worth the visit. If you request a seat at the far end of the window, you won't be disappointed with the view. It's away from the rest of the airport hustle and bustle, but it can be somewhat noisy.

Departure Lounge, Upper-Level view of the crowd

If it is people watching that you prefer to immerse yourself in, then the following restaurants can offer an excellent view of the crowd from above.

Armadillo

Armadillo offers a South Western cuisine and a view of the lower level Departure Lounge. There are some great healthy options here.

Shake-a-Hula

Shake-a-Hula is situated between Armadillo and Eat is also another location for people watching. However, the menu offers fewer healthier options if any.

Union Jacks –

Union Jacks has a less footfall noise than Armadillo or Shake-a-Hula while overlooking the lower level. The menu also offers healthy options, as it contains the same items as Jamie's Italian restaurant opposite. There is a quiet hum from the floor below. The most peaceful place to sit is on the far side away from Yo! Sushi.

Yo! Sushi –

As the upper-level platform turns the corner, Yo! Sushi offers a long view of the lower level. Music accompanies the background noise.

Viewing platforms with low footfall

If you wish to get away from the crowds before boarding, then the corridors to the gates offer a chance for quiet reflection while watching the plane loading and taxing off to the runway. These areas are a lot quieter than the main hall in the Departure Lounge. Unfortunately, there are no other viewing platforms in the North Terminal at Gatwick Airport, but you could try these gates.

Gates 45 – 55 are accessible to travellers that want to stretch their legs. There are plenty of spots where you can stop and watch the aeroplane's load.

Gates 101 –113 are extremely busy, and once up the stairs to Pier 6, there is little turning back, unless you use the lift to go down a level and then it's quite a walk. It may raise suspicion from staff who regularly travel through the corridors as the traffic flow is usually to the gate not to the Departure Lounge. Best to only use if you know you are boarding from these gates.

Corridor to Gates 557 – 574 This long corridor has views over the loading bay areas. Gatwick Airport has recently relocated some seats along the walls of the hallway. It is much quieter here than the main Departure Lounge area, and not far to walk. If you are stretching your legs, then this is an excellent viewing platform to watch the plane's load.

Relaxing the body

Massage

Massages can be very effective in relieving tension and pain in muscle and can be a powerful method for improving your travel health and wellbeing. It's great if you're feeling tired and sore from your journey and need to relax. While more research is required to confirm the precise benefits of massage, studies indicate that message is helpful in relieving anxiety, myofascial pain, insomnia, soft tissue strains or injuries, joint pain and headaches. It can prove invaluable when travelling to ward off headaches, strains and anxiety.

However, if you feel pain or have deep vein thrombosis (or symptoms of such as burning calf muscle), taking blood-thinning medications, then it might be best to discuss any massage therapy with your doctor first.

Here are a few places where you can get a massage when travelling via Gatwick Airport's North Terminal.

Public and free massage

World Duty Free Store

Rather an unlikely venue, but a little bit of pampering can do wonders. You'll find the World Duty Free stores often offer a relaxing hand massage, neck massage or a mini facial for free. All treatments are designed to last between two and ten minutes. It's a chance to relax while you are pampered. All you need to know is which counter to head towards. Here are three we found.

Dior – for a hand or neck massage
Jo Malone – for hand and arm massage
Molton Brown – for a pampering hand and arm massage

Massage Chairs

Unfortunately, there are no massage chairs located anywhere in Gatwick Airport's North Terminal.

Lounges with Spa's

Virgin Clubhouse Lounge & Spa

If you are fortunate to travel via Virgin Airlines on business or first class, then you can take advantage of their new Clubhouse Spa. Opened in January 2017, it hosts several treatment rooms offering bespoke therapies including a relaxing head massage, therapeutic back massage, seated back and shoulder massage, trigger point massage, Thai foot massage, hot stone treatments for back, feet and legs.

Access to: Reserved for Upper-Class passengers and Flying Club Gold members.
Cost per treatment: Choose one of the complimentary services or upgrade to one of the more specialised options available.
Opening hours: 7.00 am to 12.30 pm. Treatments aren't guaranteed, and appointments are available on a walk-in, first come, first served basis.
Location: After security, you'll find the Clubhouse in lounge pavilion of the Departure Lounge.

Directions: You enter the Clubhouse through a light, private corridor leading directly to the reception and concierge area.

Hotels with massage near Gatwick Airport's North Terminal

The best places for a massage before you fly is currently one of the nearby hotels. The hotels below offer fully qualified masseurs and a range of treatments. Make sure you book in advance to secure a time slot which suits your travel schedule.

Arora Hotel

The massage facilities at the Arora Hotel range from Thai massage to therapeutic massages. The hotel also offers a sauna and steam room as part of the spa. It is the most accessible hotel to get to by train or bus from Gatwick South terminal and is open to external guests (non-residents and non-members). The train ride is only 13 minutes.

Telephone: To book a massage call 07861248294 **or email on** marek@junglehealing.co.uk
Access: Available to non-members and external guests.
Cost: Massage prices range from £50 for 60 minutes to £85 for 120 minutes. Free use of the sauna and steam room. There is a twenty-four-hour cancellation policy to avoid 100% charge.
Opening hours: Advanced bookings only.

Includes: Sauna and steam room. You can also stop for lunch or coffee in their tranquil atrium before heading back to the hustle and bustle of the airport.
Additional services: There is also a gym with cardiovascular exercise machines and a range of equipment, reflexology treatments and yoga. The car park facilities are free, but if you are also staying overnight, you can also park your car while you are on your trip at the cost of £10 per day.
Location: Southgate Avenue, Crawley, West Sussex RH10 6LW
Directions: **By public transport**, it couldn't be easier as the hotel is right next to Crawley train station. There is a gate from the platform into the hotel. Buses from Gatwick Airport also stop very close to the hotel.
Train from Gatwick Airport: The easiest way is to hop on a train at the South Terminal. They run every 15 minutes until late at night. The train journey is about

13 minutes, and the tickets cost £3.20. The shuttle from the North to South Terminal is three minutes.

Bus from Gatwick Airport: Alternatively, you could catch the bus from the South Terminal (Fastway 10, Fastway 20, 400, 460). Fastway 10 and 20 stops a minute from the hotel. Depending on the route, the journey takes between 13 and 20 minutes.

If you are travelling by car head east on Airport Way onto the M23, leave at junction 10 and take the A2011 towards Crawley. At the first roundabout, take the second exit and continue on the A2004. At the second roundabout, take the first exit towards the Country Mall. Go straight through the next two sets of traffic lights, past the Country Mall on the right, and under the railway bridge. The hotel is on your right.

Alexander House Hotel & Utopia Spa

Many reviewers praise Alexander House for their excellent hospitality and relaxing massages. Set within 120 acres of English countryside, this is a place where you can really unwind before setting off on a business trip. The massages range from a 40-minute Indian Head Massage to an 85-minute full body massage. There are also body wraps to indulge yourself.

Telephone: +44(0) 1342714914 **or email** admin@alexanderhouse.co.uk
Access: Open to non-hotel guests and residents.
Cost: Individual massages range from £70 to £125, day spas from £99.00 and body wraps & scrubs between £70 to £175.
Opening hours: Daily 8 am to 8 pm

Includes: Spa days are inclusive of lunch or afternoon tea. Zen garden with outdoor hot tub and barrel sauna, as well as a collection of relaxation lounges.
Additional Services: Professional hair salon, state of the art gym and outdoor tennis court.
Location: Turners Hill, Crawley, Sussex RH10 4QD
Directions by public transport:
If you're travelling by taxi or private car from Gatwick Airport, it only takes 15 minutes. Head on down the M23 and B2110 to Siskin Avenue, turn left onto Siskin Avenue, and you'll find Alexander House Hotel and Utopia Spa on the right.
Train from Gatwick Airport It takes about 30 minutes by train from Gatwick South Terminal, then southbound on the Thameslink to Three Bridges, which takes about 5 minutes. At Three Bridges train station, walk for 3 minutes to Stop B and catch the number 84 bus to East Grinstead alighting at Fen Place Farm. It takes about 15 minutes; then it is a minute walk to Turners Hill.

Bus from Gatwick Airport takes about 45 minutes on either the Fastway 20 and then Bus 84 to East Grinstead alighting at Fen Place Farm or catch the Fastway 10 to Crawley and then Metrobus 84 to Fen Place Farm. Once you alight at Fen Place Farm, it is only a minute to Turners Hill.

Cottesmore Hotel Golf and Country Club

Described as a hidden gem near Gatwick, Cottesmore Hotel Golf and Country Clubs offer a full range of massage treatments from a back massage to an Indian head massage for the shoulders, neck and head. It is ideal if the work and travel environments place a strain on your upper body muscles. There is also a hot tub, sauna and steam room, not to mention all the other activities. Only 13 minutes from Gatwick by car, you could enjoy a full range of facilities within the health club, including treatments, personal training and fitness classes.

Telephone: 01293 528 256 **or email** spa@cottesmoregolf.co.uk
Cost: Dependent on the massage treatment with a price range from £32 for a 25-minute Swedish massage to £65 full body Decleor back massage.
Health Spa visitor rate: £15.00 (non-member), Guests (with a member) is £7.50
Access: Visitors are welcome, as well as hotel guests (complimentary). Membership is available at an annual or monthly rate. Spa Packages are also available.
Opening hours: Monday to Friday 6.30 am to 9.30 pm. Weekends and Bank holidays 8.00 am – 8.00 pm.

Includes: Swimming pool, hot tub, sauna, steam room.
Additional services: Golf course, tennis court, gym with cardiovascular and weights equipment, fitness classes and personal trainer.
Location: Buchan Hill, Pease Pottage, Crawley, RH11 9AT, United Kingdom.
Directions: The club is only 13 minutes from Gatwick Airport by car or taxi, and 1 mile from junction 11 on the M23.
By car from Gatwick Airport Head east on Airport Way, continue on the M23 to Brighton Road/B2114. Take the exit at Junction 11, take Horsham Road and Forest Road to the lodge.
By train from Gatwick Airport The train departs at Gatwick South Terminal, southbound. Go six stops to Brighton and alight at Crawley. It takes about 10 minutes. The walk from Crawley station to Forest Road takes about 25 minutes (approximately 1.3 miles). Total time by train would be roughly 1 hour.

Felbridge Hotel and Spa

Reviewers report 'total relaxation' with the massages they had at the Felbridge Hotel and Spa. Guests can choose either a half day spa treatment or longer depending on their travel schedule. There is also a fully equipped gym, boasting state of the art Technogym equipment and a team of personal trainers.

Telephone: 01342 337700 or email chakraspa@felbridgehotel.co.uk
Access: Non-residents (as part of a spa package), gym members, hotel residents
Cost: for visitors, there is a half day spa at £65. Other spa packages are also available for a six-hour duration. Each spa package also has a meal or afternoon tea inclusive. Off-peak, membership is available from £38 per month or annual membership at £400, with no joining fee. Peak membership is £55 per month.
Opening hours:
    Monday to Friday 6.30 am – 9.00 am
    Saturday – Sunday 8.00 am – 9.00 pm

Includes:

> **Minimum Half day (4 hrs) spa pass** offers full use of gym and spa facilities (sauna, steam room, Jacuzzi). Supplied with robe, towels and slippers. Also have a choice of breakfast, lunch, afternoon tea or dinner, along with one 55-minute treatment (choose full body massage, facial, manicure or pedicure).
> **Membership** includes full access to the spa, two tennis courts, complimentary induction session, fresh towels on arrival, use of robe and slippers, complimentary tea & coffee, discounts off spa treatments, products, food, accommodation.

Additional services: Personal training sessions, tennis courts, spa and swimming pool.
Location: Situated on London Road, in East Grinstead, West Sussex RH19 2BH. The hotel sits prominently on the A22 and is only a 15-minute drive from Gatwick Airport.
Directions: It is just 8 miles from Gatwick Airport. Approximately only 15 minutes by car or taxi to the airport. Head east on Airport Way. Continue on the M23. Take the A264 to London Road/A22 in East Grinstead.

Chapter 6: Wi-Fi at Gatwick Airport

Enhancing connectivity to reduce strain

Connectivity is crucial when travelling on business. Not being able to access the internet or having a poor internet connection is one of the largest stress factors for business travellers.

The inability to work en route means business executives are losing valuable preparation time, making last-minute changes to a presentation or revising sales data just before a meeting. It also means that day to day office work mounts up, making it difficult to keep up, with numerous emails awaiting attention upon return to the office. The consequences of poor connectivity over the long term can be quite disastrous for health and productivity as business people who travel predominately report lower psychological well-being than those who do not travel. It comes down to feeling one is in control of work demands and having a positive perception of one's job and career security.

Although cost is often argued as the biggest driver of corporate travel policies, business travellers actively take into account connectivity and convenience when selecting or changing their travel arrangements. On route, connectivity can be a mixed bag. While public Wi-Fi is becoming ubiquitous across cafés, transport and hotels, in reality, one can't really be sure what they're going to get until they get there.

Connectivity in the past has been a revenue stream for airports and hotels, partly based on the need for return on investment and partly based on keeping up competitor's offerings. Now it is starting to become a free or inclusive offering, seeming to show how the company is looking after their travelling customer needs. Unfortunately, free often means a poor signal, slow speed or difficult to access. This simply adds more strain to the business traveller who eventually gives up and pays for a higher standard of service.

Despite Gatwick International Airport being the second largest airport in the UK, and reportedly one of Europe's premier airports, it sadly lacks a fast, free Wi-Fi. Gatwick Airport has been reported as having the slowest service at London Airports with only 0.5 Mbps. However, there are faster speeds throughout the airport, if you know where to find them.

So, we have conducted the search for you, to see what connectivity is on offer and just how good it really is. We have found places where you can access Wi-Fi, for free as part of a complimentary service, and subscription based. We've also looked at download speeds and referred to numerous traveller's reviews to ascertain whether any 'super-fast' claim is justified.

Depending on how much time you have, the route you are undertaking and what you require a Wi-Fi connection for will determine the best place for you to connect. Below are some options for you to choose from when flying out of Gatwick Airport's North Terminal.

How to access Gatwick Airport's free Internet

There are several options to enable you to access the internet at Gatwick International Airport's North Terminal. The first being the use of the free Wi-Fi available to all airport passengers, next is via the public internet as the surf boxes scattered throughout Gatwick Airport. Thirdly, you can use a more private connection in the airport and business centre lounges. You can even access the internet en route to your next destination. Finally, you can access as a guest at a connecting hotel, within their free business areas or as a paying guest.

Gatwick Airport's free Wi-Fi

Gatwick Airport has teamed up with Boingo internet providers to offer free Wi-Fi for those who sign up as a MyGatwick account holders. When you become a MyGatwick account holder, you will receive 90 minutes free of charge, in two 45 minute instalments.

If you require more than 90 minutes, you can pay on an hourly basis with the Boingo Hotspot subscription. Boingo has over one million hotspots worldwide, so as a single account holder you can log on at anyone of their hotspots in airports, hotels, cafes, restaurants, etc. In the UK, they cover 60% of UK enplanements.

Unfortunately, reports indicate the speed of the MyGatwick Wi-Fi can be very slow and has a weak signal, so if you require a Wi-Fi connection for urgent business or to download documents, you might find the other solutions below less frustrating.

To access the free Wi-Fi, you just navigate to your device's list of available wireless networks. Click on the 'get online now' and select 'Gatwick FREE Wi-Fi'. Sign up for or log into your MyGatwick account. Click on the 'Get online' button for 45 minutes of free Wi-Fi. You can get another 45 minutes once the session is finished by repeating the above steps.

How to Subscribe to Boingo

If you're finding the capacity of the Gatwick free Wi-Fi too slow, then you can use a premium service provided by Boingo, which offers greater speed. Boingo enjoys an exclusive arrangement with Gatwick Airport. While there might be a business case for such a vast differential between the free Wi-Fi speed and the premium rate, it can be somewhat frustrating if you are in a hurry or need to access documents quickly and log onto the free Wi-Fi first. One could question the ethics of such a differential when passengers are ultimately paying for the supply through their airport fees anyway, not without standing it is reportedly the slowest Wi-Fi amongst all the London airports.

Boingo offers several price plans, including a mobile, unlimited, pay as you go, hourly, Europe, Asia or global plan. The monthly subscription gives you access to over a million other Boingo hotspots, including other international airports, with over 25 airports in the UK and 100,000 hotspots nationwide.

Prices start from £3.95 for an extra hour or £9.95 per month. For more information on price plans, click onto Boingo's website. **www.boingo.com**

Best places to connect

Public Internet

Surf boxes, marked on the airport's map as an internet zone, are available for public use and operate as a pay as you go internet access.

They are located within the North Terminal in Check-in areas level 1 and 2. There is also a printer at Check-in level 1 and 2, just in case you need to print out your flight details or ticket again. Unfortunately, the internet zones in Arrivals Hall and Departure Lounge have been removed since our last visit.

The cost is 10 p per minute for internet access, with a minimum charge of £1, and £1 per printed page. Each surf box accepts either coin or credit cards for payment.

Check-in, Level One

The Internet zone is located on the left-hand side as you walk in from the entrance, next to the escalators, just before the Easy Jet Check-in counters and by the lifts to level 2. There are four surf boxes located here and a printer.

Check-in, Level Two

Public internet access is available on level 2 of the Check-in area located just opposite the Emirates Information Counter. As you enter from the car park, walk through the entrance on the far left, and you'll find the internet zone just to the right at the end of Check-in Zones C and D, just opposite Emirates Tickets and Information booth. There are four surf boxes. A printer is also available.

Finding Wi-Fi en route

If you're short on time and need to check your travel arrangements or email work documents, then working en route to or from the airport might be worthwhile considering. As transport infrastructures are improving, so is service provision on trains and private connections. Listed below are both private and public transport options which provide free Wi-Fi.

Public transport: Train Services
Gatwick Express

In 2016, twenty-seven brand new Gatwick Express trains entered service. They were designed to 'transform the journey between London and Gatwick' by the provision of on-train Wi-Fi with power sockets to match. When we travelled on the new trains, we found the Wi-Fi signal to be heavily promoted as Free Wi-Fi and Entertainment. The signal was very strong, and the download speed fast. It doesn't offer any security for private data. However, it was straightforward to access.

Just click on the connect under your Wi-Fi settings, then click on 'add an account' and provide your details where prompted. These include your email address, gender, age, the reason for travel and if you wish to be remembered on subsequent trips.

Additional services include Evening Standard news, booking for Gatwick Express tickets in the future and flight information. Power points are also available at window seats.

Top Tip: When we travelled on the Gatwick Express the speed for download was reportedly 72 Mbps, which is faster than within Gatwick Airport. So if you have documents to download at the last minute, it might be preferential that these are downloaded en route to the airport.

Private Transport: Car rentals

Some hire car companies are now providing Wi-Fi as an add-on product to the cost of hire. Here are two of the leading companies.

Budget Car Rentals

Budget Car Rentals provides mobile Wi-Fi access with coverages across the UK and offers up to 1 GB of data per day. Simply reserve online or add to your rental at the rental station. Which is great if you're from overseas and want to save money on roaming or hotel charges. Very easy to connect, all you need to do is switch it on.

Wi-Fi offers unlimited wireless access for five devices, including laptops, smartphones, tablets and other Wi-Fi enabled devices.
Located at North Terminal in Arrivals: ground floor. Just opposite the UK and Republic of Ireland Arrivals exit.
Cost: £11.20 per day. All fees are payable at the local rental station when collecting the device. You can reserve this online when you book your car, or you can ask at the rental station.

Avis Car Rentals

Avis now offers their car hires the ability to stay connected across 12 countries in Europe when renting one of their vehicles with their Mobile Wi-Fi. Just choose 'extra' when booking online and pick Mobile Wi-Fi, or pop into the rental counter at the airport.

Avis Mobile Wi-Fi provides unlimited access to surf the web at 1 GB data per day with their wireless internet access for laptops, smartphones, tablets and any other Wi-Fi-enabled device.
Located at North Terminal in Arrivals: ground floor. Just opposite the UK and Republic of Ireland Arrivals exit.

Cost: £9.86 per day. The mobile Wi-Fi unit allows up to five devices at a time and operates on a cross-border capability which means there are no roaming charges when travelling aboard.

Private Transport: Chauffeur hire cars

Private Chauffeur cars are also now offering complimentary Wi-Fi. Here are a couple of Chauffeur driven vehicles which operate from Gatwick Airport's North Terminal which offer Wi-Fi.

EG Chauffeurs

EG Chauffeurs provides executive business travel for London Gatwick Airport. Free onboard Wi-Fi is available. Highly rated by reviewers, EG Chauffeurs received a 9.5 out of 10 rating.

Booking online: www.egchauffeurs.com
Telephone Bookings: +44(0) 207 117 2905
Email: info@egchauffeurs.com

iChauffeur

iChauffeur is a Greater London based luxury chauffeur car company and operates to and from several South East airports. Wi-Fi is available in some of the cars, so make sure this is requested when booking. Phone charges for Blackberries, iPhones and some other mobile phones are also available in the car.

Booking online: www.ichauffeur.co.uk
Telephone Booking: +44(0) 20 8400 4829
Email: info@ichauffeur.co.uk

Wi-Fi Executive Cars

Wi-Fi Executive Cars are available to hire for airport transfers to Gatwick Airport, along with other London airports. They offer complimentary Wi-Fi internet access in all their cars, as well as being equipped with in-car charger for mobile devices.

Booking online: www.WiFiexecutivecars.com
Telephone Bookings: +44(0) 01628 30 80 55
Email: info@WiFiexecutivecars.com

Wi-Fi where you can dine

For reasons described above, the restaurants and cafes in Gatwick's North Terminal all offer the free Gatwick Airport Wi-Fi. Reportedly "sometimes ok and sometimes slow". If you wish to download documents or work, then using an alternative location to access the internet might work out better for you or upgrading the supply is another option.

Arrivals, Ground Floor

There is only one option here for you to access the internet over some nourishment in the Arrivals Hall.

Costa Coffee

The signal strength in Costa Coffee was reportedly very strong, although not a very fast download speed when we visited at 12 Mbps. We also found the best locations to access emails is either down the back of the café to the far right or at the far left of the service counter.

There are also two benches at the front of the café which specifically cater for accessing the internet with power points.

Check-in, Level One
Hampton by Hilton, incorporating Starbucks

The Hampton by Hilton hotel is only a few minutes along the corridor from the Easy Jet Check-In on Level One. Here you can have a Starbucks coffee, snacks and light meals in their bar lounge and business centre area while surfing the internet. There are plenty of tables to sit at, as well as a workbench near the business area which sits up to twelve people and has plenty of power points. The Wi-Fi is complimentary.

Check-in, Level Two

There are two cafes on level two where you can access the Gatwick free Wi-Fi when dining or over coffee.

Jamie's Coffee Lounge

Here the use of mobile devices and working on larger devices is encouraged. There are plenty of places which cater for those wanting to access email. Head straight towards the main window, and just behind the service counter, you will find a workbench with power points to charge your device at the same time. At the time of our visit, we found the signal here to be good but the weaker and slower than the Nicholas Culpeper upstairs.

An additional workbench has been added to the front of the café, with plenty of power points, for diners who may wish to access the internet on their mobile device.

The Nicholas Culpeper.

When we visited, we found the Nicholas Culpeper, upstairs, to have a stronger signal and download link than Jamie's Coffee Lounge. This might be explained by the fact there would have been fewer diners accessing the Wi-Fi at the time of the visit.

Departure Lounge, Lower and Upper Level

We found during our visits the access to the Wi-Fi, both regarding signal strength and download capacity varied from restaurant to restaurant. Walking from end to end of the upper level in the Departure Lounge, the download speed ranged from 1 Mbps to 24 Mbps. As noted above, all restaurants relied on travellers accessing the free Gatwick Wi-Fi provision and didn't provide their own Wi-Fi for customers to access.

Wi-Fi where you can work

If you don't have internet access already and need a quiet place to think while accessing your emails and work, then here are a couple of places you might prefer to the main Departure Lounge areas.

Check-in, Level One
Workbench

On the right-hand side of the entrance, just past the Bureaux de Change is a workbench where you can access your emails and charge your device. There is sufficient room for ten people here, with sufficient dual power sockets available.

Regus Business Centre at the South Terminal

If you have more than 3 hours to wait at Gatwick Airport, then it might be worthwhile considering the use of Regus Express Business Centre and Lounge at the South Terminal, which is only 3 minutes by interconnecting airport terminal shuttle. You can catch the shuttle on Level One near the train station.

Regus Business Centre offers a fast Wi-Fi along with other business facilities and complimentary beverages, reportedly more rapid than the free Wi-Fi or Boingo. Also available are meeting rooms and print facilities.

Open: 6.00 am to 6.00 pm Monday to Friday.
Telephone: 0870 880 8484
Access: Open to all business travellers. Free access to Regus members.
Cost: The drop-in use of Business Centre's lounge is £8 per hour or £32 per day for non-members. **Facilities:** Document station offering print, scan and copy and free high-speed internet.
Additional Services: Free beverages, fruit & biscuits, along with kitchen facilities including a microwave, meeting rooms and shower amenities.
Location in the South Terminal is by lift just between Bureau de Change and Costa Coffee in the Arrivals area, level two. When you alight from the shuttle, walk through the entrance of the terminal, turn right at WHSmith, and you will find the lifts just before Costa Coffee. Take the lift to the ground floor and turn right upon exiting the lift.

Wi-Fi where you can relax

No. 1 Lounge

The No. 1 Lounge in the North Terminal is one of the largest lounges where you can relax and keep pace with others through the internet. When you've had a chance to lift your head up, you can take in the most extensive view of the runway. If it's work you're catching up on or have a precise email to write, then please note this is one of the busiest lounges. It would be better to head straight to the library which has dedicated desks for working on mobile devices and plenty of power points. Here there is less risk of interruption or distraction.

Wi-Fi is free and unlimited. We didn't find any customer reviews indicating problems with speed or connectivity. We found the access to the Wi-Fi relatively easy, and it was quick to register. The signal strength was strong, and the download capacity was recorded at 54 Mbps, which is far more Gatwick's free Wi-Fi download capacity when we visited other areas within the Departure Lounge.

Open: 4.00 am to 10.00 pm daily.
Access: All travellers including groups and children. Open to all those who want to use a **lounge away from the main thoroughfare.**

Facilities: There are plenty of workspaces by the window in the first section of the library, a large working desk in the centre of the room in the second section, and soft seating with tables in the remaining areas of the library room. Elsewhere, there are desks by the window in the buffet area, plenty of tables in the TV lounge seated areas, and swivel chairs with power points by the main windows with a runway view. There is also a meeting room for hire with Wi-Fi access. Lastly, there are also two internet terminals near reception with printing facilities.

Cost: Lounge entry for adults is £30 if you book in advance or £37.50 on the door without booking. If your flight is delayed and you want to stay longer, then you can buy additional hours.

Free access to: Dragonpass, Diners Club, Institute of Directors, Lounge Club, Priority Pass, Dining Club, Caxton FX.

Location: On the lower level of the Departure Lounge, after security, on route to gates 45-55 and 101 -113.

Directions: Once through security into the main Departure Lounge, turn left and follow the signs to the 'Airport Lounges'. These are situated just past the London News Company along the hallway towards gates 45 – 55 and 101 – 113. Turn right once you walk into the corridor from the Departure Lounge, and right again. Pass through the double glass doors; the No1 lounge is straight ahead.

Aspire Lounge

Open to all. However, access may be restricted in busy periods due to space constraints. When you walk in, turn left, and you'll find a dedicated quiet area with tables, and comfortable chairs with power-points suitable for working on a mobile device.

Wi-Fi is free and unlimited; however, some of the customer reviews have mentioned they have had problems with reliability and access. Others reported it was good. We found the signal strength very strong, download speed was good, recorded at 54 Mbps, but had some difficulty logging on initially when we visited the first time.

Open: Open hours are from 4.00 am to 10.00 pm, with a slight seasonal variation

Facilities: Large lounge chairs and dedicated quiet areas.

Access: Welcomes anyone who is travelling, which means it may not be the most peaceful lounge to work or relax in. Nevertheless, it is still quieter than the main Departure Lounge.

Cost: Lounge entry for adults is from £17.99 if you book in advance or £35 on the door without booking. If your flight is delayed and you want to stay longer, then you can buy additional hours.

Free access: Institute of Directors, Lounge Pass, Priority Pass members, Diners Club, Dragon Pass, Aspire Platinum membership and Vueling Airline passengers.
Location: First floor of the Departure Lounge in the Lounge Pavilion.
Directions: Turn left after security and follow the signs to the 'Airport Lounges'. Head towards gates 45 – 55 and 101 – 113, as you pass London News Company into the main hallway to the gates, you will see a corridor on your right. Go through the double glass doors and take the lift to the first floor. The lounge is located on the right-hand side.

Emirates Lounge

If you are flying first or business on Emirates Airways, then you can use the Emirates Lounge to connect to the internet. It has been recently renovated to include a business centre with new facilities, including free broadband and wireless LAN access, along with computers and laptop workstations.

Wi-Fi is available and described by past lounge users as 'Solid'.

Access for: Emirates First Class and Business Class travellers or as an Emirates Skywards Platinum or Gold member departing on an Emirates flight. One guest is allowed if travelling on the same plane.
Opening hours: First departure to the last departure.
Location: First floor of the Departure Lounge.
Directions: Head towards gate 101 – 113, as you pass London News Company, you will see a corridor on your right. Go through the double glass doors and take the lift to the first floor. The lounge in located on the left-hand side.

My Lounge

Open to all but slightly less formal than the No. 1 Lounge. My lounge offers a relaxed atmosphere suitable for managing a quick internet search or picking up last minute preparatory materials. Perhaps not the quietest airport lounge for accessing and focusing on emails or work via Wi-Fi, but still much quieter than the main Departure Lounge. There is a workbench on the left as you enter, a large communal table in the centre of the room and two free internet terminals at the front of the lounge for guest use.

Wi-Fi is inclusive of the entry fee and unlimited. Some customers have commented in past reviews that they had issues with the Wi-Fi working correctly. We found the signal strength very strong, but the connection was relatively slow when we visited.

Open: 6.00 am to 8.00 pm

Facilities: Two private rooms for relaxation. One more for light entertainment. Two computer terminals and printing.

Cost: Lounge entry for adults is £18 if you book in advance or £24 on the door without booking. If your flight is delayed and you want to stay longer, then you can buy additional hours.

Free access to: Institute of Directors, Lounge Club, Lounge Pass, Priority Pass, Diners Club

Location: in the Departure Lounge, Lower Level. After security, follow the signs for the airport lounges and My Lounge. MyLounge is situated on the left as you enter the Lounge Pavilion.

Directions: Head towards gates 45 – 55 and 101 – 113, as you pass London News Company into the main corridor to the gates, you will see a hallway on your right. Go through the double glass doors. The lounge is located on the left-hand side as you enter the Lounge Pavilion, just before the lifts.

Wi-Fi where you can sleep and shower

There are a couple of hotels located within or connected to Gatwick Airport's North Terminal where you can access the internet without much difficulty. Some hotels will also allow you to access the Wi-Fi free of charge when visiting, so don't be shy about just popping in.

Sofitel Hotel

Directly connected to Gatwick North Airport, Sofitel Hotel has over 500 rooms available, as well as a business centre.

Wi-Fi is complimentary for guests with a room. However, guests have reported a slow speed, and some mentioned having experienced issues with connecting to the free Wi-Fi. You can pay extra for faster speed or upgrade your room and receive a more rapid speed included in the price. Other reports suggest that it depends on your booking process. Apparently, if you book direct with the Sofitel Hotel or through Accor, you will get a faster Wi-Fi connection compared to booking through other online booking agents. We find this rather a strange customer centred practice if the case and concluded after reading reviews over the past year; there is a basic free Wi-Fi for guests, but you may need to pay more for a faster speed. Some reports suggested this was £15 extra at the time of review.

Telephone: + 44 (0) 1293 567070

Prices: range from £122 per night for a room, at the time of review. Day rates are £79 for a day room.

Location: The Sofitel hotel is connected to Gatwick Airport through a covered walkway on the right-hand-side of the shuttle on the North Terminal, level one.

Directions: From the terminal exit on level one, walk straight ahead to the right of the shuttle to a covered walkway sign posted Sofitel Hotel. Walk down the corridor, and you're at the entrance within 2 minutes. If you are arriving by car, you will find the entrance to the hotel on the ground floor next to the Hotel's car park. Alternatively, you can park in the Airport car park with easy access to both the hotel and airport terminal on level one.

Hampton by Hilton

Hampton is connected to the North terminal. It offers a guaranteed service which differentiates it from other hotels in and around Gatwick Airport. If you're not satisfied, they don't expect you to pay! This level of commitment has earned them high ratings on customer review sites, and in 2015 they were awarded a TripAdvisor Certificate of Excellence. There is a communal business centre next to the lobby on the ground floor.

Wi-Fi is offered free to all guests, both in rooms and at the 'work-zone' area which reportedly you can use without checking in overnight. The majority of guest comments we reviewed were extremely complimentary towards the fast speed and easy connection for Wi-Fi. They also have on offer printing of documents and photocopying services, along with light bites if you need a quick snack. When we visited, the reception was very approachable.

Telephone: +44 (0) 1293 579999

Room rates: Overnight room rates are around £136 per night, and all guests receive a complimentary breakfast, and if you are an AA member, you can also receive a 10% discount. Day rates are £69. Meeting rooms are also available to hire.

Location: The entrance to this hotel is near the Easy Jet Check-in on level one. Just follow the signs to the right of the check-in desk. You will see a sign above the entrance to the corridor for the Hampton by Hilton.

Directions: Turn right at the Easy Jet Check-in area and walk towards the end of the hall. Walk straight ahead through the entrance under the sign and follow the passage to the left. Walk through the automatic double glass doors. The total distance is about 50 steps from the Easy Jet Check-in to the hotel reception.

Premier Inn

Premier Inn at Gatwick is one of 700 value based hotels in a UK-wide chain. They pride themselves on being conveniently located at several UK airports, including Gatwick's North Terminal.

Basic Wi-Fi is unlimited and free to overnight guests and up to 3 devices. Alternatively, you can upgrade to a faster package with a maximum download of 1 GB per day. The majority of reviews we saw were not complimentary over the free Wi-Fi service, stating it was slow, or they had a poor connection. Similar comments were made on the upgraded Wi-Fi which many found was slow or suffered poor connection, while others were pleased with the link speed. One reviewer summed up his experience with "not a good option for business travellers', while others voiced their frustration and didn't feel they should need to pay for an upgrade at all as it should in their opinion be part of an essential service.

Telephone: + 44 (0) 871 527 9354
Wi-Fi Cost: There is free Wi-Fi throughout your stay for up to 1 GB per day and three devices. If you wish to download large files or stream films, then you can upgrade to an Ultimate Wi-Fi package at the cost of £5 for one day, £15 per week, £30 per month, and £150 per year. You can pay by credit card or buy a voucher from reception.
Room Rates: Room rates at the time of publication were from £62.50 per night.
Locations: Directly opposite the North Terminal drop-off point.
Directions: Simply walk outside the main entrance of the terminal on level 1, down the escalator and cross the road.

Chapter 7: Keep your mobile devices charged

Charged mobile devices reduce travel stress

Being without sufficient battery life on your phone, laptop, Kindle or any other device when you travel can cause unnecessary strain. Not being able to use your devices to work is the second highest stress factor when travelling on business. Yet, it is so easy to forget to charge before setting out, pack a charger or use the battery life up en route.

Surprises on business trips are also quite stressful. In fact, losing one's possessions is the highest stress factor when travelling on business. Anxiety is heightened now there are new security rules on travelling with devices. The UK Government's new security guidelines state that anyone flying from a UK airport is expected to be able to show that their electronic devices in their hand luggage can be switched on.

Passengers carrying devices which they cannot switch on may not be allowed to bring the device onto the aircraft. So, if your phone or other device runs out of battery life, you could be asked to either leave the device behind or not to travel until it is charged sufficiently to turn on. This new rule affects all flights leaving all UK airports, in and out of the UK, including Gatwick Airport.

Some airlines, like British Airways and Virgin Atlantic, have agreed to either keep the device for their passengers at the airport until they can collect them on their return, or forward the device to another address. However, not all airlines offer this level of customer service.

Alternatively, you can avoid the anxiety of losing your device or missing your flight, by knowing in advance where you can charge your device before queuing at the boarding gates.

At Gatwick Airport, there are a variety of locations where you can charge your device(s), although many of these places may not be immediately obvious. Even the official phone charging stations can be challenging to locate.

Also, in times of delay or inclement weather, when the airport is overcrowded, and many travellers need to charge their mobile phone, there are a limited number of phone charging stations which can become over-subscribed very quickly.

It can be frustrating as well as time-consuming to find a power point which is available to use. Even, more so if you have some critical emails or preparatory work to complete. So, we have searched Gatwick Airport's North Terminal for you.

All the locations for charging your device, which we have found, are listed below. We've included where you can charge en route, the best places when you're dining, relaxing, working, along with some of the more unusual places for when lots of people are trying to charge at once. We've also searched for fully charged battery banks and charging units should you wish to charge without using a power point.

Where you can charge in the North Terminal

Charging en route

You can now charge your mobile devices en route when travelling to and from Gatwick Airport if you are taking public transport. The following transportation has power points for charging your devices.

Gatwick Express

The new Gatwick Express trains have power points located at the window seats. The journey takes approximately half an hour, which should be sufficient time to charge your phone. There are two power points per window seat at each table so you could potentially charge two devices at the same time, depending on who is sitting next to you.

Charge while you pick up a colleague

The Arrivals Hall has recently been renovated. It now offers several power points near seats so you can charge your phone while you wait to pick up a colleague. We found power points at the following locations.

Columns in centre opposite UK & Republic of Ireland Arrivals

There are two columns here, both with a row of seats surrounding each column, which host a double power point.

Left wall in the UK & Republic of Ireland Arrivals Hall.

There are two double power points near the UK & Republic of Ireland Arrivals exit on the left-hand side wall, next to the internet terminals.

Columns in centre of main Arrival Hall area

Dual power points are located on most of the columns in the main Arrivals Hall. Unfortunately, there are no power points next to the rows of seats just outside Costa Coffee. However, there are plenty of power points in Costa Coffee, and specifically, if you are waiting for a colleague, there are two workbenches at the front of the café with four dual power points at each workbench.

Charge your devices while you wait to check-in

There are plenty of free charging points before and after security. These are mainly located on walls or large columns, along with internet zones, work benches, and some restaurants & cafes. Knowing where to charge or which café has power points you can use, saves time and resource. In times of delay, many of the power points might already be in use, so we've included some locations where they might be less obvious.

Check-in, Level One

If you are stuck in a queue waiting to check in, then there are some power points around the Check-in area, which you can utilise.

Columns just opposite the Easy Jet Check-in counter.

There are a couple of power points on the columns located just in front of the escalators, near the Easy Jet Check-in counters.

Left wall in the check-in area.

There are two sets of dual plugs on the left-hand side near the entrance to the public toilets. There are also some seats here.

Back wall, on the left-hand side of the check-in area.

There is a power-point socket by the four seats at the end.

The corridor leading to the toilets.

There is one power point in the corridor leading to the toilets at the far left-hand side.

Ladies toilet.

Yes, there's even a powerpoint here, on the wall just opposite the mirrors.

Check-in, Level Two

There are very few power points here. You may find the odd one on a column near the escalator, but we could find none between the rows of Check-in. Your best bet is to try the cafes or the internet zone (see below).

Charge your devices while you wait to board

So, you have made it to the Departure Lounge, with a little time to spare to recharge your phone. No need to worry about finding a power-point, we've done the exploring for you.

Departure Lounge, Lower Level

Unlike other airport terminals, there are not many dedicated benches where you can sit and charge your phone once you come through security, nor are there many power points within public seating areas. We needed to look very hard to discover where they were.

So, we've been out exploring and found the following accessible sockets.

The quiet area between Boots the Chemist and Dixons Travel.

An ideal place to charge is in the quiet area at the far end of the Departure Lounge. Head straight towards the largest Boots the Chemist at the far end when you enter from security. To the right of Boots is a seating area. Here you'll find power points on the columns by the windows. These are conveniently located next to the seating area, which has a low footfall being off the main thoroughfare, so you can keep an eye on your phone while relaxing.

Column opposite Boots the Chemist.

Boots the Chemist's largest of two shops, at the far end as you enter the Departure Lounge from security, has a column right outside with a power point on it.

Column opposite Dixons travel.

The larger of the two Dixons travel shops is located on the right-hand side of the Departure Lounge as you come through security, heading towards Boots the Chemist at the end. It is situated between Boots and Jo Malone. The powerpoint is on the column directly opposite Dixons travel.

By the lifts near the toilets.

Halfway down the right-hand side of the Departure Lounge between Boots the Chemist at one end and Weatherspoons' Red Lion pub at the other end are the lifts to go upstairs. You will find a power point socket here as well.

Next to Weatherspoon's Red Lion pub.

There are two power point sockets next to the exit door for Gates 557 – 574, one on either side next to a row of seats.

Column opposite security near Weatherspoon's Red Lion pub.

World of Whiskies

World of Whiskies is situated next to Dune and the Sunglass Hut. You'll find a column with power points on it behind the screen and the rubbish bins directly in front of the World of Whiskies.

Column at Kath Kidson.

The powerpoint is on the column just opposite Kath Kidson, facing the World Duty Free shop. It is visible from the seating area, so you can sit while you charge.

Gate specific power points

You will find power points along the corridors when you head to the following gates.

Passage towards Gates 45 – 55 and 101 to 113.

Gatwick's North Terminal has recently relocated some of its seating. In doing so, they have added some extra power points for you to charge your phone.

Just as you turn right into the hallway, just past the London New Company, you will notice several rows of seats to the left. Here you will find a box of six power points and another box of four power points. The columns to the right of the seating also host dual power points.

If you continue down the passage to Gates 45 – 55 and 101 to 113, you will find a complimentary newspaper and magazine rack. There are two power points on either side of the magazine rack. If you use the power point on the far side of the rack (nearest to Gates), there are also four seats.

Just before Gate 49

At the end of the passage, just before turning to walk to gates 46 – 49, there are several power points next to the chairs in front of the window.

Gate 51

Near the toilets, there are three benches (four seats per bench) with power points.

Gate 52 – 53

Four sets of power points between Gates 52 to 53.

Gate 54

Four power point on the column opposite Gate 54, with chairs next to them.

Passage to Gates 557 and 574

Not many people will bother finding power points along here. It's off the main thoroughfare, so it's an ideal place to charge when stuck in the airport due to inclement weather or lengthy delays. You'll find eight power points along the passage to Gate 557 and another five power points along the passage to Gates 572 – 574. Gatwick North Terminal has relocated some seating here as well, and you can now sit along the wall opposite the main windows and relax while you recharge your phone.

Departure Lounge, Upper Level

There are some power points also scattered around the upper level of the Departure Lounge. We found a number when we went exploring.

Outside EAT

On the right of EAT, as you come up from the stairs in the middle of the Departure Lounge on the lower level, you'll find a power point. There is another power point on the column opposite EAT.

Near Union Jacks

There is a power point socket on the column near Union Jacks Bar overlooking the World Duty Free.

Near the lift

Overlooking World Duty Free shop below is another power point.

At the top of the middle stairs

There is one power point on the right at Shake a Hula next to the workbench.

Toilets at the far end

These have a power point in the corridor outside the toilets. There are also two in the ladies' toilets. Unfortunately, we were unable to verify if the men's toilets had power points.

Charge your devices while you dine

Some cafes will actively encourage you to charge your phone and other devices while eating in their establishment. Here are some for you to choose from;

Arrivals, Ground Floor

If you are stopping for a quick bite, before travelling onwards, then try the cafe in the Arrivals hall where you are welcome to charge your devices.

Costa Coffee

There are several places you can charge your devices here. Costa Coffee has recently added two work benches at the front of their café. Each workbench seats eight and have four dual power points. If these are occupied, then there are three dual power points located at the tables along the wall on the left-hand side of the food service counter and three dual power points below the bench seats at the tables along the back wall to the left of the service counter. If these are also occupied, then try the tables at the back of the café towards the right-hand side, where there are several dual power points located.

Check-in, Level One

There are a couple of cafes on this level. However, Costa Coffee doesn't offer seating, but the Hampton by Hilton lobby does.

Hampton by Hilton with Starbucks Coffee

The Starbucks which was here has recently removed into the Hampton by Hilton bar and business centre area. It is a little gem for charging your device in peace and quiet while you have a hot beverage or a small bite to eat. You can enjoy a Starbucks coffee, snacks or a light lunch here. There are several tables which host power points next to them, either on the wall or in a floor box.

Location: The entrance to this hotel is near the Easy Jet Check-in on level one. Just follow the signs to the right of the check-in desk. You will see a sign above the entrance to the corridor for the Hampton by Hilton.

Directions: Turn right at the Easy Jet Check-in area and walk towards the end of the hall. Walk straight ahead through the entrance and follow the passage to the left. Walk through the automatic double glass doors. The total distance is about 50 steps from the Easy Jet Check-in to the hotel reception.

Check-in, Level Two

There are a couple of eateries here which welcome business travellers who need to use or charge their devices.

Jamie's Coffee Lounge

Jamie's Coffee Lounge has apparently given some thought to the needs of their customers. There is a long workbench at the front of the café with several dual power points. Ideal if you wish to have a quick coffee and bite to eat while charging your device.

For more relaxing dining, head towards the tables on the edges surrounding the cafe. They all have double power points as well. Choose one which has a red bench seat, and you'll find the powerpoints below the seat itself.

If you want a quieter area to charge and dine, then head straight to the back of the café, just behind the service counter, towards the windows, you will find several seating arrangements with power points. The workbench at the window offers six sets of double power points while seating up to eighteen diners. Just opposite this are four tables, each seating up to four people, with a dual power point per table. On the far right hand side of the tables are two smaller tables, cosy enough for two diners, with power points. If you prefer a more open space for recharging your phone, then the tables on the left-hand side with leather bench style seats have power points as well.

Nicholas Culpeper

All the tables by the wall offer power points. When downstairs, choose a table which has a blue leather bench style seat, and you find a power point just under the seat. When upstairs select a table on the left, where the power point is just under the brown leather seat.

Departure Lounge, Lower Level

The Departure Lounge, Lower Level, often gets very crowded, and the number of restaurants on the lower level where you can charge your device is extremely limited. Your best bet is to head straight to the upper level which hosts the majority of the restaurants and cafes. There is one exception:

The Red Lion Pub

The Red Lion Pub now has two narrow benches on either side of the bar area. The first bench is on the right, which seats six people and has a power point on the far left. The second bench is on the left under the stairs, and also has a power point for charging your phone or mobile device.

Departure Lounge, Upper Level

Some eateries are savvier than others. They want people to come in, even if just to recharge their mobile devices while having a quick bite to eat. This way they might encourage you to linger longer over another drink or dessert. They also tend to be those with a variety of seating options, some clearly dedicated to the lone traveller with a laptop or two diners come together for a meeting of minds.

Wagamama, by way of example, is exceptional. It offers several options of seating with power points so customers can charge their devices while dining. If you don't take offence at the noisiness of the environment, or the wait to be seated during peak times, then this restaurant is the easiest place to charge your device while dining as it offers the most power points.

All the following restaurants have power points where you can charge your mobile devices.

Armadillo

There is a power point next to the island in the middle of the restaurant. You will need to request the table next to the power point.

Comptoir Libranais

Comptoir Libranais has two dual power points near the tables next to the wall on the left-hand side.

Garfunkel's

There are some tables with power points, but not at all tables. You are most likely to find power points at the tables which have a long couch bench.

Jamie's Bakery

Jamie's Bakery has three double power points at the stalls (one at each) next to the wall.

Jamie's Italian

Jamie's Italian restaurant has power points near some of the tables.

Pret A Manger

In the outside seating area, there is one power point on the column next to the workbench, and another on the other side of the column next to the table.

Starbucks

Situated between Jamie's Italian restaurant and the toilets, just near the middle lift. Lots of people work on their devices in the front of the café, but there are no power points here. Your best bet is to try at the back of the café, near the large window. There are many tables here with dual power points.

There are five tables on the left by the front window which have dual power points below the seating. There are also four tables on the right of the window, just behind the service counter, and each table has a dual power point. If you're still stuck, and these tables are all full, then there is also a power point near the accompaniment and cutlery stand.

Union Jacks Bar

Situated opposite Jamie's Italian restaurant & bakery at the far end of the upper level has power points at their tables closest to Yo! Sushi on the right as you walk in.

Wagamama

There are several areas where power points are provided for customers in this restaurant. The long bench at the far end of the restaurant offers eight sets of power point sockets. There are also two power points at the seats near the window. There are booths on the left at the far end, opposite the window, which also has power points at each booth. Finally, the bar has two sets of double power points on three sides, underneath the bar top.

Yo! Sushi

We missed the power points on our first visits as they aren't easy to spot. You'll find power points around the conveyer belt in the middle of the restaurant. Suitable for charging small devices, but not a great place for getting the laptop out.

Charge while you work

There are several dedicated working places where you can charge your devices while you work. They range from workbenches to full business services centres in the airport.

Check-in, Level One

Charging phone/workbench

As you walk into the check-in hall from the car park or shuttle, you will find a work desk on the right-hand side, opposite the escalators, just past the Bureau de Change. There are five dual power points along with work desk for travellers to recharge their phone.

Internet surf boxes.

The internet surf boxes are located on the left-hand side of the escalators as you walk into level one from the shuttle and car park. There are two spare power points here.

Hampton by Hilton Business Centre

Hampton by Hilton offers a casual business centre for hotel and bar guests. There is an L-shaped workbench which seats twelve people, which has four dual power points on either side. When we visited, there were several business travellers working here.

There is also an open room, apparently set up for meetings, which has six power points, along with the use of other business facilities. Alternatively, some of the tables in the restaurant area are also near power points.

Location: The entrance to this hotel is near the Easy Jet Check-in on level one. Just follow the signs to the right of the check-in desk. You will see a sign above the entrance to the corridor for the Hampton by Hilton.

Directions: Turn right at the Easy Jet Check-in area and walk towards the end of the hall. Walk straight ahead through the entrance and follow the passage to the left. Walk through the automatic double glass doors. The total distance is about 50 steps from the Easy Jet Check-in to the hotel reception.

Check-in, Level Two
Internet surf boxes.
The internet surf boxes are located opposite the Emirates check-in counter. There are four power points next to the right-hand-side surf box.

Charge while you relax

Lounges are another option to charge your phone, and you can relax or catch up on emails at the same time. There are several to choose from, and if you have membership access or flying with the operator (subject to terms and conditions), then there will be no charge to visit and use the power sockets to recharge your devices. Otherwise, you can pre-book your attendance online which is usually less expensive or register on the day.

Here is a quick summary of lounges where you can charge your devices.

No. 1 Lounge
There are plenty of power points to charge devices in this room. You will find these located throughout the main lounge on the bench alongside the window by the buffet, next to tables, and on the floor next to the swivel chairs in front of the window.

The library area also has a workbench with eight power points in front of the window located in the first section, and at the desk, in the middle of the room based in the second section, there are ten power points. You can also use guest computers provided by No. 1 Lounge while you wait for your laptop to charge. Reportedly good Wi-Fi and a quiet library area away from the hustle and bustle in the main part. Also, you can book a meeting room via No1Traveller.com website. The contact details are provided below.

Open: 4.00 am to 10.00 pm daily
Contact: 08442 64 64 40 or +44(0)2032838449 or email: enquiries@No1Traveller.com
Access: All travellers including groups and children, so it might not be the quietest lounge to charge your phone, particularly during peak holiday times.

Facilities: Plenty of power points located in the restaurant area at the tables, and at the desks around the library. Phone chargers are available upon request from reception staff.

Additional facilities: Dedicated workspace, computer terminals with internet, printing, and fax.

Cost: Lounge entry for adults is £30 if you book in advance or £37.50 on the door without booking. If your flight is delayed and you want to stay longer, then you can buy additional hours.

Free access: Dragon Pass, Diners Club, Institute of Directors, Lounge Club, Priority Pass,

Location: On the lower level of the Departure Lounge, after security, on route to gates 45 -55 and 101 -113.

Directions: Once through security into the main Departure Lounge, turn left and follow the signs to the 'Airport Lounges.' These are situated just past the London News Company along the hallway towards gates 45 – 55 and 101 – 113. Turn right once you walk into the corridor from the Departure Lounge, and right again. Pass through the double glass doors; the No1 lounge is straight ahead.

Aspire Lounge

The Aspire Lounge provides charging facilities for laptops, iPads and of course phones. On the left-hand side, as you enter the door, there is the quiet zone. There are large black leather chairs with a side table and power points. There are also numerous power points next to tables around the main lounge dining area.   The Aspire Lounge also offers Wi-Fi and refreshments included in the registration price, with some healthier menu items throughout the day.

Open: Open hours are from 4.00 am to 10.00 pm, with a slight seasonal variation.

Facilities: Power points are located in the quiet area where there are work tables and at the tables. This lounge provides European and UK power sockets for guests.

Access: Welcomes anyone who is travelling. Free entry to those who are a member of the Institute of Directors, Priority Pass, Aspire Platinum membership, Vueling airline passengers, Diners Club and DragonPass cardholders.

Cost: The Aspire Lounge is comparatively less expensive than some at a minimum of £17.99 per person when booking online.   You can book through **http://www.executivelounges.com/lounges/gatwick-north-aspire-airport-lounge**

Location: First floor of the Departure Lounge in the Lounge Pavilion.

Directions: Turn left after security and follow the signs to the 'Airport Lounges'. Head towards gates 45 – 55 and 101 – 113, as you pass London News Company into the main hallway to the gates, you will see a corridor on your right. Go through the double glass doors and take the lift to the first floor. The lounge is located on the right-hand side.

Emirates Lounge

If you are flying first or business class on an Emirates flight out of the North Terminal, or a Skywards Gold or Platinum member, then you can pop into the Emirates lounge to recharge your devices.

Emirates was recently renovated to include a business centre with new facilities, with computers, laptop workstations, free broadband and wireless LAN access. In addition to power points, guests also receive complimentary hot and cold gourmet menu items. Travel reviewers have highly rated this lounge.

Access for: Emirates First Class and Business Class travellers or as an Emirates Skywards Platinum or Gold member departing on an Emirates flight. One guest is allowed if travelling on the same flight.
Opening hours: First departure to the last departure.
Location: First floor of the Departure Lounge.
Directions: Head towards gate 101 – 113, as you pass London News Company, you will see a corridor on your right. Go through the double glass doors and take the lift to the first floor. The lounge in located on the left-hand side.

My Lounge

My Lounge is open to all travellers, which clearly caters to families as well as business travellers and holidaymakers. Consequently, it can get somewhat crowded at holiday times. There are plenty of device charging points. The bench in front of the window on the left of the room has five power points dedicated to those with a mobile device. There are also power points on the columns in the middle of the room and on the far walls near the seats, along with a dual power point in both the TV room and the games room. Finally, there is a power point next to the computer terminals so you can charge and work at the same time.

Opening hours: 6.00 am to 8.00 pm
Facilities: Bench with power-points.
Additional facilities: Two computer terminals with printing via reception.
Cost: £18 per adult when booked online, and £24 when entry is purchased on the door. If your flight is delayed and you want to stay longer, then you can buy additional hours.

Free access: Institute of Directors, Lounge Club, Lounge Pass, Priority Pass, Diners Club

Location: Located in the Departure Lounge, lower level. After security follow the signs for the airport lounges and My Lounge. My Lounge is situated on the left as you enter the Lounge Pavilion.

Directions: Head towards gates 45 – 55 and 101 – 113, as you pass London News Company into the main corridor to the gates, you will see a hallway on your right. Go through the double glass doors. The lounge in located on the left-hand side as you enter the Lounge Pavilion, just before the lifts.

Where you can find a charger

It happens to the most frequent business traveller from time to time. The mad rush to leave the office or an earlier than usual start can easily result in leaving the phone or laptop charger behind. No need to despair, we have checked out Gatwick Airport's North Terminal and here are some quick solutions.

Dixons Travel

Located in the Departure Lounge, lower level, Dixons Travel have reportedly announced they will charge devices at airports. And it is free of charge!

Retailers who sell charge packs at Gatwick Airport

Running short of time and need to charge while waiting to board? The following retailers stock charge packs which you can purchase as soon as you get to Gatwick. In some cases, you can order the evening before and collect en route.

Here a quick list of charges we found at the time of review. All prices were recorded during our review. Please note that stock changes regularly and some stores may offer reduced prices to shift stock before promoting a new range.

Boots the Chemist

Boots the Chemist offer several phone charging units. You will find Boots situated in Arrivals on the ground floor, next to M & S Simply Food, and after security in the Departure Lounge on the lower level. There are two stores in the Departure Lounge.

The first is just as you come through security, on the left-hand side of the Departure Lounge. A larger Boots is at the end of the Departure Lounge, between Dixons Travel and WHSmith.

You can order online the day before and collect when you reach the airport.

Opening in Arrivals: 24 hours
Opening in Departure Lounge: 4.00 am to 8.30 pm
Telephone: 01293 569606
Website: www.boots.com

Chargers include:

Juice Micro-USB Charger £9.99. This micro USB mains charger is sturdy, compact and useful when travelling and near a UK power point.
Juice Tube Portable Charger £12.99 A rubber coated portable power bank. The charger fits easily into your pocket or bag. Provides 2,200 mAh worth of power while on the go, which is sufficient to charge an iPhone 6, Samsung S6 or mobile fully.
Juice Power Station £29.99 Extra high capacity portable power bank. Designed to charge two devices at once. Can fully charge an iPad Air or tablet at high speeds.
Juice Squash XL Power Bank £24.99 One full Juice Squash XL charge provides two charges for the Samsung S6 and over three charges of the Apple iPhone 6.
Pebble Powerpack £10.00 1800 mAh Suitable for smartphone charger and iPhone charger.
two phones simultaneously.

Case Luggage

The case is on the lower level of the Departure Lounge, at the far right-hand side from World Duty Free exit, between Accessorize and Harrods on the right. They have travel accessory items on the stand at the front of the store.

You can also pre-order via their website. A reserve and collect service is available from Case Luggage. Simply reserve the items online and then collect as you pass through the Gatwick Airport's North Terminal. We've listed items available on their website below and provided a link for you to click on to.

Opening hours: November to March 4.00 am to 8.30 pm; April to October 4.00 am to 10.00 pm
Telephone: 0129 356 9264 Email: gatwicknorth@caseluggage.co.uk

Website: http://www.caseluggage.com
Email: gatwicknorth@caseluggage.co.uk

Chargers include:

Go Travel Mobile Charger £16.66 Available from the stand outside the store. Compatible with most smartphones, mobiles & small USB devices. Available in the store.

Tumi Portable Battery Bank Swivel £85.00 2,600 mAh Rechargeable lithium battery provides extra charge for Apple iPhone or iPod. Includes a 9" micro-USB cable. 2 years guarantee. Available online.

Dixons Travel

Dixons Travel like Boots the Chemist also has two stores on the lower level of the Departure Lounge. The first is smaller, opposite the exit from security. The other is larger and located between Boots and Jo Malone on the right-hand side as you walk down to the departure gates 45 – 55 and 101 – 113.

You can pre-order items from Dixons Travel direct by phoning the Gatwick North Terminal and asking them to reserve the item for you to collect. Unfortunately, you won't be able to order any items on-line.

Opening hours: 4.00 am – 8.30 pm daily
Telephone: 01293 569737

They have several brands of portable battery chargers, ranging in capacity and price. Here is what they had in stock at the time of review.

Chargers include:

Go Travel Mobile Charger £14.99 Available from the stand outside the store. Compatible with most smartphones, mobiles & small USB devices.

Belkin 2000 mAh £14.99 Portable USB Rechargeable Battery Pack for Apple iPhone, iPod, Samsung, smartphones and MP3 Players. Designed for travellers and commuters and is equipped with a single USB port. Comes fully charged.

Belkin 4000 mAh £17.99 Portable Dual USB Rechargeable Battery Pack for Apple iPhone, iPad, iPod, Samsung Galaxy and Universal Smartphones/Tablets. Suitable for travellers and commuters, and is equipped with two USB ports to let you charge up two devices simultaneously.

Belkin 5000 £24.99 Portable in a compact, thin design. Chargers smartphone up to 1.5 times, providing an additional 19 hours of call time or 11 hours of web browsing.

Includes heat sensors, voltage and circuitry so the external battery will not overheat. 2.4 total output to fast-charge a device and a 2.0A total input.

Belkin 15000 mAh £49.95 Lightweight (340 g) power bank which fits comfortably into a pocket or bag. Recharges a smartphone up to 5 times. Comprises two universal USB A ports to deliver 3.4 A of total power quickly and safely. Can also charge smartwatches, fitness bands, headphones and speakers. 5 V 2.0 amp input to recharge quickly.

Mophie Powerstation Mini £27.95 3,000 mAh battery is equalling up to 12 hours of extra battery. Features an integrated power indication button to show current battery life and charging status.

Mophie Powerstation 6000 £44.95 Sufficient charge for two additional charges on your smartphone. Two USB ports. Priority Charging enables pass-through charging while connected to a power source. Your device charges first and then the Powerstation will recharge itself.

Mophie Powerstation Plus mini £59.95 4,000 mAh battery is equalling up to 12 hours of extra battery. Charge a variety of Apple and Micro USB devices using a built-in switch-tip cable. Features an integrated power indication button to show current battery life and charging status.

Mophie Powerstation plus 6,000 £69.95 Includes enough battery to recharge a smartphone up to two times. The 6,000 mAh battery delivers up to an additional 24 hours of charge.

Mophie Powerstation XL £69.95 10,000 mAh. The universal batty provides three additional charges on your smartphone. Two USN ports to allow multiple devices being charged at the same time.

Mophie Charge Force £89.95 10,000 mAh Look no cables! This is a wireless charge. Simply place the juice pack wireless or QI enabled smartphone on top and push a button to start wireless charging. This 10,000 mAh battery provides a smartphone up to 48 hours of extra battery time. There is also an extra USB port to charge a second device at the same time.

Mophie Powerstation Plus XL £99.95 12,000 mAh Capable of charging two tablets simultaneously.

Mophie Powerstation XXL £89.95 20,000 Provides up to 100 hours extra battery and can power up to three devices at once including power-hungry tablets.

Morphie Powerstation USB C 10000 £79.95 15 W fast charge with speeds up to £A to charge the latest C smartphone and tablets at maximum speeds. Can charge two devices simultaneously. Priority charging when connected to power source, so your device charges first, then the PowerStation battery recharges itself.

Morphie Powerstation USB C XXL 19500 £119.00 19,500 mAh High capacity battery to provide laptops with 14 hours of extra battery life. Fast charge USB -CPD input/output to send up to 30W fast-charging speeds to you USB-C laptop or other devices. Additional high-output USB A port to charge a second device simultaneously. Priority charging is allowing your other devices to charge first then to charge itself.

Excess Baggage Company

As soon as you enter the Check-in Hall, Level One, from the shuttle or car park, you will find the Excess Baggage Company on your left. They have a small selection of handy items, including Go Travel mobile phone power bank.

Location: Check-in Hall, Level One, right by the main entrance from the shuttle, just opposite London News Company, next to Costa Coffee.
Opening hours: 5.00 am to 10.00 pm
Telephone: +44 (0) 1293 734 888 or **email:** gatwick@left-baggage.co.uk
Website: www.left-baggage.co.uk

Chargers include:

Go Travel Mobile Charge 4000 mAp £24.95. Ideal for mobiles and tablets. Offers 1 ½ hours of charge. Automatic device detection. LED power level indicator.

London News Company and WHSmith

London News Company and WHSmith are located on Check-in, Level One; Arrivals on the ground floor; Check-in, Level Two, and in the Departure Lounge on the Lower Level. They have wall chargers, USB cables and ready to charge power packs to choose.

When in the Departure Lounge, head down to the larger of the three stores (WHSmith) at the far end. You'll find several battery charging units in the middle aisle.

Alternatively, you can order online and collect from the store within 2 – 3 days.

Locations: Check-in Level One, Arrivals Ground Floor, Check-in Level Two, Departure Lounge Lower Level
Opening hours: Arrivals 24 hours; After security 4.00 am to 8.30 pm
Telephone: 01293568664 and 01293 569896
Website: www.whsmith.co.uk

Available on-line

Kit Charge/Data Cable £9.99 This is suitable for charging iPod, iPhone, and iPad devices. Simply use this cable with a USB mains or in-car charger or connect to a MAC, PC or laptop to charge your other devices and transfer data.

Juice Apple Lightning Compatible Mains Charger £12.99 This charger is compact and designed to keep Apple electronic devices charged. Made for iPod and iPhone devices.

Primo PowerBank 4400 Portable Charger £13.49

Primo PowerBank 8800 Portable Charger £19.29

Available in store when we visited

SKRoss Reload £24.99 Pre-charged and ready for use.
Recharge 3,400 mAh £16.95 single USB
Recharge 4,,000 £29.95
Recharge 6,000 mAh £24.95 single USB
Recharge 7,800 mAh £29.95 double USB
Recharge 12,000 mAh £59.95 double USB
Recharge 13,600 mAh £49.95 dual USB
Recharge 20,000 mAh £49.95 dual USB
Recharge Power on the Go 4,000 mAh £29.95
Belkin 2,000 mAh £17.99
Belkin 4,000 mAh £20.00
Belkin 6,600 mAh £30.00 2USB

World Duty Free Shop

You can either shop in the World Duty Free when you come through Arrivals or in the Departure Lounge. You will find the World Duty Free shop located on the lower level of the Departure Lounge on the left-hand side of the lounge, just before you reach the London News Company, and on the right-hand side next to Accessorise. If you are short of time, you can pre-order online, email or telephone ahead to reserve items. Here is what they had in stock at the time of review.

Opening hours: Open 24 hours or **email:** customerservices.uk@wdfg.com
Telephone: 01293 507 301 for the Departure Lounge and 01293 505 851 for Arrivals

Portable battery charges available include:

GroovE Power Stick £16.65 Battery charge for smartphone 2200, comes pre-charged. Charging time 1.5 to 2 hours. Portable solar battery charges smartphones, tablets, e-readers, GPS, cameras. Also, includes a travel pouch and has an auto cut-off safety. Good reviews.

GroovE 5200 mAh £24.59 Capacity charges iPhones/smartphones up to 3 times. Portable charger for smartphones, tablets, e-readers, GPS and cameras. Pre-charged and ready to use. Super-fast output through the USB port.

GroovE Solar Charge 3600, £33.30 Comes pre-charged. Charging time 1.5 to 2 hours. Portable solar battery charges smartphones, tablets, e-readers, GPS and cameras. Also, includes a travel pouch and has an auto cut-off for safety. Good reviews.

Chapter 8: Working Productively

The art of working productively

Travelling regularly on business isn't the 'perk' as colleagues often perceive it to be. It is a responsibility and requires a return to the company to justify the time and cost. Predictably, business relationships with clients benefit from face to face meetings as a means of increasing revenue for the enterprise. According to an Oxford Economics survey, if we didn't make those long-distance meetings, we would lose 25% of our current customers and 28% of potential revenue to competitors. The Oxford Economics survey also proposed that the conversion rate of prospective customers doubles with a face to face visit and customer meetings, which accounts for one-third of business travel, and can generate a return of at least four times the investment.

So much of our business travel outcome depends on our ability to meet with clients or suppliers as well briefed, well prepared and productive representatives. As a general rule of thumb, we appoint the most productive workers to represent the company on a long-distance trip. But it's not easy being productive when travelling on business.

There are so many factors to take into account which impacts on our work time and productivity en route. In addition to the usual office-based demands which require meeting deadlines and working well with colleagues, there are further strains when we travel, such as pre-travel arrangements, anonymity, family commitments and work-life balance difficulties.

Sleep deprivation, jet-lag and travel fatigue also impact our ability to work productively, reducing our cognitive performance, impairing concentration and working memory, resulting in an attention deficit and disrupting memory recall. The average amount of sleep the night before a trip is 5 hours, usually the worst in the seven-day period before travel. With every 1 ½ hours of lost sleep, alertness declines by a third. Which effectively means you're travelling on business in a sleep deficit and only two thirds fully functional.

It's often apparent that frequent travellers feel the strain of travelling more than colleagues who remain within an office-based environment. According to research commissioned by the Institute of Travel and Meetings (ITM), frequent travellers record psychological well-being scores substantially below the norm. As mental health scores decline, so does productivity. The ITM research confirmed frequent travellers report lower productivity associated with poor wellbeing scores, and estimated frequent flyers over time will lose 9% productivity, gradually scoring in the lowest 40% of performers for wellbeing at work.

Notably, there is also a significant minority (15%) of frequent travellers who also report feeling burnt out. They convey how travel now causes them to be less effective during and right after their trip. Consequently, they become less satisfied with the outcome of their trips and are less likely to travel going forward. Even travellers who aren't feeling worn out by their frequent business trips feel there is extra stress before they even start out.

Travel stress has an enormous impact on our ability to think and work productivity. While we can attempt to manage stressful incidences and their implications, the most effective mechanism to reducing stress is to remove the stressors. Removing a business trip altogether is probably not the right course of action for companies who want to pursue relationships with their clients and suppliers and increase their revenue. However, there are many other stressors which we can remove or at least reduce their impact when travelling on business.

A recent survey reported in the Harvard Business review revealed among the worse stress factors is the inability to work when travelling. In particular, difficulty in using a laptop, lack of internet access, not being able to charge devices, and not being able to find a space to work all constitute a loss of working time. So, when our team members visit airports, they report back information on the working areas, along with connectivity and charge points for mobile devices.

By researching the best places to use a laptop, preferably near a power point socket with good internet access, we aim to support business travellers by removing the strain of not being able to work en route.

This chapter provides information on where and how to work productivity. We have researched spaces available for business travellers at Gatwick's North Terminal and listed suitable workspaces either in 'relaxed working areas' or 'dedicated working spaces' below. We have also located suitable places to hold business meetings in and nearby the airport. These are listed below the top tips on how to work productivity in 'relaxed meeting areas' or 'dedicated meeting spaces'.

Top tips for productive working

Travelling on business may be a welcome break from the office and your typical work routine, but it is also a break from accessible resources and all your other regimes as well, such as sleeping, exercising and eating. By changing your routine and work environment, you automatically change your ability to work efficiently. Attempting to work when travelling can leave you feeling emotionally and physically drained if the environment, equipment or you are not entirely up to the task.

Getting prepared for your business trip before starting out is key to a productive trip. Follow our top tips below to help start your journey off right.

1. Secure sufficient preparation time

Given that the average business traveller finds the day before a trip adds extra stress and the average sleep is only five hours the night before, then having a 'work from home' day to prepare could be a more efficient way to start a business trip than going into the office the day before.

Time can be saved by not travelling to and from the office, and this 'extra' time can be used to focus on preparation and 'banking' your sleep hours before commencing a business trip. As a result, you will find you will be more alert and better able to problem solve, decision making will be less risky, and recovery from jet lag and travel fatigue will be much quicker, particularly if you're not starting your travels in a sleep deficit.

So, if you haven't arranged a work from home day previously, then it might be time to consider how much more you could achieve before your trip if you did request such before securing your next business travel.

2. Download large documents beforehand

Connectivity is a huge issue for many business travellers, especially if airport internet access is slow, patchy or difficult to access. You never know what you're getting until you get there. So, prepare to work off-line when travelling. Make sure you download all the necessary information and supporting material beforehand, so you don't have to rely on patchy or slow Wi-Fi en route. It is far more productive to spend your time focusing on completing projects offline rather than wasting time to download additional documents that you may or may not eventually have a chance to work on during the trip.

3. Make the best use of resources available

Each airport we visit offers different facilities. There is a lack of consistency in approach for business executives. Some airports are brilliant at aligning their services to the needs of their travellers, while others are not. Generally speaking, more business-centric services come with a high volume of passengers, newly built airports or airports which have just been through a major renovation. This aside, there are several standard features, such as public Wi-Fi, power points to charge phones and private lounges for business people to use. The trick is to know what is available before commencing your journey.

Most (62%) business people want to access their emails straight away to avoid a backlog when they return to the office. So, if the airport's free Wi-Fi is reportedly patchy, then make sure you have a backup option or know how to obtain fast, more reliable Wi-Fi once you get there. You may even decide to arrange or pre-purchase backup Wi-Fi access before you depart on your journey. This way you can choose to either access the Wi-Fi available at the airport or access a more private connection.

If there are no dedicated working spaces in the airport departure lounge, which often there are not, then knowing which restaurants have a power supply near a table can be difficult, if not near impossible, to ascertain in advance. This is why we have undertaken this research for you. In general, booking an airline which has, or is affiliated with, a dedicated lounge, or even becoming a member of an international airport lounge club can work to your advantage if you are a frequent traveller.

Similarly, if you need to print something out, then knowing where you can do this can be quite a task when in a hurry. Not all airports offer printing post security, but some private lounges do have a dedicated printer or a receptionist who will kindly print or photocopy documents for you.

4. Take items which prevent strain

If it's likely you'll be working on your laptop in the airport or aeroplane, then make sure you pack some devices with you to help reduce the strain. When you are based in the office, your workspace should be ergonomically designed to prevent muscle tension, backache, neck strain and poor posture. Studies show that bending over your laptop will place extra pressure on your spine, causing muscular tension in the short term, which could lead to early degeneration.

Business travellers who often end up hunched over their laptop en route regularly feel the effects of travel fatigue as a result of muscle tension, poor posture and neck strain from poorer working practices. Consequently, this means they won't be working for long without a decline in physical health and mental performance.

Using a separate keyboard, for example, will enable you to type in a more relaxed position. It will also allow you to place your screen at eye level (albeit on books or bags) to reduce neck strain from looking downwards. Laptop stands for travelling are also available on the market, so you can adjust the height and angle of your laptop while in the plane or a terminal cafe.

Using an external mouse will also help to reduce muscle tension as your hand is not in an unnatural position when scrolling or clicking. It seems too simplistic to mention, but the number of business travellers we see who haven't paid adequate attention to their posture is staggering.

Does it improve performance? Yes, it does as it not only means you can work easier, without physical strain but also your body is telling your mind you are in charge, you're motivated and ready to work.

5. Have a downtime action plan

No, it's not an oxymoron! Having options for when it's less feasible to undertake highly cognitive work-based assignments enables you to carry out other tasks or activities en route more smoothly. These might include simple preparatory tasks or take time out to relax such as checking out a new cuisine or listening to relaxing music.

Some business travellers use this time to learn a new language via audiobook or podcast as part of their professional development. Airport timings are usually short, including waiting in line to check in, walks to the departure gates and standing around to board. While it's not feasible to get your laptop out when you're queuing, it is possible to listen to a podcast or an audiobook to learn something new.

Some business travellers include preparation tasks on their downtime list, such as confirming appointments, notifying colleagues of travel arrangements or practising their elevator speech. These are usually low-level tasks and can also be easily added to your travel downtime action plan.

Don't forget to include on your list the possibility of keeping fit. Scheduling in time to keep fit while travelling gives you the option of having more time to do more cognitively demanding tasks upon arrival. It also helps to increase your circulation and relaxes your mind, and by doing so, it aids your performance during work-related tasks later in the day.

6. Choose your workspace wisely

Everyone works differently. Some people prefer a quiet space without distraction while others desire white noise around them. There are plenty of places at Gatwick Airport's North Terminal where you can work. We've listed below the more appropriate ones we found during our visits.

Take care you choose the workspace, if you can, which suits the type of work you wish to undertake. Some cafes may be useful for quick emails or reading over your schedule. While other locations, due to lower footfall, might lend themselves better to documents demanding greater concentration or confidentiality. We've put places which are more suited to the latter under 'dedicated working spaces' and listed the cafes and restaurants under 'relaxed working areas'.

Where to find a place to work

Relaxed Working Spaces

There are many reasons why an informal working area can be worthwhile considering. Given that many travellers are travelling alone, and there is a degree of anonymity, then a little white noise and the company of others, albeit strangers, might just be what some travellers need. If the data you're working on requires greater concentration or is of a confidential nature, then you might prefer some of the other more private options we have listed after this section.

However, if you're not deep in thought, but need a few minutes over a refreshing drink or snack, and want to feel the presence of others, then you might consider these options below. We have visited them several times to check out their suitability as a relaxed, informal working space and have added some notes next to the description.

Arrivals, Ground Floor

Costa Coffee Cafe

If you have just arrived and have time before your meeting or travel arrangement, then Costa Coffee is your only choice in the Arrivals Hall. Fortunately, it has a quiet area at the back on the right which has lower footfall than the tables at the front. Despite the busy nature of the Arrivals Hall at the front of the café, this is an area where you can work without a lot of distraction. There are several tables which have power points or nearby. Failing this, there are also tables at the front of the café to the left which also have power points.

If you're not bothered by large crowds, then the front of Costa Coffee Café now has two workbenches. There is sufficient room for a mobile device, and if you're short of time while waiting for a colleague to arrive, then this provides an opportunity to check your emails with a hot beverage to hand.

Check-in, Level One

Internet zone

There are public internet terminals located on the left-hand side of the Check-in area. As you walk into the terminal, walk straight ahead towards the Easy Jet Check-in. On the left, just past the escalator are four computer terminals. You can log on to the web here or use the computer and printer to print out documents. While there isn't sufficient space to write, it is useful to pick up and respond to last minute emails without needing a device.

Hampton by the Hilton incorporating Starbucks

If you want a little gem, then this is it. It isn't very busy during non-peak hours, and there are several tables with power points. In the middle of the room, there is also a workbench which seats twelve.

As it is out of the central check-in area not many people know about it, which explains why it is populated mainly by business travellers during peak hours. It is quiet and has a low footfall. There is Starbucks Coffee and snacks, and a short menu. If it is a quick bite and a hot beverage you desire while you work, then this is a great place to frequent. There is one drawback working here; the Gatwick Free Wi-Fi was out of range when we visited.

Location: The entrance to this hotel is right near the Easy Jet Check-in on level one. Just follow the signs to the right of the check-in desk. You will see a sign above the entrance to the corridor for the Hampton by Hilton.

Directions: Turn right at the Easy Jet Check-in area and walk towards the end of the hall. Walk straight ahead through the entrance and follow the passage to the left. Walk through the automatic double glass doors. The total distance is about 50 steps from the Easy Jet Check-in to the hotel reception.

Check-in, Level Two

Computer terminals/internet zone

Similar to the Check-in area on level one, this level also offers four computer terminals with a printer. There isn't sufficient space to work on several documents, but it is adequate if you wish to access the internet and print. Cost is 10 p per minute for the internet and £1 per page to print. You'll find it located just opposite the Emirates Check-in just before zone C.

Jamie's Coffee Lounge

At first sight, this looks busy and unsuitable for a workspace. However, if you stroll around to the back of the service counter, you will find a workbench at the front window, along with some tables to the side and back of the service area. The workbench has three sections, each with six seats and dual power points for devices per section. The footfall is low and is relatively peaceful considering the high volume of traffic at the front of the restaurant.

Similar to other cafes, Jamie's Coffee Lounge has also now added a workbench at the front of the restaurant which seats ten people. So, if the crowds don't bother you, then this is another option. There is sufficient room for using mobile devices and three double power points. However, the food service counter is right behind you, so it can get somewhat noisy.

Nicholas Culpeper Restaurant

At the Nicholas Culpeper, the best option is upstairs. It is much quieter than downstairs. If you require a power point for your device while you work, then choose the tables running down the left-hand side. Otherwise, the booth tables on the right-hand side in front of the windows are also a useful spot to work. When we visited the day before schools breaking out, we found Nicholas Culpeper upstairs to be a sanctuary from the rest of the airport bustle.

Departure Lounge, Lower Level
Weatherspoon's Red Lion Pub
The Red Lion Pub is a bustling, popular eatery and pub. If you are lucky, you'll find a space in the quiet area to the left, just inside the dining area next to the windows.

There are also two workbenches. The first is on the right-hand side, against the wall and accommodates up to six people. The second is on the left-hand side of the entrance, just underneath the stairs up to the upper level. Power points are in short supply with only one double power points per workbench. Although for both workbenches you will have your back to the other guests, the noise levels here can be quite high.

Departure Lounge, Upper Level
Comptoir Libanais Restaurant
Comptoir Libanais offers a more peaceful space than many of the other restaurants on the upper level. Tables near the window at the far end of the restaurant are much quieter as they are away from the main thoroughfare. They also have power points nearby.

EAT Cafe
Eat Café is busy most of the time. There is a workbench facing into the main thoroughfare where you can rest your laptop and have a bite to eat. Unless you are superb at blocking the background noise and distractions out, this would only be suitable for work that doesn't require heavy concentration.

Jamies Bakery
Jamie's Bakery can be very busy. When it is not, which isn't very often, there is a workbench in the middle and three high tables next to the wall. The high tables have a dual power point and seat up to four. A perfect place to casually check emails.

Shake-A-Hula
Shake-A-Hula has a workbench with power-points where you can fit a laptop on both sides. However, it is noisy with lots of distractions, so casual working at best.

Starbucks Coffee House
We found several people busy at work here each time we visited. While the footfall is high at the front of the cafe, it is quieter than the other cafes on the upper level.

There are several tables and a workbench at the front of the café. Unfortunately, there are no power points for you to plug your laptop in.

However, there are several quieter spots near the window at the back of the cafe. Directly, in front of the window, there is a workbench which is large enough to fit your laptop on. Although the view isn't great, and there is a level of noise, you will have your back to the rest of the cafe.

Also, on the right, behind the service counter, there are four tables, each with a dual power point. It is much quieter here and probably one of the best informal, relaxed working areas on the upper floor. If these are full, then the tables on the left in front of the window are also an option. Although not as quiet as those on the right, they do also offer dual power points.

Wagamama Restaurant

At the far end of the room, there is a bench alongside the wall where you can sit, very anti-socially, with your back to the other diners. Similarly, there is a bench next to the window where you can get a glimpse of the runway, but it's hard to find a seat during peak times, which is near all the time. Also, be warned there is a constant hum of air-conditioning from the restaurant's units.

Union Jack Bar

Again, this seemed to be a haven for some people working on their laptops. Dual power points are located underneath two of the tables along the wall next to Yo! Sushi. However, these tables appear to be more suitable for diners than workers due to the low height of the tables.

There are also several high bench tables which are tall enough to stand at and type. But if it's a peaceful duration you are after, then seek out the long counter at the exit to the right. You will be facing the wall if you wish to work on your laptop, but it is quieter than the above options.

Dedicated public working spaces

If you require a more dedicated spot where you can concentrate more efficiently, but still prefer to have the company of others around as a 'white noise' then you might prefer the following public dedicated workspaces. Power points are also available for all options below if you wish to charge your mobile devices at the same time.

Check-in, Level One

As you enter the Check-in area on level one, you will notice a working bench on the right-hand side of the escalators, just past the Bureau de Change. There are ten spaces, all with access to an electrical socket for your laptop or device. There is a lot of foot fall here. However, you are sitting with your back to the activities taking place.

Departure Lounge, Lower Level

No. 1 Lounge

The quietest dedicated lounge space for working is the library area in the No. 1 Lounge. As you enter the room, you will see the buffet, bar and bistro on the left. Straight ahead are tables for diners, and to the right is a slightly dimmer television seating area. You might find a spot here during non-peak times. If you turn right when entering the bar area and proceed down the steps, you'll enter the library. The library is a quiet room, designated for working. You will find it split into two sections. The first section has a working bench along the window with a superb view of the runway and several power points. In the second area, there is a larger desk in the middle of the room with many power sockets where you can also work in peace and quiet. There is also a meeting room which seats eight, where you can request to work privately if it is not already booked.

There are also two computers near the reception area which are linked to the internet. If you require anything printed, then you simply send it to the front desk, and they will print it out for you.

Open: 4.00 am to 10.00 pm
Access: All travellers including groups and children.
Facilities: Dedicated workspace, computer terminals with internet, printing and fax.
Cost: Lounge entry for adults is £30 if you book in advance or £37.50 on the door without booking. If your flight is delayed and you want to stay longer, then you can buy additional hours.
Free access: Dragon Pass, Diners Club, Institute of Directors, Lounge Club, Priority Pass, Dining Club, Caxton FX.
Location: On the lower level of the Departure Lounge, after security, near gates 101 - 113.

Directions: Head towards gate 101 – 113, just past the London News Company, you will see a hallway on your right. Turn right and go through the double glass doors. No.1 Lounge is directly ahead, situated at the end.

Aspire Lounge

The Aspire Lounge has a quiet work area away from the main buffet dining zone. It is located to the left of the main entrance. There is a mix of seats with tables for you to choose from and sufficient power points for you to plug your laptop in.

Open: Open hours are from 4.00 am to 10.00 pm, with a slight seasonal variation.

Facilities: Soft, comfortable leather seats. There are no dedicated printing facilities for guests; however, if you ask the reception team, they may photocopy a couple of pages for you.

Access: Welcomes anyone who is travelling.

Cost: Lounge entry for adults is from £17.99 if you book in advance or £35 on the door without booking. If your flight is delayed and you want to stay longer, then you can buy additional hours.

Free access: Priority Pass, Diners Club, Institute of Directors, Aspire Platinum membership, Vueling Airline passengers and Dragon Pass cardholders.

Location: First floor of the Departure Lounge.

Directions: Head towards gate 101 – 113, as you pass the London News Company, you will see a hallway on your right. Turn right down the corridor, go through the double glass doors and take the lift on the left to the first floor. The lounge is located on the right-hand side.

My Lounge

While it may be a less formal lounge than the other lounges, it offers two computer terminals, printing, a large table and bench area for working. There is also a den room at the far end which offers more peace and privacy. There are plenty of power points for your laptop on the workbench.

Opening hours: 6.00 am to 8.00 pm

Facilities: Two computer terminals.

Cost: Lounge entry for adults is £18 if you book in advance or £24 on the door without booking. If your flight is delayed and you want to stay longer, then you can buy additional hours.

Free access: Institute of Directors, Lounge Club, Lounge Pass, Priority Pass, Diners Club

Location: Departure Lounge, lower level.

Directions: Head towards gate 101 – 113, as you pass London News Company, you will see a corridor on your right. Turn right and proceed down the hallway and go through the double glass doors. The lounge is located on the left-hand side just before the lifts.

Dedicated working places directly connected to Gatwick North Terminal

There are several places you can work which are accessible to Gatwick Airport by foot. The Hampton by Hilton reportedly allows non-residential guests to access their business facilities, while the Regus Business Centre poses a modest charge. If you are a guest at the Sofitel Hotel directly connected to the airport, then you can also enjoy complimentary facilities.

Hampton by Hilton

Described as an oasis at the North Terminal by one business reviewer, the Hampton by Hilton offers business services for all business travellers. Other reviewers have also noted the convenience being right next to the terminal with only a two-minute walk from check-in, and their car park if you are on an overnight business trip. Complete with everything you need from printing to complimentary computer terminals, you can conduct your business in their business centre without business lounge entrance prices. We found the reception to be very approachable and willing to help even though we weren't a hotel guest. However, we were unable to utilise the business facilities fully. Our advice is to ask at reception, and they can direct you from there.

Access: To hotel guests and business travellers.
Facilities: Business centre with complimentary printing service, express mail, fax photocopying services, computers, printer, fax, free Wi-Fi.
Additional services: Starbucks Coffee, lunch menu and car park.
Location: The entrance to this hotel is right near the Easy Jet Check-in on level one. Just follow the signs to the right of the check-in desk. You will see a sign above the entrance to the corridor for the Hampton by Hilton.
Directions: Turn right at the Easy Jet Check-in area and walk towards the end of the hall. Walk straight ahead through the entrance and follow the passage to the left. Walk through the automatic double glass doors. The total distance is about 50 steps from the Easy Jet Check-in to the hotel reception.

Regus Business Centre at the South Terminal

Regus Express Business Centre and Lounge at the South Terminal is only three minutes by direct airport shuttle. You can catch the shuttle on level one near the train station. Once at the South Terminal, you will find a workplace dedicated to those travelling on business. They operate a 'drop in' service during weekdays.

For business travellers, it offers a productive work environment with excellent facilities in a distraction-free environment.

Open: 6.00 am to 6.00 pm Monday to Friday
Telephone: 0870 880 8484
Access: Open to all business travellers. Free access to Regus members.
Cost: The use of Business Centre's lounge is £8 per hour (£32 per day). All beverages are complimentary.
Facilities: Document station offering print, scan and copy, free high-speed internet
Additional Services: Free tea & coffee, kitchen facilities with microwave, meeting rooms, showers.
Contact: 0870 880 8484
Location: There is a lift before security in the South Terminal, Arrivals area, where you can gain access to the Business Centre. The lift is situated just between Bureau de Change and Costa Coffee and will take you to the lower level where the business centre is located.
Directions: Catch the shuttle from the North Terminal to the South Terminal. When you alight off the shuttle, walk through the entrance of the South Terminal, turn right at WHSmith, and you will find a lift to the lower floor just before Costa Coffee, on the right-hand side.

Sofitel London Gatwick

This four-star hotel is directly connected to the North Terminal and offers a business centre and a Sofitel Club Lounge. Reviewers have found the hotel responsive to business needs which they have rated as consistently good.

Access: Hotel residents have use of the business centre to meet their needs. Accor cardholders also have access to the club floor and lounge.
Facilities: Computer terminals, printing and photocopier.
Additional services: Club floor and lounge with refreshments and views of the runway.
Location: The Sofitel Hotel is connected to Gatwick Airport through a covered walkway on the right-hand-side of the shuttle on the North Terminal, level one.

Directions: From the terminal exit on level one, walk straight ahead to the right of the shuttle to a covered walkway sign posted Sofitel Hotel. Walk down the corridor, and you're at the entrance within 2 minutes. If you are arriving by car, you will find the entrance to the hotel on the ground floor next to the hotel's car park. Alternatively, you can park in the airport car park with easy access to both the hotel and airport terminal on level one.

Meeting facilities

The business meeting can take many forms. Depending on the type of meeting and attendees, you can choose from several locations at Gatwick Airport. There are some informal meeting areas before and after security at Gatwick's North Terminal. We've listed the most suitable below.

If you want more private meeting rooms, then we have also listed those that you can hire within the Airport and externally close by.

Relaxed meeting areas
Arrivals, Ground Floor
Costa Coffee Cafe

Costa Coffee offers a good place for an informal meeting over a cup of coffee. The best place to go is down the back on the right-hand side. There are plenty of tables here for a quick meeting between two to four people. It is amazingly quiet even during busy days, as it is away from the main thoroughfare and doesn't have a lot of other white noise, such as air-conditioning units.

Alternatively, try the alcove just behind the food and drinks fridge, on the right-hand side. Here's it is quite tranquil, no footfall and a soft black leather couch, making it ideal for a private, yet informal meeting.

Check-in, Level One
Hampton by Hilton incorporating Starbucks, Business Centre and Bar

Hampton by Hilton has included what use to be the Starbucks Café just opposite their reception and lobby into their public space and business centre. Not only can you now order Starbucks Coffee and snacks for your meeting, but there also are more tables for a small meeting of two to four people, along with an open meeting room with a large table arranged to accommodate up to eight people.

There are not many business travellers frequenting the room, as it is tucked away in the hotel lobby area and away from the main hustle and bustle. Consequently, it is quite tranquil.

Check-in, Level Two

Jamie's Coffee Lounge

At the back of the café, directly behind the service counter, you will find a quieter space than the front or side of the café for a meeting. There are four tables with seating for four people, and two tables to the right for two to four people. All have power points next to them. If these are occupied, then there are a couple more tables to the left of the service counter. However, this area is more exposed to the airport thoroughfare.

Nicholas Culpeper

For an informal meeting with more than four people, then upstairs at the Nicholas Culpeper has a large table to the left-hand side, just to the left of the lift. There is enough seating for eight people. When we visited, there was apparently a meeting taking place.

Don't be put off by the busy downstairs. While downstairs tables were fully occupied, upstairs was quiet. There are side booths directly in front of the window upstairs, although there is plenty of light, the view is of the car park. There are also tables along the left-hand side which have power points. Both options are suitable for an informal meeting over a bite to eat.

Departure Lounge, Lower Level

Weatherspoon's Red Lion pub.

The quietest area in this pub is at the far corner, on the left, by the window. There is sufficient table space for up to four people.

Departure Lounge, Upper Level

There are very few restaurants where you can have a meeting or business discussion in a sufficiently quiet space without being overheard or interrupted by others. We only found four which might be reasonable, where the others were too busy or more suitable for dining only.

Comptoir Libanais

There is a quiet space with dining table space for four people on the left by the window.

Jamie's Bakery

We noticed business travellers were using the small benches on the right next to the wall for a quick catch up over coffee. Laptops were being used and conveniently charged by the dual power point. These stalls seat up to four people.

Wagamama Restaurant

There are four booths at the far end of the restaurant on the left which seat just two people directly opposite each other. Here, the constant noise from the air-conditioning makes it difficult for others to overhear your conversation. There are power points, but the tables are small and may not accommodate a laptop and food simultaneously.

Union Jack Pub

Meetings of a non-confidential nature comprising two to eight people are feasible in the Union Jack Pub. There are several high tables where business people were meeting when we reviewed this pub. These tall tables fit up to eight people and participants can either stand or sit to discuss work matters.

If there is only two of you, then you may find the tables on the right by the entrance, next to Yo! Sushi are a good place for a meeting. Power points are available should you wish to discuss a shared laptop presentation. The best timing is during non-peak times.

Aspire Lounge

The Aspire Lounge has a quiet work area away from the main buffet dining zone. Next to this dedicated quiet zone are several tables suitable for an informal, low-key business meeting between a couple of attendees. Alternatively, the far end of the room around the corner to the right would also be suitable for an informal meeting with some privacy.

Open: Open hours are from 4.00 am to 10.00 pm, with a slight seasonal variation.

Access: Welcomes anyone who is travelling.

Cost: Lounge entry for adults is from £17.99 if you book in advance or £35 on the door without booking. If your flight is delayed and you want to stay longer, then you can buy additional hours.

Free access: Priority Pass, Diners Club, Institute of Directors, Aspire Platinum membership, **DragonPass cardholders and Vueling Airline passengers.**

Location: First floor of the Departure Lounge.

Directions: Head toward gates 101 – 113, just pass London News Company there is a hallway on your right. Turn right down the corridor, go through the double glass doors and take the lift on the left to the first floor. The lounge is located on the right-hand side.

Meeting rooms within Gatwick's North Terminal

No. 1 Lounge

The No. 1 Lounge offers a meeting room for up to eight people. It is light and airy with plenty of natural light and a view of the runway. You can book the meeting room in advance. They offer other business services. You can also book and use the room if you are travelling solo and want more privacy than the library room next door.

Open: 8.30 am to 6.30 pm on Monday to Friday, and 9.00 am to 6.00 pm on Saturdays for meeting room availability. The lounge is open from 4.00 am to 10.00 pm

Contact: 08442 64 64 40 or +44(0)2032838449 **or email:** Enquiries@No1Traveller.com

Cost: The meeting room is complimentary to travellers who have gained access to the lounge. Meeting guests are £35 per person, and this will also include access to the lounge.

Free access: Dragon Pass, Diners Club, Institute of Directors, Lounge Club, Priority Pass, Dining Club, Caxton FX. Privium and Wexas

Facilities: Wi-Fi, computer, photocopying, printing.

Additional Services: Print, fax, scan document and desktop internet access.

Location: On the lower level of the Departure Lounge, after security, near gates 101 - 113.

Directions: Head toward gates 101 – 113, just pass London News Company there is a hallway on your right. Turn right into the hall and through the double glass doors. No.1 Lounge is straight ahead at the far end.

Meeting rooms directly connected to Gatwick North Terminal

If you prefer to conduct meetings at a nearby hotel or business centre, then there are several very close by to choose from which offer excellent facilities at reasonable rates as well as the convenience.

Hampton by Hilton

The Hampton by Hilton is only a few minutes from the check-in desks, level one at the North Terminal, which makes it a perfect location for a meeting when travelling on business via Gatwick Airport. Hampton by Hilton offers a boardroom style meeting room for 16 people. A minimum of ten people is required.

Access: For companies, business travellers and hotel guests.
Contact: On-line pricing and book system.
Telephone: +44(0) 1293 57999 **email:** LONGN_hampton@hilton.com
Facilities: Basic meeting wireless internet access, business centre, audio/visual equipment, flip chart and markers, all-day non-alcoholic beverage service.
Additional services: Complimentary car parking.
Location: The entrance to this hotel is right near the Easy Jet Check-in on level one. Just follow the signs to the right of the check-in desk. You will see a sign above the entrance to the corridor for the Hampton by Hilton.
Directions: Turn right at the Easy Jet Check-in area and walk towards the end of the hall. Walk straight ahead through the entrance and follow the passage to the left. Walk through the automatic double glass doors. The total distance is about 50 steps from the Easy Jet Check-in to the hotel reception.

Sofitel London Gatwick

This nine-storey, four-star hotel offers eleven meeting rooms ranging from six to twenty-two delegates boardroom style. The location is convenient for business travellers who have a flight to catch as it is only a short walk from the North Terminal. All rooms come fully equipped with AV equipment, tea & coffee and are available to hire to non-residents. There is also an executive boardroom for a maximum of 16 participants and several larger conference rooms.

Access: The meeting rooms are available to hire to all, and you needn't be a hotel resident overnight. If you are an Accor card holder, you can book via the Accor website and use your points.
Telephone: +44(0) 1293 567070 **Email:** SLG@Sofitelgatwick.com
Facilities: 32" LCD HDTV, projector screens, microphone, DVD player, flip charts, LCD projector, extension cords, high-speed internet, air-conditioned, in-room tea/coffee station.
Additional services: Safe deposit box at reception, copy/print service is available, menus with healthier options are also available.
Location: The Sofitel hotel is connected to Gatwick Airport through a covered walkway on the right-hand-side of the shuttle on the North Terminal, level one.
Directions: From the terminal exit on level one, walk straight ahead to the right of the shuttle to a covered walkway sign posted Sofitel Hotel. Walk down the corridor, and you're at the entrance within 2 minutes. If you are arriving by car, you will find the entrance to the hotel on the ground floor next to the Hotel's car park. Alternatively, you can park in the Airport car park with easy access to both the hotel and airport terminal on level one.

Regus Express Business Centre – South terminal

The Regus Express Business Centre is one of the best options if you want to keep your meetings close to the Airport and don't require accommodation. Regus Express Business Centre and Lounge at the South Terminal offers eleven suitable meeting rooms from two to twelve people. It is only 3 minutes by direct airport shuttle from the North Terminal. You can catch the shuttle on Level One near the train station.

Open: 6.00 am to 6.00 pm Monday to Friday.
Telephone: 0870 880 8484
Access: Open to all business travellers. Free access to Regus members to the lounge.
Cost: Cost of hire of a meeting room is from £55 per hour. Should you also need, the use of Business Centre's lounge is £8 per hour (£32 per day) for non-members. All beverages, fruit and biscuits are complimentary.
Facilities: Flipchart, high-speed Wi-Fi, AV Technician onsite, free high-speed internet, document station offering print, scan and copy.
Additional Services: Free tea & coffee, kitchen facilities with microwave, meeting rooms and showers.

Location: For those arriving from the North Terminal, there is a lift before security in the South Terminal, Arrivals area, level two, where you can gain access to the Business Centre. The elevator is situated just between Bureau de Change and Costa Coffee and will take you to the lower level where the business centre is located.

Directions: Catch the shuttle from the North Terminal to the South Terminal. When you alight from the shuttle, walk through the entrance of the South Terminal, turn right at WHSmith, and you will find a lift to the lower floor just before Costa Coffee.

Meeting Rooms within a close distance

If your preference is to meet in proximity to the North Terminal, but far enough away from the hustle and bustle, then please see the options below.

Alexander House

Reviewers have described this as the perfect place for a business meeting, particularly being so close to Gatwick Airport. The service has been pronounced as impeccable, and reviewers mention enjoying the array of meeting spaces, both formal and relaxed. There are so many meetings rooms to choose from, ranging from 8 to 40 boardroom style, including a vineyard meeting room, meeting rooms with private garden, and the lounge for a small one to one client meetings.

Telephone: +44(0) 1342 859753 **or email** sales@alexanderhouse.co.uk

Access: Open to non-hotel guests and residents.

Cost: Day delegate rates are based on the number of attendees, from £39.00 to £79.00 per person + VAT. It includes a two-course working lunch. Half day rates are also available at £55 per person + VAT

Meeting Hours: Daily 8 am to 6 pm

Includes: Use of outdoor facilities, including a tennis court and putting green.

Facilities: Free high-speed internet and parking, business centre.

Location: Turners Hill, East Grinstead, West Sussex RH10 4QD

Directions by public transport:

If you're travelling by taxi or private car from Gatwick Airport, it only takes 15 minutes. Head on down the M23 and B2110 to Siskin Avenue, turn left onto Siskin Avenue, and you'll find Alexander House Hotel and Utopia Spa on the right.

Train from Gatwick Airport. It takes about 30 minutes by train from Gatwick South Terminal, southbound on the Thameslink to Three Bridges, which takes about 5 minutes. At Three Bridges train station, walk for 3 minutes to Stop B and catch the number 84 bus to East Grinstead alighting at Fen Place Farm. The walk takes about 15 minutes; then it is a minute walk to Turners Hill.

Bus from Gatwick Airport takes about 45 minutes on either the Fastway 20 and then Bus 84 to East Grinstead alighting at Fen Place Farm or catch the Fastway 10 to Crawley and then Metrobus 84 to Fen Place Farm. Once you alight at Fen Place Farm, it is only a minute to Turners Hill.

Best Western

Best Western Gatwick Skylane Hotel is only a short-haul from Gatwick and very affordable for day meeting rooms. It offers two rooms suitable for a meeting ranging from 10 to 30 people boardroom style.

Access: Open to hotel residents and non-residents.
Contact: 0845 620 0506 or **email** venues@bestwestern.co.uk
Cost: £100 per half day.
Facilities: Wi-Fi, Natural Daylight, business centre.
Additional Services: Restaurants, car parking.
Location: Best Western Gatwick Skylane Hotel, 34 Bonehurst Road, Horley, Gatwick, RH6 8QG
Directions:
By car: From Gatwick's North Terminal, head north on Departures Road towards Coach Road, turn left onto Northway. At the roundabout, take the 2nd exit onto the A23 slip road to Redhill/Crawley. At the next roundabout, take the 3rd exit onto Brighton Road on the A23. At the following roundabout, take the 2nd exit onto Bonehurst Road. The Best Western is on your right.
By taxi: You can use the airport shuttle which is only £3 one-way transfer or £5 return journey.

Courtyard London Marriott Gatwick Airport

The Courtyard Marriott is within walking distance of the South Terminal. It has three modern meeting rooms all located on the ground floor. Access is through a spacious and light Atrium with a glass roof on top which also provides the meeting rooms with secondary natural daylight from the Atrium. Meeting room capacity ranges from 8 – 36 boardroom style. Conference space for 72 is also available

Access: Open to hotel residents and non-hotel residents.
Cost: From £80 per half day or £120 for a full day. Day delegate rate is also available at £32.00

Facilities: High-speed Wi-Fi, Business Centre with computers, copy and fax service, as well as network and internet printing, AV technician onsite, AV equipment, LCD panel, LCD projector, TV, television production service provider.

Additional Services: Free onsite parking available for delegates, wireless internet access is also available.

Contact: +44 (0) 1293 566300

Location: London Gatwick Airport, Buckingham Gate, Gatwick, England, RH6 0NT

Directions: By foot, turn right upon leaving the South Terminal building. Walk past the Hilton Hotel and follow the signs for Schlumberger House. The hotel will be on the right, approximately a 15-minute walk.

The hotel also has a shuttle to and from the North Terminal for £3 (one way). If you prefer a taxi, the estimated taxi fare is £6.50

Langshott Manor

Langshott Manor is a small restored 16th Century Elizabethan Manor house set in three acres of country gardens. It offers several boardrooms and business suites with up to minute conference facilities and natural daylight which cater from 12 to 30 delegates boardroom style.

It is very close to Gatwick Airport's North Terminal and is less than ten minutes by car or taxi.

Access: Open to hotels residents and non-residents.

Contact: 01293 780080 or **email** sales@langshottmanor.com

Cost: A meeting room is £125 per room.

Full day delegate rates from £49 +VAT person November to April & August and £59 + VAT per person May to October. Includes room hire from 8 am to 6 pm, stationery, tea & coffee, mineral water and dining option.

Afternoon Tea Meeting at £20 + VAT per person, from 3 pm to 5 pm. It includes cream tea, unlimited tea & coffee and stationery.

Facilities: Business Centre, Wi-Fi, data projector & screen, flipchart.

Additional Services: 2 private dining rooms, 3 AA Rosette restaurant, car parking.

Location: Langshott Manor Hotel, Ladbroke Road, Horley, Near Gatwick, Surrey, England, RH6 9LN.

Directions: It takes less than 10 minutes by car from Gatwick Airport. Get onto the A23, London Road from Departures Road. Follow the A23 to Ladbroke Road in Surrey. Take Langshott Wood to Langshott Manor Hotel.

SECTION THREE: Healthy Lifestyle
Chapter 9: Travel Fit at Gatwick Airport

Exercising en route

Exercise has enormous physical and mental benefits when travelling for business. It boosts your immune system, increases energy levels and improves productivity. It can also help to reduce stress, alleviate jet lag and is associated with significant mood benefits directly linked to smoother interaction with colleagues.

Exercise has also been shown to improve time management, so it's ironic that exercise is often the first thing to disappear from your itinerary when you feel time pressured.

Travel delays, client meetings, business dinners, plus handling routine work from your home location can leave you with little apparent time to work-out. However, with some advanced planning and creativity, exercise can be both a beneficial and enjoyable component of your business journey.

In this chapter, we explore resourceful ways in which you can keep fit during your business trip, from simple exercises while you queue, impromptu walking routes to enthusiastic workouts. We've tried to make these as practical as possible, involving no or very little extra equipment, and relevant to the North Terminal at Gatwick Airport by utilising the facilities that are already available to travellers passing through the terminal.

There are also helpful tips on where to find a quieter spot to do some exercises while seated and which stairwells are less populated for modest exercise. So, whether you're queuing at Check-In, just arrived or waiting to depart, there are plenty of opportunities to keep fit.

We've even included connected and nearby hotels which offer gyms, swimming pools, tennis courts and golf courses, along with shops or vending machines within the North Terminal where you can purchase spur-of-the-moment fitness items, such as fit-bits, swimwear and running shoes.

All the research has been done for you, so all you need to do is to choose which activity best suits your needs and business travel schedule, and where you prefer to exercise.

What to pack when preparing for fit business travel

You needn't pack anything extra, although if inclined you could make space in your suitcase for some lightweight equipment to use in your room. It could include a skipping rope, resistance band or even an exercise DVD to play off your laptop. You could prepare these items well in advance of your trip. Some regular business travellers have an 'essentials bag' which they keep stocked, replenishing upon return from each business trip.

We've also noted several light-weight travel items which are highly rated by other business travellers later in the chapter. We've listed some items on our website, so you can purchase them on-line either through Amazon or direct with the retailer.

More importantly, you might include a pair of walking shoes which you can wear in the airport. If you've forgotten to pack some trainers or comfortable shoes or need a new pair, then not to worry, as our consultants have researched what is available at Gatwick Airport's North Terminal. The best option they found was to head straight for JD Sports on the upper level of the Departure Lounge. They have a range of running and training shoes available for you to choose.

Workout as you go

Exercise doesn't have to involve elaborate routines, sophisticated equipment or take huge chunks out of your busy day. Working out on the go can be just as effective.

There's also plenty of opportunities to exercise as you wait to board. We have listed below some simple exercises to do when you are either sitting down waiting or waiting in the queue, and we've also added some places where you can quietly exercise where the footfall is at its lowest.

A simple pedometer can revolutionise your workout business travel experience. The human body is designed to move, not to sit all day. The easiest way to get moving is to walk, and walking is accessible to nearly everyone. It's free; you don't need special clothing or equipment, and you can do it almost anywhere at any time. A target of 10 – 12,000 steps a day is surprisingly easy to achieve when travelling, particularly if you choose to walk through airports rather than using the travellators.

With this in mind, we have devised several walking routes at the North Terminal for you to try. Our travel health consultant has explored the North Terminal at Gatwick Airport and recorded the number of steps on routes suitable from a gentle stroll to a brisk walk. So you won't need to purchase a pedometer if you haven't already got one. Although, if you wish to record your total steps when en route to reaching a target number, you could either pack one in your cabin luggage in advance or pick up a Fitbit at the airport which will monitor your steps along with other key indicators. See our list of stockers at the end of this chapter.

So, don't just sit there! Take a few moments to exercise while you wait. Here are some great tips on how and where you can make this as easy as possible.

Exercises when sitting

If flight delays result in long periods of sitting, intersperse working on your laptop with a few simple exercises to keep you feeling supple. Ease tension in your neck by relaxing your shoulders and gently dropping your head, so your right ear moves towards your right shoulder. Hold for five seconds and repeat the other side. Roll your shoulders forward five times using a gentle circular motion and then reverse the movement a further five times.

Get to work on your core during short or long-haul flights. Focus on your oblique abdominal muscles by simply lifting your right hip off the seat, hold for five seconds and lower. Do the same movement with your left hip. Repeat ten times.

These light exercises can be done anywhere when seated, but it is advisable to find a quiet place to sit, so the noise level doesn't increase your anxiety and muscle tension. If you need to relax, then use the breathing exercises in Chapter 5. Below are some quiet places we've found where you could work, relax and exercise.

Quiet places for exercises when sitting.

We checked both the check-in areas as well as the departure lounges for places to do silent exercises in and found the following are quite suitable.

Arrivals, Ground Floor
UK and Republic of Ireland Arrivals

The area in front of the UK and Republic of Ireland Arrivals exit has less traffic than the International Arrivals area. So, your best bet if you are waiting for a colleague, is to head to the left of the arrivals hall towards the UK and Republic of Ireland Arrivals exit. Here you will find two places in which you can do a few quick, quiet stretching exercises while waiting. The first is on the left-hand side on the chairs next to the internet. The second is on the chairs surrounding the columns in the middle of the hall.

Check-in, Level One
Seated areas between the Excess Baggage Company and WHSmith

There two seating areas on either side of the entrance from the airport shuttle. One is next to WHSmith and other next to the Excess Baggage Company. Each section has several rows of seats, some of which do not have any armrests. Despite a high footfall, it provides an opportunity to stop and do a couple of the simple exercises mentioned above to keep you feeling supple before checking in.

Check-in, Level Two
The area on the left-hand side of the entrance

At the far-left entrance of the terminal, as you walk from the car park into the terminal on level two, there are seats next to Emirates ticket desk and the entrance door.

The area between Jamie's Coffee Lounge and entrance

Further along, there is another small bay of chairs. These are located between Jamie's van (you can't miss it due to the huge neon sign on top) and the entrance door.

If you want a quieter, less exposed seated space, then walk towards the back, past Check-in aisles.

Behind Check-in rows B&C

Recent renovations have provided a new alcove of chairs. There are several rows of seats now located just behind check-in area. There is less footfall here and much quieter, particularly at non-peak times than the front entrance area. It is the best of all options on Check-in Level Two.

Departure Lounge, Lower Level

Between Boots and Dixon's Travel

At the far end of the Departure Lounge on the right-hand side, between Boots the Chemist and Dixon's Travel are some seats where the footfall is much lower. There are several rows of seats on the left and to the right of the staircase. It is much quieter than the main seating area in the middle of the Departure Lounge. It is also the quietest set of stairs in the Departure Lounge, so you also have an opportunity to combine seating exercises with stair exercises. Being hidden from the main thoroughfare, other exercises which require more floor room such as stretching or lunging are also possible next to the wall.

At the start of the corridor to Gates 45 to 113

To the left of the far end of the Departure Lounge, just past the escalator and WHSmith, are several rows of seats. It is quieter here than the main Departure Lounge area and offers some space for stretching and making some lunges. What's more, there are some power points so you can charge your device or listen to some music via your phone on headphones while you undertake some of the modest exercises mentioned above.

Along the corridor to the Gates 45 to 113

There are several rows of chairs along the corridors to Gates 45 – 55 and 101 to 113. These are less used by travellers waiting for their boarding gate to be called and offer a more tranquil place to spend a few moments.

Gate 51 just opposite the toilets has four seats without armrests.
Gate 53 has four seats without armrests.
Gate 54 has four sets of four seats without armrests.
The junction between Gate 50 and 49 has four seats without armrests.

Along the corridor to Gates 557 to 574

If you want to stretch and undertake a brisk walk, then head right down to the end of the corridor towards Gate 574. You find this often deserted during the day. There are some seats alongside the wall of the corridor, should you wish to take a break or do some seated exercises. The walk to the end from the entrance is approximately 300 steps.

Exercise when queuing

You can even incorporate exercise into your queuing experience at check-in or the departure gate. As you're waiting, stand up straight and gently draw your navel in towards your spine to work the deep core muscles that help stabilise the lower part of your spine and pelvic area. Hold that contraction for 10 seconds and then release, but don't be tempted to hold your breath! Continue to breathe normally throughout the exercise and keep repeating for as long as you're waiting.

By getting creative with your business travel you really can find the time to exercise. Anything that can get your muscles working in new ways and your heart pumping is guaranteed to improve your health, increase your fitness and may even indirectly help boost your career prospects too.

Walking routes around Gatwick Airport's North Terminal

If you have time to burn, then you might consider maintaining good health by walking. Not only will you burn up a few hundred calories more than if just sitting around, but you will also improve your long-term health.

Walking at a moderate intensity (slightly faster than a stroll) is quick enough to be aerobic, raising the heart rate and achieve health benefits. At this pace, you will improve your blood pressure and reduce blood sugar levels, and thereby lessen the risk of coronary heart disease, deep vein thrombosis, type 2 diabetes, stroke, asthma, osteoporosis and some cancers in the long term.

Health professionals recommend at least 10,000 steps towards better health per day. On average, most of us walk at least 3,000 to 4,000 steps anyway. What's more, it's suitable for all ages and fitness levels. You can break this up into more manageable chunks of 1,000 steps or 10 minutes if just starting to get fit.

Gatwick Airport's North Terminal is a natural walkway when you think about it. It has long corridors and halls which you can wander around for hours! So, if you can handle the moving obstacles (other people) then walking for health is an easy option to keep you healthy while travelling. All you need are some comfortable walking shoes (forgot them? – then you can get a pair from JD Sports on the upper level of the Departure Lounge, just next to Pret A Manger), a bottle of water to sip on the way, and some healthy snacks once you've finished. Water and healthy snacks available in Gatwick's North Terminal are listed in Chapter 11 and 15.

To assist you on where the best places are to walk at Gatwick's North Terminal, we've sent one of our travel health consultants out with a pedometer to find an assortment of walking routes. They have recorded the approximate number of steps (based on 40 cm stride) and distance each route is in meters for your convenience.

We've included a walk outside the terminal itself, along with several walking routes within the Departure Lounge. Unfortunately, the Arrivals and Check-in areas were too short to provide any suitable walking routes. But don't let this stop you from waiting around!

Here are some pre-planned routes for you to choose from;

Before security, outside the terminal
River Mole
Gatwick North Terminal is surrounded by woodlands, but also by many busy roads. If getting out for a walk is important for you, then there aren't many places you can head without having to cross over a couple of busy roads. One option is to enjoy a stroll through the woods. The fifteen-minute walk to the River Mole can be a quick escape if you need time out or staying overnight in one of the airport hotels. It is approximately 1300 steps (520 meters) to the river, making 2600 steps (1,040 meters) in total there and back. Allow at least 30 minutes.

The walk to the River Mole is through woodlands so the path can be muddy during the wet season. There is also plenty of wildlife – squirrels, rabbits and birds. Make sure you allow plenty of time and have secured your luggage. You can either leave it in the hotel room, use the early check-in or take it to the Excess Baggage Company on Check-in, Level One, just opposite WHSmith, for storage.

Location: On the north side of Gatwick Airport on Perimeter Road.
Access: Walk outside the terminal entrance on Level One and take the lift at the far end of the shuttle to the ground level. Walk left along the path, towards the Arrivals Road, on the opposite side from the Premier Inn. At the traffic island, cross over the road, walk to the right, but stay on the side opposite the Premier Inn. At the large roundabout, cross over Longbridge Way, and take the path on the left through the woodlands which is parallel to A23 London Road. A small brook will run between the Woodland Path and the road A23. Keep following the path through the woodlands until you come to the bridge at the River Mole.

Departure Lounge, Lower and Upper Level

Being trapped inside the Departure Lounge for at least two hours can make you a little stir crazy. So, make the most it by getting some walking in before you board your flight.

Walking Route No. 1: Window shopping (slow – moderate)

If you want to stroll through the hustle and bustle of the lower level in the Departure Lounge, then walking from end to end is approximately 120 meters or just under 300 steps.

Alternatively, if you walk around the edges of the lower level in the Departure Lounge coming back on yourself, e.g. from security exit and circle back, then this is 250 meters or approximately 620 steps.

You can add another 370 steps with a more scenic route by walking upstairs and through the restaurants on the upper floor.

In total, if you walk around the lower level and then upstairs and along the upper level, the entire distance walked is approximately 400 meters and the aggregated number of steps walked is 990 steps. Let's call it 1000 steps in a slow to moderate motion.

Walking Route No. 2: From end to end (moderate to fast)

For a longer, faster, walking pace, with fewer obstacles and distractions, then try the gates between 557 and 574. The entrance is next to the Weatherspoon's Red Lion pub. Turn left, and the walk to Gates 559 and 557 is approximately 90 metres, equivalent to 225 steps or turn right to Gate 574, and the walk is about 120 meters or 300 steps. Double this, i.e. from end to end, starting at the entrance just past Wetherspoons' Red Lion Pub, and you will have covered over 1,000 steps or 400 meters.

If it's the view of the planes you want, then this route also has one of the best views.

Walking Route No. 3: The workout number 1 (moderate to sprint!)

Late for your boarding call? Or just fancy a long, fast stroll? Getting from the Departure Lounge, lower level exit to the London News Company at Gate 103, is approximately 500 meters, or just over 1200 steps.

If no one is about, you might consider increasing your intensity by doing a round on the travellator walking the wrong way. Beware: Gatwick Airport North Terminal will not thank you for walking in the opposite direction in peak traffic, so it's something that should only be considered when it is very quiet. Whatever you do, don't walk backwards – always face the way you are travelling.

Walking Route No. 4: Workout number 2 (moderate to sprint)

Another route for a brisk stroll is to Gates 49. Unlike Walking Route No. 3, there are no stairs. From the exit at London News in the lower level of the Departure Lounge to Gate 49, there are approximately 600 steps. Travelling there and back – you will have done 1200 steps (480 meters).

There are also two travellators, so when no one is around, and you are walking back to the main departure hall, you could increase the resistance of your walk by walking the wrong way on the travellator. Although, Gatwick Airport may request you to refrain from walking in the opposite direction of the travellator.

Stairways to Heaven

Some of the most interesting places in an airport are on the upper levels, where you can visit restaurants or take a view of the runway or walkways. Airports have ample stairs and stairs are a brilliant way to exercise. In fact, climbing the stairs burns more calories per minute than jogging. Research shows that regularly taking the stairs when travelling is good for healthy bones, cardiovascular fitness and it helps weight management. It's low-impact (provided you're not hopping or jumping several at a time) and can easily fit into your travel routine.

So instead of taking the lift or the escalator, take the stairs and exercise at the same time. You can do this inconspicuously, just going up and down over and over again. Or you could try out some more strenuous exercises or faster pace.

Gatwick has several staircases, which are about 20 – 30 steps high. Some are out of the main thoroughfare, and in quiet times could be used for light exercise. There are plenty to choose from, before and post-security.

First of all, pick a staircase, preferably one of the less populated stairways at Gatwick Airport. We have explored the Check-in, Arrivals and Departure Lounge for you and listed their suitability below this section.

Then, depending on your level of fitness choose a workout. Simply start by warming up for 3 minutes by walking up and down the stairs. Then perform each exercise for 60 seconds and rest for 30 for a minimum of five minutes but no longer than 20. Cool down with 3 minutes walking up down the stairs.

Light Beginners Workout

This one is for you if you're relatively new to exercise.
- Speed walk up the stairs and back down.
- Tricep dips off the lowest step with bent knees (see instructions below)
- Step ups using the lowest step
- Plank using the lowest step (see instructions below)

Moderate Workout

This one is for you if you exercise regularly but like to take things at a steadier pace.
- Jog up and down the stairs
- Tricep dips using the lowest step with straight legs (see instructions below)
- Plank using the lowest step (see instructions below)
- Hop ups using the lowest step

Hardcore Workout

This one is for you if you work out regularly and love an intense workout.
- Sprint up the stairs and jog back down.

- Tricep dips off the lowest step as hard and fast as you can. (see instructions below)
- Hop up all the stairs and jog back down
- Press ups using the lowest step

Quick reminder on how to do Triceps Dips and the Plank using the stairs

- **Tricep dips off the lowest step with bent knees**
  Find a comfortable step at the bottom of the stairs and sit down. Roll your shoulders back and down to open up the chest, bring your hand directly underneath the shoulders with palms down onto the step. Stretch your legs out, keeping your knees bent. Pressing down on your palms, straighten your arms and lift your buttocks off the step. Then bend your elbows lowering the hips down, and then repeat and exhale while extending your elbows and lifting yourself up.

- **Plank using the lowest step**
  Face the stairs and place your hand on the second step with your elbows directly underneath your shoulders and legs fully extended. Make sure your feet are together, tuck your pelvis under, and pull your shoulder back. This should resemble a semi-horizontal press-up position. Your body should be in a straight line from your shoulders to your ankles. Breath in and out calmly. Tighten your stomach, squeeze your bottom together, then reach for the higher step, one hand at a time, and then back again. Keep your body straight at-all-times. When you are finishing, gently roll out of it. An alternative would be to lift one leg at a time and hold, then move up and down for a few movements. Then swap to the other leg and repeat.

Where are the Stairs?

We've explored the arrivals, check-in and departure halls for stairs for you to use. Here are the options available to you along with comments about their suitability.

Arrivals, Ground Floor

There is one public set of stairs in the Arrival lounge which leads to Level One. You'll find these directly opposite the Bureau de Change. During peak times and throughout the day, these stairs are in constant use. Any attempt to exercise here, even in the modest form, will be met with confusion and annoyance from other travellers using them in the opposite direction. Best to only consider using these stairs when there is low footfall.

Departure Lounge

There are four sets of stairs in the Departure Lounge going from the lower to the upper level.

The set of stairs at the end of the hall between the large Boots pharmacy and Dixon's Travel are the quietest set of stairs and least populated than the other two on this side of the Departure Lounge. There are also more steps than the other two staircases with thirty steps in total. However, there is a sharp turning halfway, so you'll need to take care if you're doing a vigorous walk as visibility is poor halfway.

The second set of stairs are the main stairs in the middle of the Departure Lounge, on the right-hand side. These comprise of two 'lanes' on the lower tier joining into one lane from halfway. These stairs are wider in girth than the other three sets of stairs. There are twenty steps in all. However, these are in constant use and remain extremely busy during the best part of the day. So only attempt to exercise on these stairs during a very quiet period.

The third set of stairs is directly opposite the far entrance into the Departure Lounge from security, situated next to Weatherspoon's pub the Red Lion. There are twenty-five steps with a break/landing half way. These are quite busy during peak times, but not as busy as the main stairs. Again, it would be better to use these only during non-peak times.

The fourth set of stairs runs right alongside the escalator in the left-hand corner of the Departure Lounge. Most people seem to prefer to take the escalator, so these stairs offer an excellent alternative to the stairs on the opposite side of the Departure Lounge which is busier. There are thirty steps in total.

Travellator Treadmill

Power walking is a fantastic way to exercise, and where better than the airport where there can be miles of free treadmill. Health professionals have recommended using travellators when no-one is around as a form of intense walking. All you need to do is hop on the travellator so that you are steadily moving against the flow of the belt to provide the resistance of a treadmill. Whatever you do, do not walk backwards! Always face the way you are travelling. You may also notice that Gatwick Airport has placed no entry signs at the end of some travellators to deter anyone walking in the opposite direction of the travellator. Although, this practice isn't discouraged in other airports.

Some common sense must prevail, and it is best done when there is no-one around so you can avoid being hit by a group of travellers coming your way. Generally, this is either late at night or during periods of extreme weather conditions when there are lengthy delays.
You will find several travellators in the Departure Lounge en route to gates 101 – 113 and gates 45 - 55.

There are two travellators are along the corridor for Gates 45 – 55. The first travellator, between Gates 52 and 53, is approximately 120 steps when walking alongside it, and the second travellator, between Gate 50 and Gate 52 is about 200 steps when walking alongside.
The next travellators en route are to Gates 101 – 113. There are two travellators between Gate 101 and 113, and each is approximately 100 steps when walking alongside.

Hotels with fitness and leisure facilities nearby

There are many hotels next to and nearby which offer fitness and recreation facilities. It is a case of knowing which one will suit your timetable and has your preferred activity, along with which hotel provides access to nonhotel guests if you're not staying overnight. So, we've researched a few for you to try out. These are listed below. We've included hotels with swimming pools, tennis courts and golf courses, as well as those with gyms.

Hotels with Gyms

The hotel gym is an ideal opportunity to keep on track with your fitness while travelling. Size, equipment and opening times can vary, but most will have treadmills, a cross trainer, a range of weights and a floor area for bodyweight training.

Check out the gym before your first workout, so you know what's available and can plan your workout accordingly. Always take a bottle of water and a towel with you and if you've got a personal trainer at home ask them to create a workout for when you're travelling.

It's essential to warm up and cool down to reduce the risk of injury. A warm-up can be as simple as a brisk walk around the room to prepare both your body and mind for exercise. The cooldown is essential to bring your heart rate back down and gently stretch out the muscles you've been working.

The best type of exercise to help increase circulation before a flight or during transit is the one you're already doing as part of your usual routine at home. Do what your body is used to doing. However, take care with high-intensity workouts during transit as if you're tired you risk further fatiguing yourself or even injury.

If working up a sweat in the gym is the last thing you want to do, then simple flexibility and stretching workout can be very effective. Wiggle your toes, rotate your wrists and roll your shoulders!

Exercise and movement kick starts your circulation freeing you from fatigue, lethargy, and slow thinking. It refreshes, revitalises and sharpens your mind.

Not sure which hotels offer a gym? There are many hotels in the Gatwick Airport and the surrounding area. Unfortunately, those in Gatwick's North Terminal and nearby South Terminal all require you to be staying at a hotel resident. There are, however, hotels that are very close by which will allow visitors to use their gym (tennis courts, swimming pools and golf courses) for a small charge or as part of membership.

We have contacted the hotels in the airport and the surrounding area to find out which have facilities feasible to use when staying overnight or waiting some time before a flight. These are listed below, starting with the nearest hotels first.

Hotels with gyms at Gatwick Airport's North Terminal

Hampton by Hilton

The Hampton by Hilton is very conveniently located at the North Terminal at Gatwick Airport and offers business travellers a small well-equipped gym with the latest equipment. It is also very generously stocked with towels and water. It isn't overused so you can get a good workout most times.

Telephone: +44(0) 1293 579999 **email:** LONGN_hampton@hilton.com
Access: Hotel guests.
Cost: Complimentary for hotel residents.
Opening hours: Available 24 hours a day. You will need your room key to gain access.
Includes: Gym comprises exercise bike, stepper, treadmill, a cable machine, dumbbell rack and yoga/gym balls. No rowing machine. Room for yoga stretches.
Additional services: Water dispenser with hot and cold options, music, towels. Snacks available at the bar.
Location: Longbridge House, North Terminal, Gatwick Airport, West Sussex, RH6 0PJ. The entrance to this hotel is near the Easy Jet Check-in on level one. Just follow the signs to the right of the check-in desk. You will see a sign above the entrance to the corridor for the Hampton by Hilton.
The gym is on the lower ground floor below reception.
Directions: Turn right at the Easy Jet Check-in area and walk towards the end of the hall. Walk straight ahead through the entrance and follow the passage to the left. Walk through the automatic double glass doors. The total distance is about fifty steps from the Easy Jet Check-in to the hotel reception.

Sofitel Hotel

General description:
The Sofitel Hotel is a luxury hotel offering business travellers a modest gym with aerobic machines. From past user reviews, it doesn't appear to get very busy but has the appropriate equipment to do the 'job'. For residents, it is ideal for a pre-flight workout or for reducing the effects of jet lag when just arrived.

Telphone: +44 (0) 1293 567070 **or email** reservations3@sofitelgatwick.com
Access: For hotel residents only. The key is held at reception.

Cost: Complimentary for hotel residents. Alternatively, you can stay in a day room and have access to the gym, along with the use of the business facilities. When we checked out the dayroom rate, the cost was £79 for a day room at the time of review.

Opening hours: Available 24 hours a day.

Includes: The gym comprises two bikes, a cross-training machine, two treadmills, free weight, fitness ball, mats, lat pull down, rowing machine.

Additional services: Business facilities, day rooms, bar, restaurant and the internet.

Location: North Terminal, London Gatwick Airport, West Sussex RH6 0PH. The Sofitel hotel is connected to Gatwick Airport through a covered walkway on the right-hand-side of the shuttle on the North Terminal, level one.

Directions: From the terminal exit on level one, walk straight ahead to the right of the shuttle to a covered walkway sign posted Sofitel Hotel. Walk down the corridor, and you're at the entrance within 2 minutes. If you are arriving by car, you will find the entrance to the hotel on the ground floor next to the Hotel's private car park. Alternatively, you can park in the Airport car park with easy access to both the hotel and airport terminal on level one. It is only 240 metres and takes about 4 minutes to walk from Arrivals on the ground floor to the hotel.

Hotels with gyms at Nearby South Terminal

Courtyard by Marriott

The Courtyard by Marriott Hotel is within walking distance of Gatwick Airport's South Terminal. The hotel welcomes business travellers and invites their residents to maintain their workout routine in their state-of-the-art gym, equipped with the latest equipment. Reviewers have found the gym to offer good facilities and overall 'better than other hotel gyms.'

Telephone: +44 01293 566300

Access: Hotel residents only.

Cost: Complimentary to hotel residents.

Opening hours: 24 hours a day.

Includes: Gym comprises cardiovascular equipment, free weights, treadmill, rowing machine, step walker and cycles.

Additional Services: Free wireless in public areas.

Location: London Gatwick Airport, England RH6 0NT

Airport Shuttle Service: £3 one way. Phone +44 844 3351802

Directions:

By walking: It is approximately a 15-minute walk. Turn right upon leaving the South Terminal building. Walk past the Hilton Hotel and follow the signs for Schlumberger House. The hotel will be on the right.

By Car: It will take approximately seven minutes to drive from the airport. Head south-west on North Terminal Approach towards Departures Road. Slight right onto Arrivals Road. Keep right to continue on Northway. Turn right towards Northway. Turn right onto Northway. At the roundabout, take the 4th exit onto Airport Way. At the roundabout, take the 2nd exit onto Ring Road. Slight left onto Buckingham Gate. Turn right to stay on Buckingham Gate. Turn right, and the hotel is on your left.

Hilton London Gatwick Airport

The Hilton has a small yet well-equipped gym for residents, featuring modern Precor equipment. It gets busy at peak times. Otherwise, it's a relatively quiet gym. The Hilton is connected to Gatwick Airport's South Terminal via a corridor, and the gym is situated along the corridor just opposite Costa Coffee.

Telephone: +44 (0) 1293 610 828 **email:** london.gatwick@hilton.com
Access: Hotel guests.
Cost: Complimentary to hotel residents.
Opening hours: 24 hours a day, access via the key holder.
Includes: Gym comprises modern Precor equipment, free weights, selection of aerobic machines, two treadmills, one bike and one elliptical machine, two multi-resistance machines.
Location: South Terminal Gatwick Airport, Gatwick RH6 0LL
In the corridor which connects the hotel with the terminal right opposite the Costa Coffee. **Additional services:** Towels are supplied. There is a water tank within the fitness room.
Directions: Simply take the shuttle to the South Terminal from the North Terminal. Walk from the shuttle to the Hotel.

Nearby hotels with gyms

Arora Hotel

Arora Hotel is the most accessible hotel to get to by train or bus from Gatwick South Terminal which is open to guests (non-residents and non-members). The train ride is only 8 minutes. If you are staying the night, then there is also an airport shuttle service. The hotel offers a very well equipped, 50 station state of the art gymnasium, along with a sauna and steam room, along with a beautiful atrium for lunch or coffee. The gym has an emphasis on cardiovascular exercise and features a range of equipment from air fan rowers to computerised treadmills.

Telephone: +44 (0) 01293 520208 **or email on** inspire@arorainternational.com
Access: Available to non-members and external guests.
Cost: Hourly pass for £4 per hour, or £10 guest pass for the day.
Opening hours: 24 hours, seven days a week.
Includes: Sauna and steam room, free WiFi.
Additional services: A lovely atrium in the hotel where you can enjoy coffee or lunch before heading back to the hustle and bustle of the airport. There is also a range of massage and reflexology treatments available. Car parking is available for £10 per day, up to 200 cars.
Location: Southgate Avenue, Crawley, West Sussex RH10 6LW
Airport Shuttle Service: The hotel provides a scheduled transport service from the airport at quarter past the hour, on a request basis with a small charge per person. The cost is £3.50 per person.
Directions:
By public transport; It couldn't be easier as the hotel is right next to Crawley train station. Buses from Gatwick Airport also stop very close to the hotel.
Train from Gatwick Airport; The easiest route is to hop on a train at the South Terminal, right next to Check-in. They run every 15 minutes, until late at night. The train journey is about 8 minutes, and the tickets cost £3. There is a private gate from platform two into the hotel grounds. To use the gate access, follow the signs to the end of the platform and press the intercom button at the gate.
Bus from Gatwick Airport; Alternatively, you can catch the bus from the South Terminal (Fastway 10, Fastway 20, 400, 460). Fastway 10 and 20 stops a minute from the hotel. Depending on the route, the journey takes between 13 and 20 minutes. The nearest bus stop is Southgate Avenue North, which is near the hotel entrance.
If you are travelling by car; Head east on Airport Way onto the M23, leave at junction 10 and take the A2011 towards Crawley. At the first roundabout, take the second exit and continue on the A2004. At the second roundabout, take the first exit towards the Country Mall. Go straight through the next two sets of traffic lights, past the Country Mall on the right, and under the railway bridge. The hotel is on your right.

Europa Gatwick Airport

Spindles Gym at Europa Britannia Lodge is ideal for frequent flyers heading out from Gatwick Airport and is only 10 minutes by car. In addition to the fully equipped gym, there is also a heated swimming pool, sauna and steam room. Hotel guests and non-resident members are welcome. This may suit those using Gatwick Airport on a regular basis.

Telephone: 01293 882 779 **or email** spindles714@britanniahotels.com
Access: Members and hotel guests only.
Cost: Spindles operates a membership for non-residents at £20 per month (pay by direct debit), and hotel guests pay £4.00 per session. Towel hire is £1.00.
Opening hours: Monday to Friday 6.00 am to 9.00 pm, Saturday & Sunday 8.00 am to 8.00 pm.
Includes: Fully equipped gym
Additional services: Heated indoor swimming pool, hot tub, sauna and steam room.
Location: Spindles Health Club, Europa Hotel, Balcombe Road, Crawley, West Sussex, RH10 7ZR
Directions: Only 10 minutes away by car or taxi.
By Car; If you are travelling by your car, then head east from the airport on Airport Way to M23. Continue on M23 to Balcombe Road/B2036. Take exit 10A from M23. At the roundabout, take the 4th exit onto Balcombe Road/B2036. The Europa Hotel is on the right.
By Taxi; ETS/Road Runners Taxis offer guests affordable transfers (£9) to the and from the airport. Contact 01293 922811.

Sandman Signature London Gatwick Hotel

The Sandman is a luxury hotel only 3 miles from Gatwick making it an ideal location for a stopover. It offers a small yet fully functional gym. Reviewers noted that it wasn't overcrowded, quiet and offered a variety of equipment. Overall, they rated it as adequate and inviting. In addition to the gym, there is a sauna, steam room, and 15-metre pool.

Telephone: 01293 561186 **or email** res_gatwick@sandmanhotels.co.uk
Access: Residents only.
Cost: Complimentary to hotel residents.
Opening hours: 9.00 am to 9.00 pm
Includes: Weights, rowing machines, running machine and exercise bike. Towels are supplied. There is also a water cooler in the changing rooms.
Additional Services: 15-metre pool, spa bath and steam room.
Location: 18 – 23 Tinsley Lane South, Three Bridges, Crawley West Sussex, RH10 8XH
Airport Shuttle Service: Doesn't offer an airport shuttle.
Directions: The Sandman is very close to Gatwick and very quick to get to by car.

By Taxi; ACE Cars has a special rate of £8.50 for Sandman Signature London Gatwick Hotel Guests. Call ACE on 01293 888 888

By Car; Nine minutes from Gatwick Airport North Terminal. Head east on Airport Way. Take exit ten from M23. Follow Crawley Avenue (A2011).

Nearby Hotels with tennis courts

Copthorne Hotel Effingham

The Copthorne Hotel is set amongst a picturesque parkland estate, just ten minutes from Gatwick International Airport. Tennis courts are open to non-hotel residents, and tennis rackets are available to hire.

Telephone: 01342 714 994
Cost: £5 per racket.
Access: Non-hotel residents and hotel residents.
Opening hours: Monday to Friday 7.00 am to 9.00 pm, Saturday & Sunday 8.00 am to 8.00 pm.
Additional services: A nine-hole golf course, a croquet lawn health club, gym, treatments rooms, sauna, steam room and 20-metre swimming pool.
Location: Situated in West Park Road, Copthorne, West Sussex, RH10 3EU the hotel is easy to get to from Gatwick Airport.
Airport Shuttle: Complimentary to hotel guests.
Directions: Just 11 kilometres away.
By car: Head east on Airport Way. Continue on M23. Take A264 to Turners Hill Road/B208 in Copthorne. At the Roundabout, take the 1st exit onto Turners Hill Road/B2028.

Cottesmore Hotel Golf and Country Club

The Cottesmore Hotel Golf and Country Club opened their two new outdoor tennis courts in spring 2016. They are accessible to visitors for a small court rental. You can also hire tennis rackets and towels, along with health club entry for a low cost which includes a gym and swimming pool. Only 13 minutes from Gatwick Airport, you can enjoy a quick match if you have 4 or more hours to spare before your outward-bound flight.

Telephone: 01293 528 256 **or email** membership@cottesmoregolf.co.uk
Cost: The visitor rate is £14 for health club entry, £7 for tennis court, £2.20 for tennis racket hire, £1 for a towel, lockers require a £1 coin.

Access: Visitors, members, and hotel guests are welcome.

Opening hours: Monday to Friday 6.30 am to 9.30 pm. Weekends and Bank holidays 8.00 am to 8.00 pm.

Includes: The use of the gym, pool, sauna, hot tub and steam room.

Additional services: Nine and eighteen-hole golf course with featured holes.

Location: Buchan Hill, Pease Pottage, Crawley, RH11 9AT, United Kingdom.

Directions: The club is only 13 minutes from Gatwick Airport by car or taxi, and 1 mile from junction 11 on the M23.

By car from Gatwick Airport; Head east on Airport Way, continue on the M23 to Brighton Road/B2114. Take the exit at Junction 11, take Horsham Road and Forest Road to the lodge.

By train from Gatwick Airport; The train departs at Gatwick South Terminal, southbound. Go six stops to Brighton and alight at Crawley. It takes about 10 minutes. The walk from Crawley station to Forest Road takes about 25 minutes (approximately 1.3 miles). Total time by train would be roughly 1 hour.

Felbridge Hotel and Spa

Described by guests as having a massive very well-kept tennis courts, Felbridge Hotel and Spa offers two newly refurbished modern tennis courts. You can either hire a room for the night (hotel residents have free access to the tennis courts) or if sufficient time allows, just hire the courts and equipment. Open to non-residents. Also available as part of membership.

Telephone: 01342 337700 **or email** chakraspa@felbridgehotel.co.uk

Access: Non-residents as part of a spa package, gym members, hotel resident.

Cost: Pay and play is available to the public for just £7.50 per hour. Equipment (rackets and balls) can be hired. Complimentary to hotel residents, members and spa package deals.

Opening hours:
Monday to Friday 6.30 am to 9.00 pm (last entry 8.30 pm)
Saturday & Sunday 8.00 am to 8.00 pm (last entry 8.30 pm)Daily adult only hours 11.00 am to 4.00 pm

Additional services: Gym, spa and swimming pool.

Location: Situated on London Road, in East Grinstead, West Sussex RH19 2BH. The hotel sits prominently on the A22 and is only a 15-minute drive from Gatwick Airport.

Airport Shuttle: A taxi shuttle service is available on demand 24 hours a day. The cost is £12.50.

Directions: It is just 8 miles from Gatwick Airport.

By car; Approximately only 15 minutes by car or taxi to the airport. Head east on Airport Way. Continue on M23. Take the A264 to London Road/A22 in East Grimstead.

Nearby hotels with swimming pools

Europa Gatwick Airport

Spindles Gym at Europa Britannia Lodge offers an indoor heated pool, along with sauna and steam room. It's only 10 minutes by car. Non-residents are welcome as part of a membership package. If you are a frequent user of Gatwick Airport, then membership could inspire a swim here to relieve the travel strain on a regular basis. A taxi service is available from the airport if you're not already passing on your way to Gatwick Airport.

Telephone: 01293 882 779 **or email** spindles714@britanniahotels.com
Access: Members and hotel guests only.
Cost: Europa operates a membership for non-residents at £20 per month (pay by direct debit), and Hotels guests pay £4.00 per session. Towel hire is £1.00.
Opening hours: Monday to Friday 6.00 am to 9.00 pm, Saturday & Sunday 8.00 am to 8.00 pm
Includes: Hot tub, sauna, and steam room.
Additional services: A fully equipped gymnasium.
Location: Balcombe Road, Gatwick RH10 7ZR
Directions: Only 5 miles away and 10 minutes by car or taxi. The hotel is not far from junction 10A of the M23.
By Car; If you are travelling by your car from Gatwick Airport, then head east from the airport on Airport Way. At the roundabout, take the 1st exit onto M23 heading to London. At the roundabout, take the 2nd exit onto the M23 slip road to Brighton. Merge onto the M23, at junction 10A, take the B2036 exit, at the roundabout, take the 4th exit onto Balcombe Road.
By Taxi; ETS/Road Runners Taxis offer guests affordable transfers (£9) to the and from the airport. Contact 01293 922811.

Felbridge Hotel and Spa

Felbridge offers an indoor heated swimming pool, spa pool, steam room and sauna. Adult only swim time is between 11.00 am to 4.00 pm. Felbridge is a four-star hotel, only a 15-minute drive from Gatwick Airport. Best travelled to by car, as public transport would involve several changes and take approximately an hour. Reviewers have rated the swimming pool as immaculate, relaxing and of high quality, but can be busy in the morning.

Telephone for bookings: 01342 337700 **or email** chakraspa@felbridgehotel.co.uk
Access to: Non-residents as part of a spa package, free to gym members and hotel residents.
Cost: Half day spa £65. Other spa packages are available for a six-hour duration. Off-peak membership is available from £38 per month or annual membership at £400, with no joining fee. Peak membership is £55 per month.
Opening hours:
   Monday to Friday 6.30 am to 9.00 pm (last entry 8.30 pm)
   Saturday & Sunday 8.00 am to 8.00 pm (last entry 8.30 pm)
   Daily adult only hours 11.00 am to 4.00 pm
Includes: Half day spa package includes full use of spa facilities (sauna, steam room, Jacuzzi and gym). Supplied with robe, towels and slippers. Also have a choice of breakfast, lunch, afternoon tea or dinner, along with one 55-minute treatment (choose full body massage, facial, manicure or pedicure). Membership includes access to gym, tennis courts, discounts on food, treatments and accommodation.
Additional Services: Fully equipped gym and outdoor tennis courts.
Location: Situated on London Road, in East Grinstead, West Sussex RH19 2BH. The hotel sits prominently on the A22 and is only a 15-minute drive from Gatwick Airport.
Airport Shuttle: A taxi shuttle service is available on demand 24 hours a day. The cost is £12.50
Directions: It is just 8 miles from Gatwick Airport.
By Car: Approximately only 15 minutes by car or taxi to the airport. Head east on Airport Way. Continue on M23. Take the A264 to London Road/A22 in East Grinstead.

Sandman Signature London Gatwick Hotel

http://www.sandmansignature.co.uk/find-hotels/gatwick/
The Sandman is a luxury hotel just a stone throw from Gatwick making it an ideal location for a stopover. It has a 15-metre pool, steam room and spa bath. Reviewers have commented on how lovely, clean and warm the pool was. Recent refurbishment has been noted by some of the guests as well. Power showers were also noted as an excellent facility post-swim.

Telephone: 01293 561186 **or email** res_gatwick@sandmanhotels.co.uk.
Access: Residents only.

Cost: Complimentary to hotel residents.

Opening hours: 9.00 am to 9.00 pm.

Includes: Towels and water cooler in changing room.

Additional Services: Spa bath, steam room and gym.

Location: 18 – 23 Tinsley Lane South, Three Bridges, Crawley West Sussex, RH10 8XH

Airport Shuttle Service: Doesn't offer an airport shuttle.

Directions: Only three miles from Gatwick, so the journey is relatively short.

By Taxi; ACE Cars has a special rate of £8.50 for Sandman Signature London Gatwick Hotel Guests. Call ACE on 01293 888 888

By Car; 9 minutes from Gatwick Airport North Terminal. Head east on Airport Way. Take exit ten from M23. Follow Crawley Avenue (A2011)

Nearby hotels with golf courses

Cottesmore Hotel Golf and Country Club

Cottesmore offers 27 mature golfing holes in 207 acres of beautiful Sussex countryside. Only 15 minutes from Gatwick. It provides both a nine-hole course for a quick game, suitable for beginners and complete golfers and an eighteen-hole championship course which played host to Sussex Open Championship in 2006. Both courses offer featured holes. Visitors are welcome, along with their guests. If you're a frequent flyer on business and enjoy a game of golf, then a membership or corporate membership might be worthwhile considering.

Telephone: 01293 528 256 **email:** accommodation@cottesmoregolf.co.uk

Cost:
> **Griffin Course, 18 holes**
> **Monday to Thursday** £32
>> After 11.00 am £27
>> After 1.00 pm £23
>
> **Saturday & Sunday** £30
> **Phoenix Course 9 holes**
>> Monday to Friday £12
>> Saturday & Sunday £14
>
> **Phoenix Course 18 holes**
>> Monday to Friday £14
>> Saturday & Sunday £15
>> **Annual Membership** is £1210 plus £100 application fee and includes the use of health club.

Access: Visitors are welcome, along with members and hotel guests.

Opening hours: Weekdays 7.00 am, weekends tee off 6.30 am.

Includes: Pro shop is available for purchasing items and is open from 7.15 am on weekdays to 6.00 pm, and 6.15 am on weekends to 6.00 pm.

Additional services: Health club with gym, swimming pool, steam room, hot tub and tennis courts.

Location: Buchan Hill, Pease Pottage, Crawley, RH11 9AT, United Kingdom

Directions: The club is only 13 minutes from Gatwick Airport by car or taxi, and 1 mile from junction 11 on the M23.

By car from Gatwick Airport; Head east on Airport Way, continue on the M23 to Brighton Road/B2114. Take the exit at Junction 11, take Horsham Road and Forest Road to the lodge.

By train from Gatwick Airport; The train departs at Gatwick South Terminal, southbound. Go six stops to Brighton and alight at Crawley. It takes about 10 minutes. The walk from Crawley station to Forest Road takes about 25 minutes (approximately 1.3 miles). Total time by train would be roughly 1 hour.

Copthorne Hotel Effingham

The Copthorne Hotel is set amongst a picturesque parkland estate, just ten minutes from Gatwick International Airport. It offers a par 2/3 9-hole golf course. Reviewers have highly rated the course as well maintained.

Telephone: 01342 716 528 **email:** enquiries@effinghamparkgc.co.uk

Cost: £12 for nine holes of golf and £17 for 18 holes of golf

Access: Non-hotel residents can access the golf course.

Opening hours: Monday to Friday 7.00 am to 9.00 pm, Saturday & Sunday 8.00 am to 8.00 pm

Includes:

Additional services: Two floodlit tennis courts, a croquet lawn health club, gym, treatments rooms, sauna, steam room and 20-metre swimming pool.

Location: Situated in West Park Road, Copthorne, West Sussex, RH10 3EU, the hotel is easy to get to from Gatwick Airport.

Airport Shuttle: Complimentary to hotel guests.

Directions: Just 11 kilometres away.

By car: Head east on Airport Way. Continue on M23. Take A264 to Turners Hill Road/B208 in Copthorne. At the Roundabout, take the 1st exit onto Turners Hill Road/B2028

Retail Therapy

There are several shops within the North Terminal which stock items to support fitness. However, these stores only stock a limited range, and it might require some shopping around before you find the items for your exercise preference. So, we've done some research for you, and have listed various items and where to find them below. In some instances, you may need to pre-order items either online or by phone, with the intention of picking them up when you pass through the terminal.

Boots the Chemist

There are several Boots the Chemist at Gatwick's North Terminal, including one before security (in the arrivals hall) and two within the Departure Lounge. You can pre-order online and collect either from Boots the Chemist within the North Terminal Departure Lounge or before security at Unit 2 near M&S Simply Food, opposite Costa Coffee on the ground floor, post-exit from Customs and Excise.

Opening in Arrivals: 24 hours
Opening in Departure Lounge: 4.00 am to 8.300 pm
Telephone: 01293 569606
Website: www.boots.com

Some of the products they stock include;

Activity fitness bands

   Fitbit Charge 2 Heart Rate & Fitness Wristband £119.99 Includes PursePulse heart rate, multi-sport modes and connected GPS. Track all day activity, exercise and sleep, while making the most of your entire routine with smartphone notifications.

   Fitbit Blaze Fitness Super Watch £149.99 Provides steps, distance, active minutes & calories burned, workout states, along with measuring sleep. Also provides PurePulse continuous heart rate, displays calls & texts and music control. Syncs with iPhone, Android, windows, Mac+PC and is water resistant.

   Fitbit Alta HR Special Edition £149.99 Provides steps, distance, calories burned and active minutes. Smarttrack auto exercise recognition, PurePulse continuous heart rate, auto sleep tracking, silent alarm, call, text and calendar alerts. Syncs with iOS, Android, Windows, Mac and PC.

   Garmin Vivofit 3 Activity Tracker Black £89.99 Features include step counter, sleep monitor. Compatible with iPhone 4S or later and most Bluetooth Smart capable Android devices.

Garmin Vivosmart HR Activity Tracker £139.99 Features include wrist heart rate, move bar, smart notifications, steps, sleep monitoring. Works with iPhone 4 S or later and Android devices.

Garmin Vivoactive HR Activity Tracker £239.99 Features include SkyWatch application, AccuWeather Minute Cast widget, vivoactive HR XL and water rating up to 50 metres.

TomTom Fitness Tracker Small £129.99 Tracks body composition (body fat and muscle mass), monitors heart rate, counts steps, calories burned, distance walked, active time and sleep time.

Pedometers

Tanita PD – 724 Axes Pedometer £24.99 Includes neck strap. Includes step counter, distance measurement, calorie consumption and total walking time.

Dixons Travel

Dixons Travel is located within the Departure Lounge, lower level, on the right-hand side of the Departure Lounge. In fact, there are two stores. The larger one being right down the far end next to Boots the Chemist and the smaller store being up near Wetherspoons Pub next to World Duty Free.

Dixons Travel offers some activity trackers. Orders can be placed by phoning Dixon's Travel direct at their Gatwick North Terminal store. They would be able to check and reserve your product for you. Unfortunately, you may not be able to order all the items listed below online. They do select products to feature on their website which you can reserve and pick up when passing through the airport.

Opening hours: 4.00 am to 9.00 pm daily
Phone number: 01293 569737
Website address: www.dixonstravel.com/london-gatwick/north

Some of the activity trackers they stock include:

Garmin Vivofit 3 £47.99 black and regular. Features include; IQ motion detector, daily step goal, move bar and progress tracking.

Garmin Vivosport £129.00 Slate colour, medium size. Features include; built-in GPS, heart rate variability tracker (HRV), and daily fitness monitor. Comes in a slim and vibrant design.

Garmin Vivoactive 3 £219.00 Features include: smartwatch connects to your smartphone for notifications and messages, preloaded health trackers and sports apps, downloadable apps, faces and widgets to personalise your smartwatch. Connect to compatible Android or iOS smartphone.

Michael Kors Grayson Smartwatch £290.00 Features include; notifications for email, text and built-in fitness tracker. Voice activation from Google Assistant. Large stainless-steel bracelet and a fully round-shaped case with a touch-screen dial.

Fossil Q Venture Smartwatch £229.00 Full round digital display, with multiple features which include customisable faces and apps, discreet notifications and info at a glance. Compatible with phones running Android 4.3 or iOS 9.0

Fitbit Alta £85.00 Is a customisable fitness tracker. Features activity monitoring and workouts.

Fitbit Alta HR Black £109.00 Features include; built-in heart monitor, step counter, distance covered and calories burned

Fitbit Charge 2 Black large £89.00 Features include PurePulse heart monitor, multi-sport tracking to monitor running, gym sessions, yoga and more. Also comes in a small size.

Fitbit Blaze £137.00 Tracks activities throughout the day, monitors sleep, progress and goal setting. GPS tracking to support route, run time, distance, pace and elevation. Also offers next level instruction and coaching to improve performance and target attainment.

JD Sports

JD Sports is located in the Departure Lounge, Upper Level, just between Pret A Manger and the Sunglass Hut. If you have forgotten your fitness items or gym clothes, then JD Sports stock some essentials, including swimwear and goggles, gym clothes, yoga mats, skipping ropes and foam rollers. If you want to run while away but have forgotten your kit, then JD Sports stock includes well-known brands to replace all your necessary gear.

Unfortunately, unlike Boots, JD Sports does not offer click and collect from stores within airports. You can, however, view their products online before visiting the store.

Opening in Departure Lounge: 4.00 am to 8.30 pm
Telephone: 01293 223016
Email: customer.service@jdsports.co.uk
Website: www.jdsports.co.uk

Some of the products they stock include;

Activity Trackers

Garmin Vivosmart Activity Tracker £200.00 Includes tracking movement on steps, distance, calories, heart rate and intensity when you train. You can also receive texts, calls, email and social media alerts on the go!

Swimming

Swimwear, including shorts, Speedo swimming briefs, swimsuits.

Goggles

Speedo Aquapulse Goggles £13.00 Designed for maximum comfort, fit and vision. Ideal for swimmers who wish to train or keep fit. Ergonomic soft seal for enhanced comfort.

Speedo speed socket goggles £23.00 A classic racing goggle featuring advanced dual shot injection construction, double head strap that boasts an exceptionally secure fit for racing. Anti-fog lenses with UV protection.

Zoggs Fusion Air Googles £12.00 Undistorted vision with a larger frame for a more comfortable fit. 180 degrees of peripheral vision and anti-fog to control clarity with UV protection.

Michael Phelps Googles (dark lens) £25.99 High-performance goggles, distortion-free 180-degree range vision. The lenses offer 100% UV/UVB profession with scratch resistance and anti-fog treatment. Hypoallergenic and latex free.

Caps

Speedo Fastskin 3 Swimming Cap £27.00 Features include IQfit Profile and designed using accurate head mapping data to create optimum comfort, hydrodynamic performance and ease of use.

Speedo Plain Moulded Swim Cap £5.00 Features 3 D moulded silicone.

Tennis

Tennis attire, including tops, shorts, shoes, balls.

Tennis rackets

Babolat Pulsion 102 Tennis Racket £50.00 Graphite composite frame construction. Lightweight design.

Babolat Pure Aero French Open Roland Garros Tennis Racket £210.00 Features include FSI spin technology for spin, bigger gaps between strong for more flexibility and bite on the ball. Graphite/Tungsten material.

Head IG Heat Pro Tennis Racket £99.99 Super light-weight racket uses Innegra fibres. It has an oversized head and is easy to swing which is ideal for recreational play or beginners.

Babolat Drive 105 Strung Tennis Racket £120.00 Features include Cortex technology and a 105 sq cm head size to generate more power on ball impact. Ultra-lightweight.

Wilson Open 23 Tennis Racket £17.99 Features include a C-Beam construction to ensure stability and solid power. The Airlite Alloy construction to provide lightweight and strength. Extra length on the racket for implosive play on overhead shots and serves.

Running

Running attire, including leggings, shirts, shoes, socks, hats, gloves

Nike Lightweight Smartphone Armband with a wallet inside £25.00 Made with stretch material for fit. Also features transparent window that is touchscreen compatible.

Nike Lightweight Running Backpacks £85.00 Features include multiple compartments, sectioned structure for organised storage, stabilised construction to help reduce bounce when running, ventilated back-pane, adjustable strap for fit and hydration pocket for water storage.

Hotel Room Travel lightweight equipment

Foam rollers

Nike Textured Foam Roller £30.00 Features a thick, ridged surface for increased flexibility and range of motion.

Yoga

Nike Yoga Kit £30 (include mat, block and yoga strap) Complete with foam yoga mat, a lightweight yoga block and yoga strap.

Nike yoga mat £23.00 3mm yoga mat comes with straps for ease of carrying.

Skipping ropes

Karakai Digital Jump Rope £6.00 Adjustable jump rope with a digital indicator on one of the handles.

Nike Speed 2.0 Jump rope £13.00 Part of the Crosstown Running range.

Chapter 10: Acquire some fresh air and sunshine

Sunshine and fresh air are often forgotten ingredients to business traveller's life. Yet, having time outside every day is highly germane to frequent business travellers. Just ten to fifteen minutes outside can have a significant impact on traveller's health. In addition to enhancing physical health, being outdoors can also aid mental wellbeing, including relaxation, happiness and perceptions of greater vitality.

Business travellers are often in a hurry to find a spot inside to catch up with emails and contact colleagues before check-in or get through security as quickly as they can. As soon as you are inside the airport's check-in area, you may notice a distinct lack of any botanical elements. Once through security, this does not improve, and it is near impossible to get outside, except if walking to the plane across a tarmac. Airport terminals are typically perceived as just bricks and mortar, frequently resembling aircraft hangars with a rather sterile environment. Yet, it's the green outdoor constituents which people visually associate with vitality. Without greenery, the traveller's mood lowers, the crowd appears to hover closer, and the atmosphere gradually depresses.

Stopping a while outside before entering the terminal has it's advantageous, firstly the air which is circulating tends to be fresher. While some airports are located near woodlands away from inner city suburbs, other airports may offer a terrace or garden area. Where-ever there is nature, there is usually better air quality, as plants contribute oxygen to the surrounding environment. Breathing in oxygen where the air is less stale brings greater clarity to the brain. Stale air is often shared air, recycled with lower oxygen, higher carbon dioxide content. Our brain uses a large proportion of the oxygen circulating in our blood, so stopping outside a crowded terminal or stepping out every now and again may help raise the oxygen levels circulating in your body and provide more lucidity of thought.

Secondly, sunlight is also essential for good health. Health professionals are discovering the sunshine may have a greater array of health-giving properties than they previously realised. A lot of this is to do with the sunlight stimulating the production of several vital hormones. These contribute to our physical health, including bone mass, muscle strength, possibly immune functions and blood pressure, while simultaneously enhancing our happiness, energy and sleep-wake cycle.

For the business traveller, many of their ailments, such as fatigue and depression, can be improved with a short duration soaking up the sun's rays. Unfortunately, for many of us, most of our time is spent inside a terminal or in transit. The benefits of stopping outside for ten to fifteen minutes unquestionably outweigh the long-term health problems associated with insufficient time alfresco each day. Here are some of those benefits explained with direct relevance to the business traveller.

Enhanced happiness

Sunshine is believed to improve your happiness by increasing the release of serotonin in your brain. Serotonin, frequently referred to as the happy hormone, is associated with boosting mood and helping a person feel calm and focused. It is also a precursor for our sleep hormone, melatonin.

Health researchers believe there may be a biochemical link between the lack of sun, increase production of melatonin (the hormone which triggers sleep), a decrease in serotonin and dopamine (which affect our mood) and seasonal affective disorder (SAD).

The symptoms reported during periods of little sun exposure include depression, fatigue, trouble concentrating, anxiety, irritability, lack of interest in normal activities, increased need for sleep, social withdrawal, greater appetite, weight gain and a craving for carbohydrates, particularly sugary foods. Low levels of serotonin in population studies found a higher risk of SAD (seasonal affective disorder).

Improves your sleep and reduces jet lag

Sunlight stimulates your master body clock and maintains your circadian rhythm to keep the body in homoeostasis (equilibrium). When sunlight hits the eyes, the cells in the retina signal your brain triggering a response in your master body clock, resetting your body's rhythm and keeping it 'on schedule' for the release of hormones which control sleep/wake cycle, aid digestion and regulate metabolic processes.

Sunlight will cause the production of melatonin (your sleep hormone) to decrease, and the release of cortisol (your alert hormone) and serotonin to occur. The sleep-wake cycle is contingent on morning sunlight to help you sleep at night. When exposed to sunlight or brilliant artificial light in the morning, your nocturnal melatonin production will also start sooner in the evening, and you go to sleep more easily at night.

Makes you more active and alert

Serotonin and melatonin levels are interlinked, driven by daylight and darkness. Regular sunlight exposure will increase the serotonin levels in your body, making you feel more active and alert. It is normally produced during the day and converted to melatonin in darkness. Melatonin regulates sleep and brings the onset of sleep faster. Having lower levels of melatonin during the day gives you more get up and go.

Melatonin production has seasonal variations and is produced for a longer duration during winter than in summer. Whereas high melatonin levels correspond to short days and long nights, high serotonin levels in the presence of melatonin reflect long days and short nights. This is why during summer you may need less sleep but still feel livelier.

Hence, it is valuable, even in winter, to ensure you have some sunlight each morning, as having lower levels of melatonin and increased levels of serotonin during the day you may feel you have more get up and go. So, if you are travelling during the daytime, make sure you get some sunlight en route, particularly in the morning, and that you avoid bright light in the evening.

Better still, if you're travelling long haul, then use one of the jet-lag apps mentioned in Chapter 2: Coping with Jetlag, to find the right sunlight time for you based on your journey schedule and destination.

Chronic fatigue moderation

Another benefit is that our body creates vitamin D from direct sunlight. Not getting sufficient Vitamin D from the sun is one hazard of frequent travel. Some research shows an association between low vitamin D status with little sun exposure, as well as seasonal disorders and chronic fatigue syndrome. It is unclear at present just how vital the connection with vitamin D is, and there is a lack of research to establish a firm conclusion.

While you can also obtain vitamin D from your diet by including oily fish, eggs, meat, fortified cereals, soya milk and spreads, getting sufficient sunshine each day has the other health benefits as mentioned here. If possible, it is best to get both sources of vitamin D each day. During winter, you may also need a vitamin D supplement.

Reduces aches and pains

Vitamin D is vital for the regulation of calcium and phosphorus within our bodies, and subsequently essential for healthy bones and muscular activity. Its primary function is to absorb calcium into our bones. Vitamin D deficiency can manifest itself with aching in the bone and muscles due to thinning of the bones and muscular weakness.

Insufficient vitamin D intake affects almost 70% of the European and US population and around 50% of the population worldwide. This pandemic is attributed to lifestyle and environmental factors which reduce exposure to the sunlight. In the UK, approximately 40% of adults have a low blood status during winter.

Business travellers who spend most of their time inside terminals and travelling may be at higher risk of having a low vitamin D status. Ultraviolet B (UVB) of sunlight stimulates the production of the vitamin under the skin. In fact, some estimates report ninety percent of our vitamin D is produced by contact with the sun. This makes it essential for business travellers to seek the sun wherever they can.

Exercise, especially load bearing such as a walk outside, supports calcium reabsorption as well. In fact, exercising outside provides an enormous benefit for bone health. For more information on exercises, you can do while travelling, refer to Chapter 9. We've also listed places for you to get outside just below this section.

Lower blood pressure and cardiovascular disease

Business travellers tend to have higher clinical symptoms of cardiovascular disease, including higher blood pressure. Being outdoors more often may help to lower blood and pulse pressure.

Getting outside and smelling the aroma produced by nature promotes relaxation. A few minutes of deep breathing could help you to relax, reduce your anxiety, remove the tension in your muscles, reduce your heart rate and subsequently lower your blood pressure.

Improved immunity

So, if you've been cooped up on the journey to the airport or realise you're about to spend hours in close quarters with other travellers, then take the opportunity to step outside for a few minutes before commencing the next phase of your journey. From here on, you're about to share the same air, carrying the same germs and contaminants, with thousands of other passengers.

When in proximity to others you are exposed to all sorts of impurities. Fresh air will fill your lungs and help to dilute and remove airborne toxins. What's more, mild exercise, such as a walk outside, can raise your immune system by increasing your 'killer cells' (neutrophils, monocytes and macrophages) which act in your first line of defence against infection. Like all living cells, these attacking cells are oxygen dependent and need oxygen to function if they are to kill and destroy bacteria, viruses and germs.

While some research suggests both UVA and UVB radiation can have a direct effect on immunity, the relationship isn't entirely clear, but it would appear direct sunlight may help raise immunity by also increasing the activity of white blood cells. Other research suggests vitamin D might have a role to play in immunity. Population studies show that those experiencing a range of immunity diseases tend to have low vitamin D status. However, clinical trials show little effect of additional supplementation, inconsistent results for various immunity-based conditions and a lack of evidence.

The most gratifying approach is to ensure you get sufficient sunlight and a balanced diet containing plenty of vitamin D regardless of any existing conditions.

Getting sufficient sunlight and vitamin D

According to the World Health organisation, you only need about 10 – 15 minutes of sunlight on your arms, hands and face to enjoy the vitamin D boosting benefits of the sun. When combined with a walk, it's an excellent way to remain alert and productive. Gatwick Airport has some peaceful places where you can venture out and catch some sunlight. You'll find these calmer places listed below. The UK is notorious for low sunlight levels during winter, so be prepared to get some sun at your destination as well!

Where ever you are, be sure to choose the time of day relevant to the season. The sun is usually at its strongest between midday and 4 pm. The summer sun may be too intense during these hours, while in winter interaction after mid-day might be more beneficial while the sun is at its strongest.

If sunlight isn't readily available or the light is too weak on the days you travel, then you could consider using a light therapy which is used as a treatment for mild SAD and to help regulate your sleep/wake cycle. Doctors and psychologists can provide guidelines on how to use a light therapy box to the maximum effect. You will find some light boxes listed available to order and collect at Gatwick Airport's North Terminal in Chapter 2: Coping with jet-lag.

Another course of action is to ensure you have sufficient Vitamin D in your diet regardless. Seventy percent of Americans and Europeans (including British) are estimated to have a low intake of vitamin D, with 40% of UK adults having a low blood status during winter months. As a business traveller, the odds are you could have a low status if you haven't been out and about during your trip days.

The recently revised UK recommended intake of vitamin D for adults is now 10 ug per day, and Europe has just set their recommended adequate intake to 15 ugs per day, to help health professionals encourage European consumers to make healthier diet choices. The higher recommended amount set by the EU takes into account the higher latitudes where sunshine hours are less, and where the sun is weaker, which typically results in limited levels of synthesised vitamin D. The USA has a similar value.

Overall, whichever country you spend your time in, the combination of getting more sunlight and a balanced diet will help raise your vitamin D status, particularly if it is low due to a demanding business travel schedule. If you are not consuming sufficient vitamin D during winter and spring or periods of low sunshine, then you should also consider taking a vitamin D supplement.

To help you choose foods with good sources of vitamin D, we have listed the menu items at the cafes and restaurants in Gatwick Airports North Terminal, which contain ingredients that are high in vitamin D. Adequate vitamin D is essential for bone health and muscle strength. Although, health claims for vitamin D to cure fatigue or SAD isn't currently approved; it is important to include sources of vitamin D in your diet anyway, particularly when sunlight is more scarce. We've listed menu items for you in the final section below.

Sunny spots at Gatwick's North Terminal

Gatwick is surrounded by a green belt assortment of pastures, thicket and woodlands. The rural location has a sparsely populated area which also helps to maintain satisfactory air quality. In fact, Gatwick Airport has very low levels of pollutants surrounding the airport and has reportedly never breached UK or EU annual air quality limits. It is one of the largest airports in the world, yet one of the freshest airports and reported cleanest aircraft fleets in Europe.

Unfortunately, the access to green spaces outside the North Terminal is a bit of challenge as Gatwick is enclosed by several busy access and main roads. The best way to enter nearby parklands is either by walking north, which takes about 10 minutes or by catching a shuttle to the South Terminal and then walking to the nearest park area, which also takes about 10 minutes.

Alas, unlike some newer airports, there also is no greenery inside the North Terminal. Although there are plenty of viewing passages, the view is restricted to the loading bays, runways and terminal buildings. So, if you are keen to get some fresh air or to take in a landscape view, it's best to do so before you progress through security.

We've done some searching and found some locations which you may find worthwhile venturing to.

Just outside

On Check-in Level 2, just outside Jamie's Coffee Lounge and the Nicholas Culpeper Restaurant, there is a promenade between the car park and the airport entrance. You can catch some sunshine here on a summer's day. However, there are no plants, and the nearby view is entirely comprised of hotels, Gatwick shuttle terminal and the car park opposite.

Just inside

Just inside the entrance on Check-in, Level Two, to the left when you enter, next to the Emirates ticket and information counter, is a bay of seats in front of the window. The full glass framed windows provide sunlight and warmth on a winter's day, so you won't need to endure the cold weather outside. Although it won't be sufficient to synthesise vitamin D, there is a greater feel-good factor here than other seating areas within the airport.

River Mole

The River Mole runs along the Perimeter Road north of Gatwick Airport. It stretches all the way from the River Thames at Hampton Court, where it is a tributary, and flows around Gatwick Airport to Horsham. The river boasts the highest diversity of fish species of any river in England. On a warm summer's day, you will find residents fishing along its banks. You may also notice some wildlife such as rabbits, birds and squirrels, as you proceed along the path to the river, through the woodlands. It should take about 10 – 15 minutes (1300 steps) to reach the bridge over the River Mole.

Please note, the walk is along a dirt track which may become muddy during rainy periods, so make sure you are wearing comfortable outdoor shoes and have placed your luggage into early check-in or at the Excess Baggage company if needed.

Location: On the north side of Gatwick Airport on Perimeter Road.
Access: Walk outside the terminal entrance on Level One, and take the lift on the left, at the far end of the shuttle to the ground level. Walk left along the path, towards the Arrivals Road, on the opposite side from the Premier Inn. At the traffic island, cross over the road, walk right, but stay on the side opposite the Premier Inn. At the large roundabout, cross over Longbridge Way, and take the path on the left through the woodlands which is parallel to A23 London Road. A small brook will run between the Woodland Path and the road A23. Keep following the path through the woods until you come to the bridge at the River Mole.

Riverside Garden Park

Originally part of Horley Common, this former farmland is now an attractive public open space, occupied by rich woodlands and grassy glades. It hosts a human-made lake and is a favourite walking area for residents with their dogs. There is also a cycle path to get to and from Gatwick Airport, and residents are often seen fishing in the Gatwick Stream which runs through it. It's best to catch a shuttle to the South Terminal and then walk through the Garden Park. The walk takes about 10 minutes.

Location: Opposite Gatwick South Terminal on the North side of the Airport Way main road.
Access: Take the shuttle to the South Terminal. On the left-hand side of the shuttle (when facing the shuttle), at the far end there is a stairway which leads to ground level outside. Take the steps down to the ground level, turn right, cross over Caledonian Way, and keep going for roughly 50 steps until you come to two

underpasses. Walk towards the underpass on the right; signposted "Sussex border path 1989 #2" and "Car Park B". Keep walking on the path, which goes through the underpass, and eventually towards a second underpass, which goes under the Airport Way. Keep going until you reach the human-made lake. You'll find some benches here to sit at overlooking the lake.

Church Meadows

Church Meadows is a public open space which has been left undeveloped. It is within half hour walking distance from the airport and comprises meadow land and grassed open spaces. It is located on the western edge of Horley, adjacent to the A23 opposite Gatwick Airport. The meadow and grassland have some spectacular wildflowers which bloom during summer and is frequently used for picnics. The River Mole runs along the western edge where you might spot another resident fishing.

Location: Northeast of Gatwick Airport, situated on the north side of Brighton Road which runs adjacent to the A23 on the east side of Gatwick Airport. The meadow is south-west of St. Bartholomew's Church.

Access: If you go by car, travel along the A23 and take the third exit on the right at the round-about onto Brighton Road. The Meadows are on the left-hand side. If you walk, then it's easier if you use a navigation app to source walking directions, such as Google Maps.

Where to find good sources of vitamin D

There are many restaurants, cafes and retail shops which stock menu items with ingredients which are a good source of vitamin D. Making sure you consume at least one serving each day of foods which are a good source of vitamin D can be rather pleasurable. This is especially true if you enjoy oily fish (such as salmon, tuna or trout) or caviar, eggs and cheese.

You'll find the retail shops and cafes in Arrivals and Check-in areas have packaged items available all day, so you can quickly grab an item and continue with your journey at any time.

The same is also true If there is insufficient time before your flight to enjoy a meal, as there are also plenty of grab and go options which you can take with on board the plane. Restaurants tend to open until early evening (8.30 pm), but Starbucks Cafe offers items all day.

Boots the Chemist

Boots the Chemist is located on the lower level of the Departure Lounge and in the Arrivals Hall. There are two Boots the Chemist shops in the Departure Lounge. The nearest one to the security exit is the smaller. They stock a limited range of food items which contain a good source of vitamin D. The store at the end of the Departure Lounge offers a greater range of items.

Opening in Arrivals: 24 hours
Opening in Departure Lounge: 4.00 am to 8.300 pm
Telephone: 01293 569606
Website: www.boots.com

Grab and Go Snacks include;
Egg and Spinach 88 g One free-range hard-boiled egg and fresh spinach.
Prawn and Salmon Sushi 126 g Prawn Mayonnaise and re pepper California Roll, Smoked Salmon Nigiri, King Prawn Nigiri, Smoked Mackerel Hosomaki and surimi and Edamame Bean California roll.
Smoked Salmon Sushi Snack 66 g Smoked salmon California roll, smoked salmon hosomaki, cucumber hosomaki.
Large sushi 244 g
Spicy Tuna California Rolls 135 g 6 tuna, lime and coriander California rolls with a shichimi and sesame seed coating. Soya Sauce provided in a separate bottle.

Arrivals, Ground Floor
Costa Coffee

If you have just arrived and will be setting off on the next part of your journey soon, then you can also pick up a quick sandwich and hot beverage from Costa Coffee anytime. Here are a couple of prepacked items which are good sources of vitamin D.

Location: Situated on the left as you exit from International Arrivals.
Opening hours: 24 hours

Grab and Go Items include:
Free Range Egg Sandwich 342 kcal (1435 kJ)
Smoked Salmon and Soft Cheese Sandwich 388 kcal (1627 kJ)

Tuna Nicoise Salad 219 kcal (914 kJ)
Tuna Melt Panini 470 kcal (1976 kJ)
Scrambled Egg & Mushroom Muffin 298 kcal (1252kJ)

Marks and Spencer

M & S Simply Food at Gatwick North is a small supermarket store offering packaged food items which you can take on board with you. There are several items which contain good sources of vitamin D. If you choose a fresh item, then ensure you eat it soon after purchase to avoid any unwanted traveller's tummy.

Open: 24 hours
Location: Ground floor, between Boots the Chemist and Costa Coffee.

Grab and Go Items include:

Salmon & Prawn Nigiri Three king prawn and two Lochmuir salmon nigiri with soy sauce.
Free Range Egg & Spinach Protein Pot 105 g Two cooked free-range eggs and spinach. Per portion 152 kcal (633 kJ)
Oak Smoked Salmon & Egg Protein Pot Boiled egg, smoked salmon and spinach. One portion packet is 106 kcal (442 kJ)
Egg and Avocado Protein Pot 140 g. This pot contains boiled free range eggs, quinoa and avocado with parsley and light soy sauce. Per portion 185 kcal (776 kJ)
Honey Smoked Salmon & Lentil Salad Honey smoked Lochmuir salmon with black lentils, peas, sorghum and kale salad with a fromage frais and mustard dressing. Per portion: 253 kcal (1063 kJ)

Check-in, Level One

The options are limited in the Check-in area, but we have found a couple for you to try.

Hampton by Hilton incorporating Starbucks

Hampton by Hilton offers a bar menu 24 hours a day and provide a couple of options for you to choose. You can also arrive for breakfast, from £7.50, and opt for a hot meal which includes poached, boiled or scrambled eggs.

Open: Bar Menu is 24 hours, and Hot Breakfast 6.00 am to 10.00 am
Location: The entrance to this hotel is right near the Easy Jet Check-in on level one. Just follow the signs to the right of the check-in desk. You will see a sign above the entrance to the corridor for the Hampton by Hilton.

Items include:
Salmon Fillet Salad Tossed mixed salad leaves with cucumber, sliced red onion, tomatoes & croutons with lemon and French dressing.
Baked Potato with Tuna Mayo served with salad and coleslaw.

Check-in, Level Two
Jamie's Coffee Lounge
At the front windows, near the entrance, on Level two is Jamie's Coffee Lounge. You can't miss it as they've parked a van alongside it, inside the terminal. Famous for great tasting food, most of the items here are prepacked so you can quickly grab and take them with you.

Although there is a limited range here, you will find Jamie's food is very filling, and as they are based on healthy eating guidelines, they generally hit the target for providing healthier food options.

Locations: Next to Nicholas Culpeper at the front entrance.
Opening hours: 24 hours

Salmon Salad Pot: Hot smoked salmon, beetroot, fennel rocket, lemon yoghurt, lemon spinach, grapes, dill, olive oil, balsamic vinegar, thyme, mustard seeds, sugar and salt

Departure Lounge, Lower Level
Caviar House & Prunier
This could be a good excuse to treat yourself to a little extravagance. Oily fish and caviar are good sources of vitamin D. Unfortunately, the lower-fat menu items, such as shell-fish, crustacea and white fish only contain a trace amount. The following menu items include ingredients which are good sources of vitamin D.

Open: 4.00 am to 8.30 pm
Location: Middle of the lower floor, opposite Lacoste and Dune, just before World Duty Free at the far end.

Menu Items include:
Scrambled Egg & Scottish Smoked Salmon
Scrambled Egg & Balik Smoked Salmon

Scrambled Egg, Balik Smoked Salmon & Caviar
Caviar including Prunier Caviar, Prunier Saint James, Prunier Paris and Caviar House Selection.
Tuna Tartare Comprised freshly diced tuna, served with avocado, crispy onions and a citrus, soy sauce. Hold the soy sauce if you want to reduce the salt content.
Tsarina Blini topped with crème Fraiche, served with Balik smoked salmon and 10 g of Prunier caviar.
Fillet Tsar Nikolaj The tender part of Balik salmon, carved from the rear fillet.
Balik Sliced Salmon Original or Gravlax.
Balik Delight Either Discovery (a tasting platter of Balik smoked salmon) or Tartar (Balik salmon fillet finely chopped and seasoned.
Smoked Salmon & Shrimps Balik smoked salmon accompanied by succulent tiger prawns.
Scottish Smoked Salmon Finest Salmon from the pure waters of Scotland.
King Crab & Caviar King crab legs accompanied by a spoon of Prunier caviar.
Lobster & Caviar Either whole or half lobster served with 20 g Prunier caviar.
Seafood Platter A combination of smoked salmon, Balk gravlax, Balik tartar, shrimps, king prawn and oyster, accompanied by caviar.

Departure Lounge, Upper Level
Armadillo Restaurant
You can opt for eggs and salmon style dishes as part of their all-day brunch or choose one of the following main meals comprising of ingredients containing a good source of Vitamin D.

Open: 4.00 am to 8.30 pm
Location: Next to the balcony, opposite Garfunkel's.

Breakfast Items include:
Avocado Southwest Free-range scrambled eggs, smashed fresh avocado, red chilli, fresh watercress, pico de gallo salsa and a toasted muffin.
Full Works Open Omelette Free range 3 egg open pan omelette, rainbow peppers, tomato, mushrooms, fresh parsley, jack cheese, pico de gallo salsa. You can also add smoked salmon.
Free Range Eggs Any Style choice of fried, scrambled or poaches free range eggs on toast.

Main meal items include:

Chopped Chef Salad containing diced chicken, hard boiled free range egg, blue cheese, radish, tomato, cucumber, tortilla strips, charred corn, fresh herbs, cumin and sweet onion vinaigrette.

Pan Roast Salmon Fillet, served with pickled beetroot, mooli, carrot and charred corn. Served with green rice.

Comptoir Libanais

Comptoir Libanais offers mainly lamb and chicken dishes on their menu. While lamb and chicken contain a small amount of vitamin D, salmon is a better source with at least five times the amount.

Open: 4.00 am to 8.30 pm
Location: At the back of the Upper floor, opposite stairs at far right.

Breakfast items include:

Smoked Salmon & Scrambled Eggs Scrambled eggs and smoked salmon on sourdough toast, sprinkled with pomegranate seeds.

Eggs on Toast Scrambled or fried eggs on brioche or sourdough toast.

Folded Omelette Plain Freshly made to order. Three egg omelette served with roasted vine tomato.

Shakshuka with Feta Slow cooked tomatoes, red onions and peppers mixed with parsley, coriander and garlic. Topped with a baked egg and crumbled feta, served with warm pita bread.

Sirine Vegetarian Breakfast Two falafels, two eggs scrambled, avocado, halloumi cheese, vine tomato, olive and garnished with mint leaves, zaatar and sumac.

Main meal items include:

Pan Roasted Salmon served with vermicelli rice, harissa sauce, pickles, fattoush salad and garnished with pomegranate seeds.

EAT

There are many salads and sandwiches at EAT Café which contains foods with good sources of vitamin D. Items with excessively high salt contents have not been included, or we've indicated which accompaniment can be avoided to reduce the total amount of salt or excess fat.

Open: 4.00 am to 8.30 pm
Location: In the middle of the back of the upper floor, next to the public toilets.

Breakfast items include:

Poached Egg, Jarlsberg and mushroom crusty roll. 332 kcal (1389 kJ)

BBQ beans, poached egg & ham hock Breakfast pot of poached egg, smoked ham hock served with BBQ beans. 334 kcal (1397 kJ)

BBQ beans, poached egg, avocado & Feta cheese Breakfast pot of poached egg, avocado mash and feta served with BBQ baked beans. 389 kcal (1628 kJ)

Scottish Smoked Salmon & Avocado in a freshly baked baguette. 369 kcal (1544 kJ)

Free Range Egg & Tomato British free-range egg mayonnaise and tomato, served within a freshly baked baguette. 371 kcal (1552 kJ)

Grab and Go Items include:

Free Range Egg & Chilli Greens A whole free-range egg served with edamame beans, peas, spinach, chilli and lemon juice. 116 kcal (485 kJ)

Hot Smoked Salmon & Sour Cream Rye with cucumber, dill and capers. 447 kcal (1870 kJ)

Hot Smoked Salmon & Greens A Nicoise salad made with Scottish hot-smoked salmon, parsley potatoes, capers, plum tomatoes, green beans, hard-boiled egg and salad leaves. Hold the Balsamic dressing. 461 kcal (1929 kJ)

Smoked Salmon & Egg Fit Box with dressing Smoked salmon served with egg, chargrilled garlic and chilli broccoli, spinach and salsa verde dressing. 202 kcal (845 kJ)

Crayfish, Avocado & Free Range Egg Salad Mixed salad leaves with crayfish tails, avocado and free range egg. Hold the dressing. 388 kcal (1623 kJ)

Ham Hock and Egg Salad A protein packed snack bowl with mixed leaves topped with a free-range egg and ham hock served with Dijon mustard dressing. 342 kcal (1431 kJ)

Chunky Free Range Egg Sandwich Freshly baked malted bread filled with free range egg mayonnaise. 403 kcal (1686 kJ)

Tuna Mayonnaise & Cucumber Sandwich Tuna mayonnaise and thick sliced cucumber served on malted granary bread. 365 kcal (1527 kJ)

Smoked Salmon & Soft Cheese Freshly baked malted bread filled with peppered soft cheese and Scottish smoked Salmon. 367 kcal (1535 kJ)

Garfunkel's Restaurant

Garfunkel's offers several items which may contain a good source of vitamin D. However; we could not locate any nutritional information, so are not able to fully assess all possible items. Choose from these menu items to add foods with a good source of vitamin D to your diet.

Open: 4.00 am to 8.30 pm

Location: At the back of the Upper Floor, opposite Armadillo.

Breakfast items include:
Smoked Salmon & Scrambled Eggs Smoked salmon with scrambled eggs, served with brown toast.

Scrambled Eggs on Toast Freshly made with three eggs, served with brown toast.

Garfunkel's Omelette A freshly cooked omelette made with three eggs served with two hash browns, grilled tomato and pea shoots.

Main Meal items include:
Omelettes Choose from a plain omelette, a single filling omelette and a double filling omelette.

Veggie Frittata Packed full of onion, sliced mushrooms and roasted pepper.

Tuna Mayo Toastie Tuna mayonnaise, red onion & Applewood smoked cheddar cheese.

Pret A Manger

Pret A Manger offers one of the largest selections of menu items with ingredients which are a good source of Vitamin D. What's more, they are already packaged and can be taken on board your flight as a takeaway option.

Open: 3.00 am to 8.30 pm
Location: Next to the escalator at the far end of the Upper Floor.

Grab and Go Items include:
Egg & Avocado Protein Pot A handful of fresh spinach topped with diced avocado and British free-range eggs. This pot provides 224 kcal (925 kJ)

Egg & Spinach Protein Pot. Two British free-range boiled eggs and a handful of fresh baby spinach leaves. Per 99 g serving 104 kcal (437 kJ)

Smoked Salmon & Egg Protein Pot Scottish smoked salmon and a free-range egg with baby spinach. Served with a lemon wedge and seasoning. This pot provides 134 kcal (560 kJ)

Tuna Nicoise Salad Classic salad made with pole and line caught tuna and sliced free range egg. Also has a cluster of baby plum tomatoes, Kalamata olives, cucumber and fresh salad leaves. With dressing 309 g serving provides 469 kcal (1948 kJ). Without dressing 259 g serving provides 176 kcal (738 kJ)

Sesame Salmon & Black Rice Roasted salmon coated with sesame seeds paired with black rice, served with long-stem broccoli, pickled cabbage & carrot salad, edamame beans and a pot of zingy green dressing. This salad provides 369 kcal (1541 kJ)

Sandwiches

Cracking Egg Salad Sandwich A sandwich with an Italian twist. Chunky egg mayo with slices of tomato and fresh wild rocket. Sandwich provides 375 kcal (1575 kJ)

Free Range Egg Mayo Sandwich Free-range eggs are boiled and chopped chunky, mixed with free-range mayonnaise, cracked black pepper, and celery salt is added, along with a sprinkle of mustard cress. Sandwich provides 367 kcal (1542 kJ)

Tuna and Cucumber Sandwich Pole & line caught skipjack tuna mayo with spring onions, chopped capers, a touch of anchovy paste and a squeeze of lemon with sliced cucumbers. The sandwich provides 540 kcal (2268 kJ)

Scottish Smoked Salmon Sandwich Scottish smoked salmon sandwich with lemon juice and seasoning on granary bread. Sandwich provides 421 kcal (1761 kJ)

Pole & Line Caught Tuna and Rocket Baguette Mashed skipjack tuna with mayonnaise, spring onion, chopped capers, anchovy paste, a squeeze of lemon spooned on to malted bread with thick slices of cucumber, fresh rocket and seasoning. This baguette provides 540 kcal (2259 kJ)

Free-range Egg Mayo & Roasted Tomato Baguette Free-range egg mayo with roasted tomatoes. This baguette provides 447 kcal (1880 kJ)

Free-range Egg Mayo & Avocado Baguette Chunky free-range egg mayo with freshly sliced avocado and a twist of seasoning. This baguette provides 571 kcal (2390 kJ)

Mediterranean Tuna Flat Bread Pole and line caught skipjack tuna mayo with spring onion, chopped capers, a touch of anchovy paste and a squeeze of lemon on flatbread with added Greek Kalamata olives, baby leaf spinach, tomatoes and red pepper. This flatbread provides 539 kcal (2262 kJ)

Hot Items

Mexican Egg & Bean Toasted Tortilla Pret's version of Huevos Rancheros. A toasted free-range egg, avocado, feta, Mexican-style beans and a handful of fresh coriander in a kibbled rye wrap. This tortilla provides 403 kcal (1687 kJ)

Tuna Melt Toastie Generous chunks of pole & line caught tuna with Greve cheese, red onion and a dab of mayo in between two slices of our 7-seeded bloomer bread. This toastie provides 552 kcal (2318 kJ)

Starbucks

If it's just a quick sandwich, then Starbucks offers several products which contain good sources of vitamin D. They are prepared daily, making them a good option for taking on board the flight with you.

Open: 24 hours
Location: In the middle of the upper floor next to the public toilets.

Grab and Go Items include:

Smoked Salmon Bagel Hand cured west coast Scottish salmon made on top of a malted bagel with cream cheese. This bagel provides 472 kcal (1975 kJ)

Sure as Eggs is Eggs Sandwich. A double-decker egg sandwich comprising creamy seasoned free-range egg mayonnaise, topped with sliced hardboiled eggs and crisp, peppery cress, served on malted brown bread. This sandwich provides 388 kcal. (1621kJ)

Tuna Panini Pole and line caught tuna flakes with mature cheddar, mayonnaise-Bechamel sauce, Mozzarella, spring onion, chives and sweetcorn in a panini. This panini provides 496 kcal (2075 kJ)

Scrambled Egg & Mushroom Muffin This muffin provides 298 kcal (1252 kJ)

Hot Breakfast Box

Super Scrambled Eggs, Tomato and Spinach Creamy scrambled eggs served on a bed of spinach leaves, with slow-roasted tomatoes and topped with a sprinkling of mixed seeds. This hot box provides 211 kcal (882 kJ)

Yo! Sushi

Asian food always comes at the price of high salt. Aim for menu items which contain oily fish, including caviar, eggs and pork-based dishes, as these are higher in vitamin D than other menu items, and choose items which have no added sauces or seaweed as an ingredient so to restrict the salt content. We have picked some items for you which are lowest in salt, based on the nutritional information provided.

Open: 6.00 am to 8.30 pm
Location: In the corner of the upper floor at the far end.

Rolls

Salmon Dragon Roll California roll topped with fresh salmon, shichimi powder and spring onion. 192 kcal (803 kJ)

Spicy Tuna Roll Chopped yellowfin tuna, spicy sriracha and rayu chilli oil nori roll with shichimi powder. 106 kcal (444 kJ)

YO! Roll Fresh salmon, avocado and Japanese mayonnaise roll with orange masago. 144 kcal (602 kJ)

Dynamite Roll Salmon, avocado and rayu chilli oil topped with sriracha, mayo and spring onion. 197 kcal (824 kJ)

Maki

Salmon Maki small nori roll filled with fresh salmon. Four pieces. 126 kcal (527 kJ)
Tuna Maki Small nori roll filled with fresh tuna. Four pieces. 119 kcal (498 kJ)

Nigiri

Tamago Nigiri Rice block topped with sweet and light egg omelette and nori. 262 kcal (1096 kJ)

Salmon Nigiri Rice block topped with fresh-cut salmon and a touch of wasabi. 99 kcal (414 kJ)

Albacore Tuna Nigiri Rice block topped with quick-seared albacore tuna topped with truffle ponzu and spring onions. 95 kcal (397 kJ)

Sashimi

Salmon Sashimi Fresh cuts of thick sliced salmon with mooli and lemon. 140 kcal (586 kJ)

Tuna Sashimi Thick cut slices of yellowfin tuna, with mooli and lime. 106 kcal (444 kJ)

Salmon & Yuzu Salsa Sashimi Thinly sliced salmon served up with a yuzu & ponzu dressing. 104 kcal (435 kJ)

Salmon Selection Two slices of sashimi and two pieces of maki and nigiri all on one plate. 220 kcal (920 kJ)

Albacore Truffle Ponzu Sashimi Lightly seared tuna with a truffle ponzu dressing. 72 kcal (301 kJ)

Temaki

Salmon & Avocado Temaki Hand roll with nori wrapped rice cone with fresh salmon, avocado, mayo and toasted sesame seeds. 163 kcal (682 kJ)

SECTION FOUR: Healthy Traveller's Fare
Chapter 11: Hydration

Hydration helps to keep you healthy

Making sure you have adequate hydration when travelling on business is well worth considering. Even mild dehydration (1 - 5%) can induce thirst, lethargy, discomfort, increased pulse rate, fatigue, irritability, impatience, and reduced concentration, meaning you are not performing at your best when you work and travel. Dehydration also increases the risk of more severe conditions, such as high blood pressure, DVT and respiratory conditions when flying.

Unfortunately, business travellers are more susceptible to becoming mildly dehydrated than office workers. The rationale is quite simple. It's mainly to do with decreased fluid intake and increased output. When you travel, your usual routine is interrupted, and you may not consume as many drinks throughout the day as you would when at your desk or home. Tight travel schedules mean you focus on meeting business travel arrangements and forget to drink before and during the journey. Then there's a lack of access to your customary beverages, and the usual preferred choice of drink becomes more hit and miss, depending on what you enjoy and if you know where you can find it.

On top of this, due to travel schedules and lack of availability, you probably don't eat the same foods which would typically contribute to your fluid intake. On average, the food you usually eat would supply a litre of fluid to your daily intake. If you eat less of the foods which have a high water content, such as yoghurt, soups, casseroles, vegetables and fruit, than you normally would, then your fluid intake from food could easily be halved.

Then there's the loss of body fluid. Business people are more likely to drink alcohol when travelling than when they are office based. If you have had any alcohol the night before or en route, then your body may have increased its urinary output, as alcohol is a diuretic. It happens as a result of the alcohol inhibiting your brain receiving messages about your internal fluid concentrations. Consequently, it reduces the secretion of hormones that help control your body's fluid balance and causes you to excrete too much water. Thus, it can lead to mild dehydration.

There is also the environment you're travelling in which affects your body's requirements for fluid. The loss of water from your body increases at high altitudes coupled with an increased rate of breathing and a drier atmosphere. Indeed, you may find the air on the plane much drier than normal contributing to an increased loss of water from your respiratory tract as you breathe, plus there is the moisture loss from your skin. The humidity on the plane is a lot lower than other environments and set at 10 to 20 per cent compared to your office, which is typically set at 30 to 65 percent. In fact, the level of humidity can be drier than the Sahara Desert, causing you to lose more fluid than normal.

Finally, there is another type of loss, which up to 60% of international travellers suffer from; the dreaded traveller's tummy. It is particularly common for business travellers whose gastrointestinal tracts may be sensitive to changes in cuisine, although more so for those who journey to areas with poor water and food hygiene. If the water loss from diarrhoea or vomiting is severe, then electrolytes may also be lost, making flying less enjoyable and potentially unsafe. Severe diarrhoea and vomiting may be better remedied with electrolyte solutions or treatment under medical supervision.

Each of these factors contributes to reduced fluid intake and increased output. So, if you're not replenishing your body with sufficient liquids and foods while travelling, you may begin to suffer from symptoms of dehydration.

It's better to stay well hydrated

The savvy business traveller needs to be mindful of their body's water requirements. Water is essential. It is the major constituent of the body and supports many functions including transporting oxygen, glucose and various other nutrients, removing waste products, acting as a lubricant to your joints, supporting your immune system and regulating your body's temperature.

All of which are relevant to maintaining a healthy body and mind for business travel. If you don't consume sufficient water, you will notice an increase in thirst and several other unwelcome side effects. It is important to get the right amount of fluid to be healthy, fit and productive. Here are the main benefits of remaining well hydrated.

Reduce the likelihood of traveller's fatigue

Fatigue is one of the common symptoms of dehydration. Even at 1% loss of body fluid, you start to feel tired. One percent fluid loss for an adult could be a little as two cups of water (400 ml). When combined with the cramped environment and the inability to rest en route, drinking insufficient amounts of fluids will significantly add to the strain of travel that you may already be experiencing. To help prevent the onset of undue fatigue, make sure you stay well hydrated and avoid alcohol.

Staying alert and productive

Tiredness, impaired concentration, lack of motivation to move, lethargy and general malaise are all symptoms of mild dehydration. If you feel tired, cranky, moody, unable to focus or have a headache, then you will be less likely to function at your best, particularly if your concentration has declined. Worse still, you might end up offending your business contacts unwittingly with an abrupt or less considerate response. The best way to stay hydrated when working is to keep a glass or bottle of water handy and sip constantly.

Preventing traveller's colds

Sitting in an environment with low humidity and circulating air, could leave you more susceptible to catching a respiratory infection, such as a cold. Humidity keeps your airways moist, which helps the mucosal lining to trap any germs that might enter. If the air is too dry, then the mucus can't do its job, allowing viruses or bacteria to enter your bloodstream more quickly. On top of drinking sufficient fluid, you might consider a saline nasal spray or eye drops.

Lessening traveller's constipation

One of the main reasons why business travellers could suffer from constipation is inadequate fluid intake. It is usually a result of your body needing to retain water if you haven't had sufficient to drink. Becoming mildly dehydrated will increase the likelihood of constipation as the body needs to reabsorb any fluid to maintain a water-electrolyte balance. Constipation will also contribute to traveller fatigue, discomfort when travelling and increased irritability.

There are three essential components to aid digestion and prevent constipation. These encompass adequate hydration, plenty of fibre in the diet and movement. Hydration and fibre work together. Fibre absorbs water to create a softer stool to ease the transit of waste through your intestines. However, it will give up the water if needed. It's important to make sure you consume plenty of cereals, fruit and vegetables during your journey as these will provide both fibre and liquid.

Reducing jet lag

Dehydration can contribute to the feelings of jet-lag. Business travellers who journey across several time zones may feel tired and out of sorts due to the disruption of their body clock. Being dehydrated could add further fatigue.

Moreover, dehydration may also make it harder to adjust to a new rhythm as it can disrupt homoeostasis, the delicate balancing act for various internal processes. Drinking sufficient fluids throughout your destination's daytime may also help to readjust the body clock by re-establishing routine.

Lowering the risk of Deep Vein Thrombosis (DVT)

When we don't consume sufficient water, our body compensates through a series of actions so it can keep our blood circulating to our tissues with its supply of oxygen and nutrients. This includes sending messages to induce thirst and releasing hormones to prevent further loss of water in the urine. Also, when at high altitudes, the body may also increase red blood cell production to circulate oxygen around more efficiently.

Dehydration causes blood vessels to narrow and blood to thicken. This in turn makes the blood flow much slower, raising the risk of blood cells and other constituents sticking together, increasing the risk of blood clots. As your body becomes dehydrated, your heart has to work harder to pump thicker blood through the vessels, increasing the risk of deep vein thrombosis. Drinking sufficient water may help the blood to circulate more efficiently.

How much should a busy traveller drink?

To keep hydrated when travelling, health experts recommend aiming for a cup of water (200 ml) each hour. If in doubt, check the colour of your urine. It should be a pale tint of yellow. Anything darker than a light lemon or straw colour and you could probably do with a top-up of fluid.

It does not include the alcoholic variety, as alcohol is a diuretic and will serve to dehydrate you further. If you do have a glass of wine or beer, then consider a low alcohol variety, diluting it with tonic water or taking a drink of water to match each time.

Dietitians also recommend reflecting on how often you go to the toilet during the day. If your urine is a light yellow, there's sufficient volume, and you are going every two to four hours, then you're likely to be well hydrated. If you have gone from morning to mid–afternoon without a toilet break (eight hours), then you probably need to drink more.

Which fluids are best?

Fluid intakes include a variety of drinks, such as tea, coffee, milk, fruit juice, smoothies, etc., along with food. However, it is important to choose any alternative to water wisely as, although they all provide fluid and some nutrients, they may also contain calories, sugar and other less desirable substances. Drinking calories is an easy way to gain weight, and if the drink is high in sugar, then it can also have other harmful effects such as dental decay. Some drinks are also acidic, causing additional damage to the tooth enamel as well if drunk too often.

While drinking water is an excellent choice, as it won't provide calories or damage your teeth, there are other drinks which are equally, if not, more efficient at hydration. However, variety and moderation is a good rule of thumb. So choose your hydration method according to your requirements, tastes and travel plans.

Milk

Milk, for example, is an excellent hydrator. However, you wouldn't want to drink eight glasses a day as you might be consuming excess calories and saturated fat. Nor would you want to carry a bottle of milk around with you due to its perishable nature. Nevertheless, if you've been running on empty during your journey, you might like to consider rehydrating, while simultaneously consuming your dairy quota for the day, by drinking milk before boarding the plane. Advantages can outweigh the negatives, as bottled milk is usually less expensive than bottled water, and contains essential nutrients such as calcium and B vitamins. As an alternative to water, this is as good as they get. Therefore, we've listed some outlets for you to purchase milk further down this chapter.

Fruit juice

Fruit juice is slightly more hydrating than water. Juice also classifies as one of your five recommended portions of fruit and vegetables per day. But only one a day, not several, should be counted towards your five a day. Fruit juice may contain several fruits juiced together. As they are no longer in a whole form, the fibre contents are less intact, and sugars are now free to interact more with the enamel on your teeth. Along with calories, fruit juice is also acidic and will damage the enamel. Overall, you will be consuming the calories of several pieces of whole fruit in one glass with a high sugar and acidic content.

Hence, it is better to avoid drinking fruit juice between meals and more than once a day. One other option could be to dilute the juice. This can make it more efficient as a hydrator and less damaging to your health.

Smoothies

Smoothies may contain several different fruits and vegetables, and due to their mix and pulp constituents, smoothies are often promoted as nutrient-dense. However, they are also frequently energy-dense! Some airport smoothies can be as high in calories as a meal (more than 400 calories in one drink). Similar to fruit juice, they are acidic and contain free sugars which can be potentially harmful to your teeth. Also, there can be a rapid uptake of sugar into your body so a large smoothie can have a similar effect to a sweet dessert.

We've listed smoothies and fruit juices in our Chapter 14 on Five a Day. Although they contribute fluid to your diet, they also constitute a fruit and vegetable. The advice from health experts is to limit both fruit juice and smoothies to a combined total of 150 ml, which is usually much less than many of the fresh juice and smoothies now offered at most airports.

Tea and coffee

Tea and coffee also contribute to the fluid intake and can help to rehydrate, but they also contain caffeine. Despite popular belief, coffee and tea which contain caffeine in modest amounts, do not have a significant diuretic effect. While, research indicates very strong coffee may promote excretion, mild tea and coffee, served with milk, has been found to be slightly more hydrating than water. However, the caffeine is a stimulant and can adversely affect sleep. According to the WHO, caffeine is best avoided four to six hours before sleep when travelling and if caffeine is drunk during the daytime, small amounts of mild coffee every two hours or so are preferable to one large, strong cup as a single dose.

Hot chocolate and malted milk

It really depends on the brand as to how much sugar and caffeine are present in hot chocolate. Most commercial chocolate powders and café made hot chocolates and malted milk are high in sugar. For this reason, they are better consumed as a treat or a replacement for a dessert.

Caffeine is present in cocoa. However, in some branded hot chocolate powder it is minuscule, with a teaspoon only containing 2 mg of caffeine, making it suitable as an evening drink after a meal. Some research suggests hot chocolate made with milk may help induce sleep. Hence, it might be worth considering bringing your own sachet and adding it to a cup of hot milk on the flight. Hot malted milk with no caffeine is another good option.

The choice of which beverage to have will ultimately come down to taste, availability and most importantly, variety. Whichever you choose, it's worthwhile to stay well hydrated.

How much fluid is too much?

Drinking excessive amounts of fluids is not okay either, and too much water can in some instances be dangerous. Although it is scarce, it can be achieved by an excessive amount of fluid intake in a short period. Some bloggers, who aren't qualified, have suggested one litre an hour! Not only is this impractical (imagine everyone taking 12 litres on a 12-hour journey) but it is also very irresponsible, as too much water can be fatal. If you are passing urine very frequently and your urine is clear, you may be drinking more than you need. Aim for a lemon or straw colour urine output.

Eight easy ways to keep hydrated when travelling

You may feel that consuming sufficient fluids is easier said than done, particularly when on the run to meet travel arrangements. However, it can be easily managed so it fits in with your travel routine and fluid availability.

Here are eight straightforward ways of ensuring you are adequately hydrated when travelling without a lot of fuss.

1. Prepare before you start out

Don't start your trip already thirsty as this is a sign you may already be deficient in your fluid intake. Make sure the day before you travel you have had plenty to drink. You will be able to tell by the colour of your urine the night before if you need to consume more before going to bed. If your urine is darker than a pale tint of yellow (lemon or straw colour), then drink a non-alcoholic beverage before going to bed. Milk is better at hydrating than water and research suggest it is also good at helping to induce sleep, has a better satiety value and contains more nutrients.

Overnight, while you are asleep, your body is still working, and you will continue to excrete water through your lungs when you breathe out. So make sure you have a drink as soon as you get up in the morning before setting out on your journey. The same rule applies – check the colour of your urine when you first get up. If it is darker than a pale tint of yellow, then you could do with having a drink with your breakfast or before leaving.

2. On route to the airport

Don't forget to take a bottle of water with you when you are driving or en route to the airport. If you aren't in the routine of grabbing a bottle just before you leave, then make a note to put a bottle in your hand luggage when you pack.

3. Sip little and often

The best way to keep hydrated is to sip little and often. If you drink a lot of water in one go, it may pass through your body quite promptly. Water will be quickly absorbed into the bloodstream, causing the blood to become too dilute. Your kidneys will immediately start to regulate the concentration of your blood, and it will excrete any inundation relatively quickly to get rid of excess.

Hence, the best way to keep hydrated is to sip the water over your journey's duration, rather than a lot infrequently.

4. Eat foods with a high-water content

Not all the fluid we consume comes from what we drink. On average, just under a litre will come from the food we eat. So remember to choose food high in water whenever possible. This could include your favourite fruit, yoghurt, salads, spaghetti, rice, soups, fish, sauces and even desserts such as ice-cream or sorbet. If you are unsure whether these foods are supplied on board, then take a piece of fruit or pick up a fruit bowl in the terminal before departure. We've listed where to find whole fruit and fresh alternative options in Chapter 14.

5. Stock up before you board

More and more airports are offering a greater selection of drinks and food, both before and after security. Many terminals will provide a range of outlets after security which sell bottles of water. Some airports will have water fountains conveniently located near the Departure Lounge toilets which you can use to fill up an empty bottle. Others may also have a row of water bottles which are freely available or for a small donation.

Whatever you do, try to grab a bottle of water before making your way to the boarding gates. Although there might be chilled bottled water in the vending machines near the gates, it is often more expensive than buying from the retail outlets in the main Departure Lounge. At Gatwick, you can purchase a 500 ml bottle of water for half the price of those stocked in the vending machines.

6. Take what is offered

All drinks provide fluid, so take the drinks offered (non-alcoholic that is). For general guidance, most health professionals recommend around eight to ten glasses a day; that's about a ½ to 1 cup an hour. However, you are en route, and this might mean you need to make a little more effort to counter the effects of not following your usual pattern of consumption, a longer day and a drier environment. So try to aim for a cup an hour.

If the airline offers you juice, tea or coffee, then use this as an opportunity to keep hydrated. Contrary to popular belief, the diuretic effect of caffeine when in tea or mild instant coffee is insignificant and doesn't offset hydration. It's better to take what is offered than to go without for fear of going to the toilet more often. In reality, you will be excreting more fluid through your respiratory tract while on board, and this may help counteract the need to go more often.

7. Avoid alcohol

There is always an exception. Unfortunately, alcohol is one drink best to avoid. Alcohol will have a significant diuretic effect, which means you will be going toilet more often mid-flight. In addition to increasing the fluid loss from the body, it also impairs your ability to sense the early symptoms of dehydration. If you do consume the odd glass, then you should consider drinking more non-alcoholic drinks to counter the loss of fluid. Health experts recommend for every glass of wine or spirits to have a glass of water. You could also select the lower alcohol option, including beer or cider, on a flight or try a diluted version of wine.

8. Avoid high salt foods

Many airlines compensate for a loss of taste when flying at high altitude by adding more salt. Unfortunately, a high salt intake will raise your blood pressure. If you consume more sodium than your body needs, then your body will need to regulate the concentration. A high salt diet alters the sodium balance and causes your kidneys to remove less water, which in turn raises blood pressure. Unfortunately, frequent business travellers reportedly have a higher blood pressure than non-frequent travellers. So it is better to avoid foods high in salt than it is to try and consume yet more fluid.

We all know that foods high in salt include salted nuts and crisps, but some airlines are now also offering boxed snack options to purchase. Not only are they often high in salt, but they are also low in the water, such as crackers, olives, pate spread, and savoury snack packets, and have a high energy content (some are equivalent to 500 calories per box). These probably should be avoided as well as the other high salt items previously mentioned. Better to have an apple or sandwich than a dehydrated snack box.

Best places to find water in the airport

Drinking water en route is a great way of reducing travel fatigue, not to mention healthier than many other drinks as it contains no sugar which can damage your teeth. If you don't like the taste of plain water, then there are plenty of places where you can obtain sparkling, sugar-free flavoured, bottled water at Gatwick's North Terminal.

The price of bottled water varies in the North Terminal of Gatwick Airport. You won't be able to take bottles of water through security with you when you go into the Departure Lounge, which is a shame as water can be more expensive once you have passed through security. Hence, you will need to re-stock once through security. You are, however, usually allowed to take an empty bottle through to refill on the other side.

You will find water at the following places.

Free water

Unfortunately, we were unable to find a water fountain anywhere in Gatwick Airport's North Terminal, which is unusual as many airport terminals now have public water fountains. Nor were there any free bottles of water when you pass through the terminal.

However, Yo! Sushi does offer unlimited refills of water when you dine in their restaurant, after an initial glass price of £1.30. Yo! Sushi promotes a Zero Waste Society and aims to help save 1.7 million bottles a year from hitting the bins. You might be able to fill the empty bottle you've brought through with you, on the premise, it's all part of saving the planet and akin to their avowed corporate social responsibility.

Bottled water

Vending machines

Vending machines are located en route to the departure gates and within the boarding lounges.

Please note: water is more expensive from the vending machines at Gatwick Airport's North Terminal than from retail outlets and some cafes in the main Departure Lounge. The cost of a bottle of water out of a vending machine is £2.00 per 500 ml bottle.

Retail shop deals

The large chain stores on the lower level of the Departure Lounge offer various deals on bottled water. Please see list below for quantity and price;

Boots the Chemist

Boots is one of the best deals in the airport. Boots offer two 750 ml bottles of water for £2.00 which is less expensive than buying from WHSmith and other retail outlets.

They also offer
Evian 750 ml bottle at £1.30
Brecon Carreg 1 litre bottle at £1.25
Brecon Carreg 750 ml bottle at £1.15
Brecon Carreg 500 ml bottle at £0.60
Smart Water 800 ml bottle at £1.20 or
Smart Water 600 ml bottle at £0.95

London News Company

London News Company offers several brands of water at various prices. Head here if you have a long-haul flight as the largest bottle we found is a 1.5 litre Buxton at £2.29, at the time of review. London News also offers two 750 ml bottles of water for £3.

Another deal to watch out for is the free 750 ml bottle when purchasing the Sunday Times or Independent newspapers

Other bottles available are
Buxton 500 ml bottle at £1.79
Buxton 750 ml bottle is £1.89.
Evian 750 ml bottle is £2.19

But you will pay less for a 750 ml bottle at Boots and Starbucks.

Smart water retailed at 600 ml for £1.80 and 850 ml water for £2.19, which is somewhat more expensive than Boots the Chemist (at nearly twice the price).

There are also some boutique brands of water. Fit Water 500 ml by Glucozaide is £1.99, Sugarfree Well Hydrate 500 ml is £2.49 (or 2 for the price of 3 at the time of review), and Glacier Smart Water 600 ml at £1.79. All of which are more expensive than your average bottle of water.

M&S Simply Food

If you are continuing your journey within the UK, then M&S Simply Food offers the lowest price for bottled water. M&S Simply Food is just opposite the International and Domestic Arrivals exit. The cost for a 500ml bottle of water is £0.70 and for a 750ml bottle of water is £0.85.

World Duty Free Shop

You can also pick up a bottle of water when you purchase your duty-free items. A 750 ml bottle of water costs £1.30

Restaurants and Cafes

Cafes tend to offer bottles of water at a lower price than restaurants and vending machines. In fact, some more trendy restaurants sell some of the most expensive bottles of water. Which is surprising considering they tend to boast their offerings as conducive to a healthy lifestyle. Maybe they are, but some restaurants request you to pay a higher price for the privilege of the fundamentals in life.

Arrivals, Ground Floor
Costa Coffee
500 ml bottle is £1.40 or £1.75 for 750ml.

Check-in Level One
Costa Coffee
500 ml bottle is £1.40 or £1.75 for 750ml

Hampton by Hilton
A 500 ml bottle of water is £2.25.

Check-in, Level Two
Jamie's Coffee Lounge
500 ml bottle of Bleu still or sparkling water is £1.50

The Nicholas Culpeper

330 ml Strathmore sparkling or still water is £2.35

Departure Lounge, Lower Level

Weatherspoon

500 ml Strathmore spring water (spring or sparkling) is £2.20

Caviar House & Prunier

500 ml bottle is £3.00

Departure Lounge, Upper level

Pret A Manger

500 ml bottle of water is 99p or 750 ml bottle is £1.50

EAT

500 ml bottle is £1.00 or £1.69 for 750 ml bottle of Harrogate water.

Yo! Sushi

If you need a bottle to match your takeaway sushi, then a 500 ml bottle of water is £1.30, available from their sushi takeaway fridge. As mentioned above, they also offer unlimited water as part of their Zero Waste Society once you've bought your first glass for £1.30.

Jamie's Bakery

500 ml bottle of Bleu water is £1.50.

Shake-A-Hula

500 ml Strathmore still or sparking water is £1.65 or £1.95 for 750 ml.

Starbucks

500 ml bottle for £1.65 or 750 ml bottle for £1.95

Jamie's Italian

330 ml is £2.00 or £3.95 for 750 ml.

Union Jack's Bar

330 ml is £2.00, £3.95 for 750 ml.

Wagamama's

330 ml bottle for £2.10 or £3.95 for 750 ml.

Comptoir Libanais

330 ml for £2.25.

Armadillo

330 ml still or sparkling is £2.35

Garfunkel's

330 ml still or sparkling is £2.40

Lounges

Water is complimentary in all lounges. You'll find bottles of water (usually 500 ml) in the fridge or service area or jugs of fresh iced water.

Milking it further

Hydration experts have recently investigated popular beverages, such as water, milk and juice, to examine which stay in the body the longest and provide greater potential hydration. They compared each beverage against water and found that milk (fat-free, semi-skimmed and whole milk) remained in the body longer than water, thus potentially providing a greater hydrating effect.

The rationale is based on the research evidence and deduces that as milk contains various nutrients and electrolytes (such as sodium and potassium), it causes a slower emptying from the stomach. It is this slow emptying which also delays the production of urine. So, if you're going on a long flight and are worried about access to the toilet, you might be smarter to drink milk as it has a higher hydration index.

In addition, to its hydration effects, milk also provides valuable nutrients such as protein, calcium, iodine and some B vitamins. The good news is that milk, unlike juice, won't cause tooth decay. However, don't forget that milk has more calories than water, so be careful not to overdo its consumption otherwise you may unwittingly add more energy to your diet than you need to. Full-fat milk contains saturated fat, so choose semi-skimmed or skimmed milk if you like to drink it as a frequent contributor to your diet.

Where to find milk at Gatwick's North Terminal

If you wish to have a quick drink of milk just before boarding, then your best bet would be either the retail outlets or the private lounges where milk is freely available. Restaurants and cafes rarely list milk as one of their beverage options on their main menu but will serve it if requested.

We've listed both retail and catering establishments which we've found to stock or offer milk on their main menu below. In general, milk is at least half the price of water when purchased from the retail shops.

Retail Shops

M & S Simply Food (before security)
M&S Simply Food 568 ml is £0.49

Boots the Chemist
Yeo One pint (568 ml) is £0.59
Carvendale One pint (568ml) is £0.65

WHSmith and London News Company
Freshman's milk One pint (568 ml) is £0.85 (skimmed, semi-skimmed and full fat was available at the store located at the far end of the Departure Lounge).

Restaurants and Cafes

Unfortunately, restaurants and cafes do not tend to offer glasses of milk on their menu. While some restaurants and cafes do provide milkshakes and smoothies made with yoghurt, we haven't listed these due to their added or free sugar content.

Costa Coffee

When requested, we were charged £1.10 for a regular size hot milk.

Nicholas Culpeper Pub

A glass of milk is £1.20.

Wagamama

A glass of milk is £1.30.

Chapter 12: Brilliant breakfasts at Gatwick's North Terminal

Not having breakfast is a sure-fire way to start your journey feeling weary. According to the British Dietetic Association, one in three of us still regularly miss breakfast, and this is usually due to time pressures in the morning or not feeling hungry when setting off so early in the day. Still, we all need to break our overnight fast so we can refuel for the activities ahead. Substantial research evidence shows having breakfast is related to performance, particularly being able to concentrate on the day's tasks before us and our mood, along with weight control, improving glycemic control, managing jet-lag, reducing the risk of cardiovascular disease, blood pressure and diabetes. All these issues we now know affect business travellers more than nine to five office-based workers.

It makes sense to refuel as your body has, after all, still been working overnight. In fact, it's been quite busy repairing and renewing torn or old tissues and attending to your vital processes while you've been asleep. During this time, your body has been using up energy throughout its fasting state. You've relied on the energy supplied from the meal you had the evening before and then your liver's short-term storage of glycogen. However, your liver's storage runs low after 12 hours and will gradually become totally depleted, so unless you start to refuel it will need to take more drastic action to create glucose to feed your brain and vital organs. In the meantime, you may begin to feel mentally and physically drained.

Breakfast doesn't just top up our energy supplies to keep us going until lunchtime. It also contributes vital nutrients to our overall diet, making it more complete. The fewer daily meals you have, the less likely you will consume sufficient nutrients in the right balance for your wellbeing, particularly including fibre, B vitamins and essential minerals such as iron and calcium. Research using national health and nutrition surveys show non-breakfast eaters have higher energy and fat intakes while the likelihood of consuming all the food groups lessened, with a decline in vitamins and mineral intakes.

Research also shows that eating a healthy breakfast facilitates better control of our weight, with growing evidence that breakfast eaters tend to weigh less than breakfast skippers. Having a healthy breakfast can reduce hunger during the day, lessen cravings for snacking on cakes, biscuits, chocolate and crisps on board a flight, and prevent overeating at the next properly available meal. If losing weight is your goal, then dodging breakfast to save calories doesn't work very well either as those who eat a healthy breakfast lose weight more successfully.

It isn't just a weighty issue. There's more to breakfast than meets the eye. The good news for frequent flyers who may be susceptible to cardiovascular disease and diabetes is research also shows an association between having breakfast and a lower risk of hypertension, plasma cholesterol and blood glucose among healthy adults. This is where components of a healthy breakfast may have a beneficial effect on reducing blood pressure, along with plasma cholesterol, lipids and diabetes.

So, the type of breakfast is a crucial determinant. For example, fibre from oats in porridge and muesli has been shown to be effective in reducing blood pressure, total cholesterol, LDL cholesterol, blood lipids and the incidence of diabetes. Whereas insoluble fibre found in whole grains and wheat has been linked to reduced incidence of cardiovascular disease, coronary events, cancer and diabetes. While potassium, found in most foods, although unusually high in bananas, dried fruits such as apricots, milk and yoghurt, is known to regulate blood pressure, with higher levels being associated with lower blood pressure. Calcium from dietary sources, such as milk, yoghurt and dairy product alternatives, may also have a beneficial effect on blood pressure.

Not having breakfast is also linked to chronic stress. Where chronic stress is related to evening eating choices and overall empty calories in the diet of breakfast skippers, breakfast eaters' dietary intake does not appear to be affected by chronic stress. Research has also found that breakfast eaters have an overall higher diet quality with whole grains, fruit, fibre, less empty calories, calcium, potassium and folate being included. Whereas, breakfast skippers who reported stress had higher sugar and saturated fat intakes. It is reasonable to deduce that business travellers who don't have breakfast at the start of their journey are not eating as well due to chronic stress. So, if you are feeling the strain of travel on a regular basis or just feeling somewhat burnt out by it all, then changing your routine by stopping to have a good breakfast might be that fork in the right direction.

Lastly, if you are flying long haul, then having breakfast aids to realign your circadian rhythms. Eating breakfast helps to inform your master body clock that it is now time to get up. It does this by signalling through your biological processes, such as the secretion of digestive juices to break down your food and peristalsis (movement of the gastrointestinal tract) which sends signals back to your master clock. Eating a light breakfast can help reduce the effects of jet-lag by helping to synchronise your digestion tissues and organs to a new time zone faster. So, if you are flying long-haul, remember to adjust your meals times to include breakfast at your destination's breakfast time.

What constitutes a healthy breakfast?

To get the full benefits of breakfast, it shouldn't be just any old breakfast, but one which consists of many, if not all, the main food groups. Ideally, breakfast should supply between 20 – 25% of your nutritional requirements, in keeping with the British Dietetic Association recommendations, and include carbohydrate foods (starchy whole grains), dairy, fruit or vegetables and protein sources. Business travellers also need to ensure they have adequate fluids at breakfast time.

Carbohydrate foods

Starchy foods, such as bread, cereals, porridge and muesli are all quick and easy options. They provide B vitamins, fibre and are often fortified with other vitamins such as iron and calcium. If you choose ready-made cereals, then choose those that are whole-grain to ensure a good source of fibre, low in salt and not coated in sugar. Having a selection of starchy foods during the week will not only add variety to your regime but also will add different types of fibre and nutrients to your diet. Oats, for example, are high in certain types of soluble fibre which is beneficial to travellers susceptible to high blood pressure, diabetes and cardiovascular disease. Fibre from whole grain cereals is also useful for business travellers to help prevent constipation and reduce the risk of bowel cancer.

Fruit and vegetables

Fruit and vegetables at breakfast are the perfect opportunity to boost your 5-a-day. Fruit, such as mashed bananas, dried berries and stewed apples can be added to your cereal to enhance the fibre and vitamin C content in your diet, along with other valuable nutrients. Even a small serving (150 ml) of pure juice will constitute one of your 5-a-day servings. If you prefer, you can add frozen berries or banana to yoghurt or milk to make a smoothie. Another option is to include vegetables on top of your toast. Sweated mushrooms, grilled tomatoes, baked beans, mashed avocado and hummus are all great alternatives to sweet condiments. More useful tips on how to incorporate fruit and vegetables into your breakfast can be found in Chapter 14.

Dairy products

Dairy products constitute one of the main food groups which you should include in your daily food intake. Milk and dairy products are good sources of high-quality protein, calcium, iodine and B vitamins, making them vital contributors to a healthy diet. Milk provides proteins which are often in short supply from other food groups and calcium is more readily absorbed from dairy products than other sources. Milk can also be one of the main contributors of iodine in the diet.

While the trend over the last few decades has been to decrease whole fat milk consumption and increase semi-skimmed milk or non-dairy alternatives such as soy or almond milk, the consumption of dairy products has been declining overall in the average diet. Consequently, concerns have been raised regarding consumers who miss dairy products from their diet altogether are now at risk of not consuming all the protein, iodine and calcium they need to maintain muscle mass, hormonal functions and healthy bones. For business travellers who may frequently experience traveller's diarrhoea and avoid dairy products during such periods, a low intake of dairy can pose a shortfall in calcium intake which may increase the risk of osteoporosis and poorer bone health over time.

Individual milk proteins also have a broad range of other potential health benefits. While full-fat dairy products tend to raise cholesterol due to their saturated fatty acid content, we know that low-fat dairy products, which retain the high-quality protein, not only contributes to a reduced saturated fat intake but can be helpful in other ways. Studies are showing the consumption of low-fat dairy products may play a beneficial role in the treatment and prevention of obesity, type 2 diabetes and heart disease and there is some evidence which suggests milk plays a role in preventing some cancers. Considerable research shows that low-fat dairy products with the fullness of milk proteins can improve satiety, help to reduce food intake and regulate blood glucose. For example, low-fat Greek yoghurt has a higher percentage of high-quality milk protein than traditional yoghurt and can enhance satiety, along with aiding steady blood glucose levels.

In short, breakfast is the opportune time for business travellers to increase their consumption of low-fat dairy products which will raise their protein, calcium, iodine and B vitamin intakes along with providing many other health benefits.

Protein

Protein from meat, fish, eggs, beans and other non-dairy sources are also important sources which can help increase satiety while delivering an array of vital nutrients.

Such nutrients differ from dairy products and can include iron, vitamin D and other B vitamins. For this reason, non-dairy protein ideally needs to be incorporated in addition to rather than a substitute for dairy products in your daily diet.

Meat, fish, dairy and eggs have all the protein (made up of various amino acids) you need in sufficient amounts. While beans, wheat, grains and nuts offer protein, some amino acids might be in a limited quantity. So, if you do not include meat, fish or eggs in your breakfast, then protein from a variety of sources can be used complement each other. For example, the combination of baked beans on toast, whole grains with dairy, or yoghurt with nuts/seeds, peanut butter on toast, and pita and hummus, complement each other and will supply all the amino acids you need.

Preliminary research also suggests that the type, timing and distribution of protein throughout the day are important to aid satiety, glucose control, muscle growth and repair. If you spread your protein sources out to each meal time, studies suggest you will feel fuller for longer reducing the desire to eat high sugar, fat and salty snacks between meals. Ideally, if you can combine protein sources with high fibre sources, then you will indeed have a winning combination to increase satiety.

Although it isn't essential to have non-dairy proteins at breakfast every day, it can also add variety. If you wish to incorporate meat, fish or eggs, then choose low-fat cooking methods such as boiling, grilling or poaching instead of frying. Food options could include boiled eggs, grilled kippers, baked beans and grilled lean meats. It is better not to order sausages, bacon, hash browns and black pudding when flying as high fat and high salt meals aren't particularly compatible with travelling, especially if journeying frequently or long haul.

Drinks

Always remember to incorporate a drink as part of your breakfast routine. Overnight, your body has still been working, and you've been expelling fluids from your lungs, as well as in perspiration and through urine. Not having sufficient fluid can reduce your concentration, make you feel fatigued and impatient. When you travel, your usual routine is interrupted, and you are less likely to consume as many fluids as you would usually if working in an office or from home.

Being well hydrated can enhance your concentration and performance. Water, milk, juice, tea and coffee all supply fluid. So, make sure you include a drink as part of your breakfast. See Chapter 11 for more information on how to hydrate.

Putting all this together

If you put all this together, a serving of whole-grain carbohydrate, dairy or high calcium food with a portion of fruit would provide roughly 300 calories. The addition of a little protein will increase satiety and raise the energy content to 400 calories, which is approximately 25% of the total daily intake for women and 20% for men. However, don't go for any old protein. Some protein is higher in value than others, such as eggs and Greek yoghurt, while others are high in saturated fat and salt, such as sausages, bacon and black pudding.

Cooked breakfasts

A cooked breakfast can still be part of your travelling. However, a traditional fry-up is often near 1000 calories (approximately half your daily calorie requirement). In some of the restaurants we reviewed at Gatwick North Terminal, a cooked breakfast was over 1200 calories. In sharp contrast, breakfasts which include healthy leaner proteins cooked with minimal added fat are only a quarter to a half of this calorific value. A plain egg omelette, for example, is approximately 230 kcal, while a grilled kipper with grilled tomato and mushrooms is 350 kcal and baked beans on wholemeal toast is only about 250 kcal.

Restaurants also tend to add extra salt, oil and sugar as they are inclined to have a greater emphasis on taste rather than health. You can modify the fat, salt and sugar content by substituting one item with a vegetable or fruit. So, for example, the hollandaise sauce on an eggs benedict can be replaced with mashed avocado, porridge with mixed dried fruit instead of sugar, pancakes with berry compote or mashed banana instead of syrup, and baked beans instead of sausages or bacon.

Living life to the full doesn't mean going without, it just means making the best choices possible.

Top tips for achieving a healthy breakfast when travelling

It's not always feasible to get to the airport in time for breakfast, and there may not be much on offer when you arrive early, so you might need to adopt a more proactive approach to ensuring having a breakfast en route. Some of our tried and tested suggestions below are well worth a try in these instances.

Nor might it be feasible to select an item from a menu which has been reviewed by our Registered Nutritionists and Dietitians. Menus change on a regular basis, and although we aim to update our guides every six months, sometimes restaurants choose to alter their menus in between our visits. So, we've also included couple quick tips which will see you through a hurried journey when you're not able to select a known healthier option.

Breakfast on the go

If you're catching an early flight, then enabling yourself to have something en route might be the only realistic option for beginning your journey with a timely breakfast. Many airport cafes and restaurants are not fully open until the first flight has departed. Some airport lounges also chose not to open until after the first flight has boarded.

So it's a good idea to prepare your cupboard and fridge with easy to snatch items the day before. It could include a carton of juice or a bottle of water; individual pieces of cheese, a boiled egg or a punnet of yoghurt; muesli, rye or oat biscuits; banana, a piece of citrus fruit or a trail mix of dried fruits and nuts.

You might consider it worthwhile making a quick grab item the night before. For example, a whole grain roll with low-fat cream cheese or smoked salmon; an egg sandwich; or a whole grain bagel with scrambled egg and ham; or a homemade Bircher can all be made the evening prior, ready to go in the morning.

Crispy cereal and nut coated banana chunks

For a quick solution before leaving home, try pouring your muesli or crush your favourite cereal into a plastic bag which has a seal. Add a peeled banana broken into chunks and coat the chunks with cereal. Bananas are not only an excellent source of fibre but also contain potassium, which helps to lower blood pressure. For greater effect, you can also add some chopped nuts which will also provide some protein. High in complex carbohydrate, an added source of protein, fortified with vitamins and minerals, this is a brilliant breakfast when in a hurry. You can, of course, have the dry mix ready the night before and take a banana with you to peel when you get to the airport or en route.

Don't forget to pack a throwaway spoon or folk if finger food is deemed inappropriate.

Purchase a portable cereal container

Food containers which allow you to keep dry and wet foods separated are also worth considering, especially if your journey is via train or not far from the airport. Some containers are now designed to keep cereal and dairy apart until you are ready to mix the two items together. For example, you can separate muesli from the yoghurt or dry cereal from milk until you have reached the airport or en route to the airport. Some containers come with their uniquely sized spoon included.

Beware of hidden sugars in fashionable 'healthy' breakfasts

Brilliant breakfasts are those that taste great. But beware of those full of hidden sugars which caterers add. This is particularly true when a breakfast has become a popular 'health' option.

Greek Yoghurt, granola and compote is a perfect example. Most cafes, retail outlets and restaurants now offer this as either a grab and go item or an alternative to a traditional breakfast on their menu. When made at home, you can control the amount of sugar which you add. However, when purchased at airports, the compote, yoghurt and granola can all have added sugar. So much so that most items we reviewed in retail, cafes and restaurants in Gatwick North Terminal contain the equivalent of five to six teaspoons of sugar. While some of this is naturally present, such as lactose in milk or fructose in the fruit, a lot of it has been added, usually in the form of honey or syrup. Any form of sugar which isn't naturally present is still classified as added sugar, including honey and agave syrup.

To choose to a lower sugar option, select one with only granola or compote but not both. Better still, purchase a fresh fruit salad and add yoghurt or purchase porridge and add fresh fruit. Porridge and whole fruit can be purchased at some cafés such as EAT, Pret A Manger or Starbucks, and restaurants such as the Red Lion pub.

Aim for at least five grams of fibre

If you start the day with fibre, you'll be more likely to reach the recommended amount of fibre per day (30g/adult). Not only will it help keep you regular reducing the risk of bowel cancer, but it will also keep you feeling fuller for longer by slowing down the digestion of your breakfast, at no additional cost to calories and less discomfort.

You can get five grammes in just a medium-sized portion of muesli, two slices of wholegrain toast, three Weetabix, eight ready to eat prunes or a medium portion of baked beans.

Café and restaurant menus featuring good examples of fibre include porridge with banana, five-grain oatmeal, and avocado on rye. If you're stuck for choice, then most restaurants will make whole grain toast which you can then add either vegetable such as mushrooms, tomatoes and even a banana on top.

Choose a winning combination option

Excellent breakfasts are those which combine complex/starchy carbohydrate, such as porridge, cereals, or wholemeal toast, with protein, such as dairy, fish, peanut butter or eggs, which improves satiety. This means it takes longer to digest and slows digestion and absorption down, leaving you feeling satisfied without making you feel discomfort from being overfilled.

It's easier to do this when at home but harder when in transit. So, here are a couple of tried and tested examples of what you can pick up quickly at the airport.

- Egg and mayo sandwich, preferably wholegrain or rye bread.
- Yoghurt and banana smoothie.
- Smoked salmon on a whole-wheat bagel
- Boiled eggs, spinach and oatmeal or rye crackers (Boots the Chemist or Marks & Spencer).

And a couple of side combinations from the menu. Most restaurants offer at least two sides which you can combine.

- Fresh fruit and yoghurt
- Baked beans and wholemeal toast
- Poached egg on rye toast
- Top your peanut butter on whole grain toast with a banana.
- Smoked salmon and granary toast

Delayed reaction

Lastly, if eating first thing isn't your thing, then try to eat within two hours of getting up. A late breakfast is still a breakfast! You could start with something simple, like a piece of cheese and an apple, and gradually build it up over time. Once you begin to have something on a regular basis, you will become accustomed to food eaten at a particular time, and your body will begin to secrete digestive juices in anticipation. Over time, you can bring this forward a little so that your body is ready earlier in the day.

Where to find brilliant breakfasts

We've explored the breakfasts on offer at Gatwick Airport's North Terminal, and we've selected some great breakfast options for you below. These include breakfast meals which are light in calories for those either about to catch their flight and will eat again soon after boarding and those who want to lose weight, along with breakfast meals where the next meal might be at least 5 – 6 hours or not needing to reduce their daily calorific intake.

Here is a summary list of where to head.

Arrivals, Ground Floor

Costa Coffee

Costa Coffee is ideal for quick 'grab and go' options, especially if you have just arrived at Gatwick Airport as it is next to the Arrivals exit. It is one of the few cafes here which are open 24 hours. There are also places to sit at the back and to the right of the café which are away from the main thoroughfare.

Location: Situated on the left as you exit from International Arrivals.
Opening hours: 24 hours

Cold breakfast options;
Whole Bananas 51 kcal (217 kJ)
Whole Apples 43 kcal (183 kJ)
Fresh Fruit Salad Pot A pot provides 45 kcal (190 kJ)
Organic 0% Fat Greek Style Yoghurt A pot provides 67 kcal (286 kJ)
Free Range Egg Sandwich Sandwich provides 342 kcal (1435 kJ)

Hot breakfast options;
Wholegrain Porridge – Gluten Free Per portion 231 kcal (969 kJ)
Instant Oat Porridge Per portion 294 kcal (1240 kJ) sugar content is 16 g
Halloumi & Roasted Pepper Focaccia Focaccia provides 411 kcal (1724 kJ)
Goats' Cheese & Sweet Chilli Chutney Panini This panini provides 447 kcal (1883 kJ)

M&S Simply Food

Conveniently located near the Arrivals exit, business travellers can shop in here for refrigerated breakfast options. There is plenty of fresh fruit, along with plain yoghurts and prepared pots of mixed cereal, fruit and mixed yoghurt items.

While many of the muesli, yoghurt and fruit combination pots and the Birchers have several forms of sugar added, the new range of quinoa-based yoghurt and fruit pots tend to rely on the natural sweetness of the fruit incorporated.

Open: 24 hours
Location: Opposite the Bureau de Change and next to Boots the Chemist

Grab and Go Breakfast Items include;

Pineapple, Melon & Grape 51 kcal (218 kJ)

Banana & Berries 96 kcal (405 kJ)

Purely Pineapple 190 g Per portion 87 kcal (367 kJ)

Melon and Grape 210 g Per portion 90 kcal (380 kJ)

Greek Style Yoghurt Unsweetened natural yoghurt made with milk. One pot serving contains 186 kcal (776 kJ)

Greek Yoghurt with Fresh Banana, Almond & Honey Granola Fat-free Greek-style yoghurt, banana, an almond and honey granola. The pot provides 220 kcal (925 kJ)

Strawberry Quinoa Yoghurt Pot Strawberry compote, quinoa and fat-free Greek-style yoghurt topped with mixed seeds. Per portion: 171 kcal (718 kJ)

Mango Quinoa Yoghurt Pot Mango compote with fat-free Greek-style yoghurt and quinoa, topped with pomegranate seeds, pistachio nuts and dried coconut. Per portion: 162 kcal (684 kJ)

Mango & Passion Fruit & Greek Style Yogurt Snack Pot Greek-style natural yoghurt with mango and passion fruit compote. Ready to be mixed. Serve as a breakfast or snack. Per pack 198 kcal (823 kJ)

Check-in, Level One

Hampton by Hilton

The Hampton by Hilton offers an oasis amongst the departing chaos at Gatwick Airport's North Terminal when it is at its busiest during the day. If you don't have a private lounge membership or need to have a breakfast meeting with colleagues who aren't flying with you, then this is an excellent secluded spot. It's tucked away from the main check-in area so to provide a sanctuary for business travellers.

Starbucks Coffee use to preside here just opposite the hotel's reception. However, it was recently incorporated into the bar and business area of the hotel's ground floor, next to the hotel reception. There is also a breakfast buffet which non-guests can access at the cost of £7.50. For hotel guests, the breakfast is complimentary, included in their room rate.

Open: Continental Breakfast 4.00 am to 10.00 am. Hot Breakfast 6.00 am to 10.00 am.

Location: The entrance to this hotel is next to the Easy Jet Check-in on level one. Just follow the signs to the right of the check-in desks. You will see a sign above the entrance to the corridor for the Hampton by Hilton. Follow the passage for roughly fifty steps, and you come to the hotel reception.

Buffet includes: Continental breakfast with a selection of cereals, bread, yoghurts and toast. After 6.00 am there is also a hot food selection.

Check-in, Level Two
Jamie's Coffee Lounge

You can't miss this coffee lounge. It's the one next to the van with a giant neon sign. The food here is freshly made each day. You can take away or eat on the premises before journeying through security. You won't miss breakfast here, as it is open all day.

Unfortunately, no nutritional information was available at the time of reviewing. We did notice, however, that this is one of the few places which offered a yoghurt mix without additional sugar. Hence worthy of inclusion.

Open: 24 hours
Location: Level two, next to Nicholas Culpeper at the front entrance.

Cold Breakfast options;
Superfood Blueberry Pot Blueberries, banana, almonds, yoghurt, chia seeds, vanilla essence.
Strawberry Pot Strawberries, banana, almonds, yoghurt, chia seeds, vanilla essence.

Nicholas Culpeper

Named after the 17th century English Herbalist and Physician, the chefs here understand that fresh ingredients can make all the difference to perceived taste and quality. This restaurant offers a variety of both hot and cold options for those seeking a healthier breakfast.

Open: 4.00 am to 8.30 pm
Location: Level two, In the front of large windows as you travel upon the escalator from level one.

Cold breakfast options

Bircher Muesli with Banana and Honey 'Rude Health' muesli served with fresh banana slices. Greek Yoghurt and Golden Honey (ask for no honey to reduce added sugar content).

Fresh Fruit Salad Served with fresh mango, pineapple, strawberries and pomegranate.

Granola 'Rude health' granola with fresh strawberries, pomegranate, Greek-style yoghurt & honey. (ask for no honey to reduce added sugar content).

Hot breakfast options

Porridge with Banana, Strawberries & Honey (don't add the honey if you wish to reduce the sugar content).

Scrambled Eggs on Toast Served with toasted bloomer bread. Ask for granary bloomer bread to increase fibre content.

Egg White & Spinach Omelette Served with slow roasted tomato & pea shoots.

Smashed Avocado on Toast Served with fresh mango, chilli, lime & coriander served on toasted bloomer bread. Ask for granary bloomer bread to increase fibre content.

Departure Lounge, Lower Level

Caviar House & Prunier

Caviar House & Prunier has been at Gatwick North's Terminal for over 15 years and continues to offer luxury dining. Breakfast is simply an extension of its excellent cuisine. No nutritional information was available at the time of review.

Open: 4.00 am to 8.30 pm
Location: Middle of the Departure Lounge, next to World Duty Free, on the lower level.

Hot breakfast options

Scrambled Egg & Scottish Smoked Salmon
Scrambled Egg & Balik Smoked Salmon
Scrambled Egg & Balik Smoked Salmon & Caviar

Red Lion Pub

The Red Lion Pub is one of the few restaurants which offers their customers an informed choice, by placing nutritional information on their menu. Although this just includes calorific information, it at least supports their clientele who want to choose according to their energy needs. The pub is busy most of the time but particularly handy if your flight is likely to depart from gates 557 – 574.

Location: Right-hand corner of the Departure Lounge as you exit from security.
Open: 3.00 am to 8.30 pm

Cold breakfast options

Berry Breakfast Bowl Crunch Granola, pumpkin seeds, Greek-style yoghurt *Hold the honey*, acai & blueberry compote, strawberry, blueberries and chia seeds. Per portion 375 kcal (1569 kJ)
Fresh Fruit Bowl A selection of fresh fruit Per portion 175 kcal (732 kJ)

Hot breakfast options

MOMA Porridge 100% natural, low fat, gluten free Porridge. Per portion: 256 Kcal (1071 kJ)
With Banana Per portion: 446 Kcal (1866 kJ)
With Fresh Blueberries Per portion: 274 Kcal (1146 kJ)
With raisins, goji berries, hazelnuts, pistachios Per portion: 369 Kcal (1544 kJ)

Departure Lounge, Upper Level
Armadillo Restaurants

The Armadillo serves South-West American cuisine. There are some great breakfasts on offer here. While no nutritional information was available at the time of review, we did find a couple of healthier options for you to try.

Open: 4.00 am to 8.30 pm
Location: On the upper level overlooking the main Departure Lounge, just above World Duty Free opposite the exit from security.

Cold breakfast options

Sunshine Granola Sundae Greek-style yoghurt, Rude Health granola, mango compote
Fresh Fruit Bowl Selection of fresh fruit.

Hot breakfast options

Wholesome Porridge with strawberries, blueberries, pumpkin seeds (no need for the honey!)
Side Orders of toast and scrambled eggs.

Brekkie Burrito Filled and grilled soft tortilla, rainbow peppers, free-range scrambled eggs, jalapeno, melted jack cheese, pico de gallo salsa, mushrooms and hot chipotle sauce.

Avocado Southwest Free-range scrambled eggs, smashed fresh avocado, red chilli, fresh watercress, pico de gallo salsa and a toasted muffin.

Full Works Open Omelette Free range three egg open pan omelette, rainbow peppers, tomato, mushrooms, fresh parsley, jack cheese and pico de gallo salsa.

Free Range Eggs Any Style Choose scrambled or poached free range eggs on toast.

Comptoir Libanais

Comptoir Libanais offers Middle Eastern cuisine in both informal dining and takeaway style. The location is straight ahead and up the stairs on the right, as you come out of security exit. No nutritional information was available at the time of review, so we've selected the best-described healthier items from the menu.

Open: 4.00 am to 8.30 pm
Location: On the upper level to the far right of the Departure Lounge.

Cold breakfast options

Homemade Granola with Yoghurt. Granola made with oats, nuts, seeds, cardamom, cinnamon and dried cranberry.

Hot breakfast options

Feta, Avocado, Cherry Tomato & Olives on Toast Cherry tomato, avocado and olives on sourdough toast, topped with crumbled feta and hommos.

Smoked Salmon & Scrambled Eggs Scrambled eggs and smoked salmon on sourdough toast, sprinkled with pomegranate seeds.

Eggs on Toast Scrambled eggs on sourdough toast.

Folded Omelette Plain Freshly made to order. Three egg-omelette with a roast tomato.

Feta Cheese Wrap A wrap filled with egg, feta, potatoes, mushrooms, fool moudamas and tomatoes served with a side of labneh yoghurt.

Shakshuka with Feta The classic dish made with slow-cooked tomatoes, red onions and peppers, mixed with parsley, coriander and garlic. Topped with a baked egg and crumbled feta. Served with Pitta.

EAT

This long-founded speedy café offers some great grab and go options. Although their birchers are lower in sugar than the majority of other cafes, these still provide a higher total sugar content than other available options. So, we have not included these in the list below. Instead, we have included a dairy-based option and a couple of wraps, which together provides a nutritious breakfast, inclusive of several food groups.

Alternatively, if you prefer a hot option, we've included a couple of their new dishes, in addition to porridge, for you to try.

Open: 4.00 am to 8.30 pm
Location: Situated at the back, mid-way along the upper balcony in the Departure Lounge.

Cold Breakfast Options
Bio-Live Berry Pot Bio-live yoghurt served with berry compote. Per serving: 136 kcal (569 kJ)
Chunky Houmous Wrap Chunky houmous & onion mix with fresh cucumber and spinach wrapped in a kibbled rye tortilla wrap. 377 kcal (1577 kJ)
Houmous & Falafel Wrap Falafel mixed with harissa houmous, chickpeas and spinach wrapped in a kibbled rye tortilla wrap. Per Portion 477 kcal (1996 kJ)

Hot Breakfast Options
Classic Porridge Simple porridge made with Scottish oats, slowly simmered with British milk Per portion: Regular 213 kcal (896 kJ), Small 137 kcal (573 kJ)
Porridge with Banana Scottish oats slowly simmered with British milk, topped with banana Per portion: Regular 234 kcal (987 kJ) Small 162 kcal (678 kJ)
Poached Egg, Jarlsberg & Mushroom Crusty Roll Crusty roll filled with poached egg, Jarlsberg cheese and sliced roast mushrooms. Per portion: 332 kcal (1389 kJ)
Avocado Sourdough Toast Lightly toasted sourdough bread topped with fresh avocado mash mixed with a little lemon juice. Per portion: 338 kcal (1414 kJ)
BBQ Beans, Poached Egg & Ham Hock Breakfast pot of poached egg, smoked ham hock with BBQ beans. 334 kcal (1397 kJ)
BBQ Beans, Poached Egg, Avocado & Feta A tasty breakfast pot of poached egg, avocado mash and feta served with BBQ baked beans. 389 kcal (1627 kJ)

Garfunkel's Restaurant
Garfunkel's offer dishes from around the world with a distinctive British, European and American influence. Breakfast is a soft mix of traditional and modern cuisine styles. No nutritional information was available at the time of review.

Open: 4.00 am to 8.30 pm

Location: Between Comptoir Libanais and Armadillo restaurants on the upper level of the Departure Lounge.

Cold breakfast options

Fresh Fruit Bowl. A selection of mixed fruit topped with fresh strawberries and pomegranate seeds.

Granola Bowl. Greek style yoghurt with granola topped with fruit and pomegranate seeds (ask for no honey to reduce the added sugar content).

Hot breakfast options

Porridge Made with either soya, semi-skimmed milk or water and topped with Summer Berry compote or apple and cinnamon compote.

Avocado on Toast Smashed avocado, mango, coriander & lime salsa with a hint of fresh red chilli, served on toasted bread.

Smoked Salmon & Scrambled Eggs Smoked salmon with scrambled eggs, served with wholemeal toast. (Hold the butter.)

Scrambled Eggs on Toast Freshly made with three eggs, served with wholemeal toast. (Hold the butter.)

Egg White Omelette Freshly made with spinach and red onion and served with smashed avocado with mango, coriander, chilli and lime, a grilled tomato and pea shoots.

Pan Hash Cubed potatoes, mixed peppers, mushrooms, tomatoes, spinach, and spring onion, with Neapolitan sauce, a sprinkle of chilli flakes and topped with a fried egg.

Jamie's Italian

Jamie Oliver created his menu based on healthy eating guidelines, great taste and dining in a casual Italian style. So, it's not surprising there are several menu items which are apt if you fancy a healthier, relaxed breakfast. His Italian restaurant is situated on the upper level of the Departure Lounge at the far end.

Open: 3.30 am to 8.30 pm

Location: Upper Level, just opposite Yo! Sushi and Wagamama.

Hot breakfast options

Proper Porridge With either fresh market berries or banana & toasted coconut or stewed bramble fruit. (no need for added sugar, golden syrup or honey)

Eggs Your way Scrambled, poached or boiled on toast

Scrambled Eggs & Smoked Salmon Smoked salmon, free-range eggs & Glasgow potato scones.

Omelette Gordon Bennett Two free-range eggs cooked with poached haddock, crème Fraiche, a squeeze of lemon and Westcombe Cheddar.

Pret A Manger

This chain café offers the most extensive selection of healthier breakfast options we could find in the North Terminal. You can either sit-in or grab and go. Items are made fresh each day. The range of tastes is impressive; from traditional baked beans with a poached egg to modern day healthy oats. Not all Birchers, granola and porridge, matched our meticulous healthy guidelines, so we've only listed those that do.

You will find the porridge here comes with optional toppings. We reviewed the analysis and just, so you know, the berry fruit compote offered less than a teaspoon of intrinsic sugar, mainly fructose within the fruit, and therefore is not considered an added sugar. In contrast, the honey topping provides 5 ½ teaspoons of (free) sugars per portion and is classified as an added sugar. The recommendation is to reduce free sugars (those added to food) to less than 5% per day, which is no more than a total of 6 teaspoons per day. So, the choice is obvious, if you wish to have a sweet topping without excessive amounts of added sugar, then opt for the fruit compote.

Open: 3.00 am to 8.30 pm
Location: Far left-hand corner on the upper level, next to the escalator.

Breakfast items to select from include;

Apples, Bananas

Pret's Proper Porridge British jumbo oats, simmered milk to make a creamy, delicious porridge, naturally low in fat. Per portion: 242 kcal (1017 kJ)

Porridge Topping Compote Fruity Compote made with strawberries, blackcurrants, blackberries, raspberries and redcurrants, slowly simmered in a pan. Per 25 g serving: 24 kcal (101 kJ)

Mango & Banana Sunshine Bowl Blended mango and banana, with a splash of coconut milk, a dash of turmeric, topped with granola (gluten-free), blueberries and coconut chips. Per 168 g serving: 253 kcal (1042 kJ)

Free-range Egg Mayo & Roasted Tomato Breakfast Baguette Chunky egg mayonnaise and roasted tomatoes in a freshly baked, breakfast-sized baguette. Per portion 309 kcal (1300 kJ)

Breakfast Egg & Avocado Baguette Chunky free-range egg mayo and sliced avocado in a freshly baked baguette. Per portion 366kcal (1533 kJ)

Breakfast Salmon and Egg Scottish smoked salmon with chunky egg mayo in a breakfast sized baguette. Per portion 339 kcal (1426 kJ)

Additional Grab and Go Items:

Cracking Egg Salad Sandwich Chunky egg mayo with slices of tomato, seasoning and fresh wild rocket. Per portion 375 kcal (1575 kJ)

Free Range Egg Mayo Sandwich Boiled, chopped free range eggs mixed with mayonnaise, cracked black pepper and celery salt, sprinkled with mustard cress. Per portion: 367 kcal (1542 kJ)

Scottish Smoked Salmon Sandwich Scottish smoked salmon sandwich with lemon juice and seasoning on granary bread. Per portion: 421 kcal (1761 kJ)

Chakalaka Wrap A vegan recipe of spicy, African-inspired chakalaka beans topped with a dollop of dairy-free coconut yoghurt alternative, filled with freshly sliced red pepper and roasted butternut squash, finished with a handful of spinach. Per baguette: 340 kcal (1425 kJ)

Starbucks

Starbucks has a selection of grab and go, both hot and cold healthier breakfast options for you to choose. They recently introduced their hot box selection, which includes Super Scrambled Eggs. They also appear to be expanding their range of porridge and have now added a Five Grain Oatmeal.

Fortunately, this café is open 24 hours so you can get your breakfast at any time!

Open: 24 hours

Location: Halfway along the upper level of the Departure Lounge, next to Jamie's Italian restaurant.

Cold breakfast options

Banana 108 kcal (448 kJ)

Berry Crunch Made with Greek-style yoghurt and a mixed summer berry compote topped with a crunchy baked honey oat Granola. Per portion: 250 kcal (1051 kJ)

Fruit Mix Sweet mango, diced kiwifruit, juicy pomegranate seeds and blueberries. Per portion: 72 kcal (301 kJ)

Smoked Salmon Bagel Each bagel is 472 kcal (1985 kJ)

Vegan Wrap with Falafel & Slaw Sweet potato falafel with mixed peppers, rainbow slaw and a tomato salsa dressing. A wrap provides 261 kcal (1096 kJ)

Sure as Eggs is Eggs Sandwich, This sandwich provides 388 kcal (1621 kJ)

Hot breakfast options

Classic Porridge Wholegrain porridge with milk and an optional topping dried fruit and seed mix. Per portion: 303 kcal (1275 kJ)

Five Grain Oatmeal (Gluten Free) An oatmeal porridge made with soya and coconut cream, with oats, golden linseed, quinoa, red & wild rice and a touch of cinnamon. Per portion: 285 kcal (1191 kJ)

Super Scrambled Eggs, Tomato & Spinach Egg Box Creamy scrambled eggs served on a bed of spinach leaves, with a mixture of fresh and slow-roasted tomatoes and topped with a sprinkling of mixed seeds. Per portion: 211 kcal (878 kJ)

Tomato, Mozzarella & Red Pesto Panini. Mozzarella with slow-roasted tomatoes, red pesto, sliced tomatoes and basil in a panini. Per portion: 432 kcal (1810 kJ)

Wagamama

Wagamama has a lot to offer: a fantastic view of the runway, lots of charge points for your devices and now it has several healthier breakfast options as well. Unfortunately, there wasn't any nutritional information was available at the time of review, so we've selected some possible healthier choices for you based on their description.

Open: 4.00 am to 8.30 pm
Location: At the far end of the upper balcony at the back.

Cold breakfast options

Fruit and Yoghurt Bowl Creamy yoghurt topped with pineapple, kiwi fruit, apple, pear, passionfruit, blueberries and lime, sprinkled with raisins and goji berries

Crunchy Granola Bowl Toasted granola and creamy yoghurt topped with pineapple, kiwi fruit, apple, pear, passionfruit, blueberries and lime, sprinkled with a mix of toasted seeds, goji berries and raisins.

Smoothies

Banana Smoothie Banana, apple and passion fruit juice blended with plain frozen yoghurt.

Mango and chilli mango blended with plain frozen yoghurt and a touch of chilli

Hot breakfast options

Avocado on toast A lightly dressed mix of avocado and chopped tomato served on a slice of toasted wholemeal bread topped with two free-range poached eggs.

Yashi okonomiyaki A Japanese-inspired omelette made with shiitake mushrooms, red cabbage and leek, dressed with traditional Japanese sauces and garnishes.

Lounge breakfast options

For business travellers who wish to escape the hordes of tourists during breakfast, which is usually when Gatwick North is at its busiest, the lounges can offer both tranquillity and a healthy breakfast.

No. 1 Lounge

The No. 1 Lounge is an excellent choice for a healthy business breakfast or breakfast meeting before boarding a plane. In addition to a healthy breakfast to be had, there are plenty of tables and places to relax or catch up on your emails prior to departure. The lounge serves a continental buffet breakfast and made to order breakfast items before 11.00 am.

Open: 4.00 am to 10.00 pm, breakfast until 11.00 am.
Breakfast:
Continental buffet items include: Greek yoghurt with toppings, cereals and fruit salad.
Made to order items include: Beans on toast, kedgeree, toast and porridge.
Cost: Lounge entry for adults is £30 if you book in advance or £37.50 on the door without booking. If your flight is delayed and you want to stay longer, then you can buy additional hours.
Access: All travellers including groups and children.
Free access: Dragonpass, Diners Club, Institute of Directors, Lounge Club, Priority Pass, Dining Club, Caxton FX.
Location: On the lower level of the Departure Lounge, after security, near gates 101 - 113.
Directions: Head towards gate 101 – 113, just past the London News Company, you will see a hallway on your right. Turn right and go through the double glass doors. No.1 Lounge is directly ahead, situated at the end.

Aspire Lounge

The Aspire Lounge offers a basic continental breakfast, which is ideal if this is your usual and don't wish to be tempted by additional items you wouldn't normally have at home. There is also a quiet area which you can use to recharge your batteries after an early start.

Open: Open hours are from 4.00 am to 10.00 pm, with a slight seasonal variation. Breakfast is served between 0.400 am, and 11.00 am.

Breakfast:

Continental buffet items include: selection of cereals, fresh fruit and yoghurts.

Hot Breakfast Items: Scrambled egg in a fresh crusty roll.

Cost: Lounge entry for adults is from £17.99 if you book in advance or £35 on the door without booking. If your flight is delayed and you want to stay longer, then you can buy additional hours.

Free access: Priority Pass, Diners Club, IOD members, DragonPass, Aspire Platinum Membership and Vueling airline passengers.

Location: First floor of the Departure Lounge.

Directions: Head towards gate 101 – 113, as you pass the London News Company, you will see a hallway on your right. Turn right down the corridor, go through the double glass doors and take the lift on the left to the first floor. The lounge is located on the right-hand side.

My Lounge

My Lounge has made a conscious effort to be modern and healthy with their breakfast options. There is a variety of healthier cold options along with healthier hot options to choose from. You can join others at the main table for breakfast or eat solo at the workbench and individual tables.

Opening hours: 6.00 am to 8.00 pm, breakfast before 11.00 am

Breakfast:

Continental buffet items include: muesli, yoghurt with various toppings, fresh fruit and fruit salad.

Hot Options include: Porridge with different toppings, e.g., dried fruits or raspberry compote or

Boston Beans with crispy bacon bits.

Cost: Lounge entry for adults is £18 if you book in advance or £24 on the door without booking. If your flight is delayed and you want to stay longer, then you can buy additional hours.

Free access: Institute of Directors, Lounge Club, Lounge Pass, Priority Pass, Diners Club.

Location: Departure Lounge, lower level.

Directions: Head towards gate 101 – 113, as you pass London News Company, you will see a corridor on your right. Turn right and proceed down the hallway and go through the double glass doors. The lounge is located on the left-hand side just before the lifts.

Chapter 13: Embracing healthier meals when travelling

Regular healthier meals with a low energy density are an apt choice when frequently travelling on business. Heavy, energy-dense meals can cause you to feel uncomfortable en route, and more importantly, they can impact on your long-term physical health and mental wellbeing. In contrast, regular lighter meals comprising a low energy density can help sustain your energy levels, provide you with the essential nutrients as part of a balanced diet and are superior in the long-term for maintaining your weight and lowering the risk of serious disease. As a business traveller, deciding on suitable meal choices can be pivotal to your performance and wellbeing.

We endure all sorts of changes to our normal daily routine when travelling on business, and it is certainly a disruption to our usual work patterns, as well as our lifestyle choices. Frequent flying regularly means leaving our familiar meals behind and replacing them with a new set of foods en route, including airport eateries. Even if you are in the habit of eating healthily at work and home, when it comes to travelling all your efforts can swiftly take flight leaving you feeling besieged by obscure airport fare.

Often, we neglect to take into account our changing nutritional needs; usually, due to reduced activity levels, meals become either irregular or too frequent if travelling long-haul and adapting to a new time zone. If experiencing a high degree of stress already, then travel fatigue, additional work pressures and anonymity make it easy to lose any residue resistance to the readily available and universally less healthy food options. Concurrently, it's often difficult to decipher from short menu descriptions of what might be the healthier choice, and nutritional information is not usually conveniently accessible.

Unfortunately, business travellers have been reporting a poorer health status than their office-based colleagues for some time now. Research began in the 1940's started to show changes in human physiology as a result of flying. Subsequent research has demonstrated that as the number of trips increases for the business person, so does the body mass index, blood pressure, blood cholesterol and lipids, making the business traveller more at risk of cardiovascular disease, cancer and diabetes. These conditions are all influenced by what we eat. Those who often fly long haul also have a higher likelihood of sleep deprivation which may lead to additional hormonal and physiological changes increasing the risk further of cardiovascular disease, diabetes and cancer.

It's not surprising those regularly flying may have a higher body mass index when you consider what is typically on offer at an airport. The meal options which are plentiful usually comprise of a high energy density (high calorie per gram of food), as typically they are high in fat, such as burgers and fries, pizza, fried fish with chips, stir-fries, lasagne and curry. Even items marketed by a restaurant as 'healthy' can be relatively high in energy, including those which contain ingredients such as healthy oils, full-fat cheese or sugar alternatives (honey, agave syrup and fruit juice).

In contrast, substantial research shows diets comprising low energy dense foods help people to maintain a lower body weight. Foods of low energy density are mostly foods which are high in fibre and water content, such as whole fruit, vegetables, stews, soups and whole grains, along with lean meats and low-fat dairy products. Compared to high energy dense foods, lighter in energy foods are often less readily available in airports and en route.

Crucially, research shows people tend to consume the same weight of food each day, but not always the same amount of energy. The consistency of volume forms a feedback mechanism which helps to inform us when we are either full or satisfied. This has important implications when choosing menu items. Eating foods low in energy density allows you to reduce your energy intake without reducing the amount of food you consume. The mechanisms for controlling hunger and maintaining feelings of satiety, fullness and satisfaction, may be intricate. However, they are essential for long-term weight control. In comparison, research also shows those who seek to eliminate a particular food group or reduce only their portion size may have a greater feeling of hunger and dissatisfaction which will reduce their desire to control their intake.

What's more, choosing foods lower in energy density can result in a more balanced approach to achieving an enhanced traveller's nutritional status. If you select menu items which are less energy-dense (low in fat and sugar yet higher in fibre and water), then the high calorific ingredients will be replaced with other nutritious ingredients. So, a diet of equal weight can be of greater nutrient value as well as less energy-dense.

Although body weight is one of the key risk factors for cardiovascular disease, cancer and diabetes, there are other factors as well, such as blood pressure, cholesterol, glucose and lipid levels. Some of which are temporarily influenced by flying. However, if you fly long-haul regularly (over six times a year), physiological changes affected by time zones, cabin environment, etc. may become more long-term.

Avoiding foods high in saturated fat, sugar and salt is more significant to the business traveller than the office worker. When business professionals fly on business, their blood pressure may already be raised due to the increased anxiety to get there on time, delayed flights and queuing, not to mention any additional work pressures they're already experiencing. If they have uncontrolled high blood pressure, high altitudes may induce greater fatigue. It applies in particular if a business traveller already has a blockage in their arteries, as the heart needs to work harder to pump sufficient oxygen around the body. The effort by the heart will further increase if the business traveller is also overweight.

Consequently, if the business traveller is not taking medication to regulate hypertension, then cutting down on salt in the long term and avoiding it when flying will help to reduce blood pressure. Likewise decreasing the saturated fat in their diet will help lessen the likelihood of building up deposits in the arteries. Additionally, if the business traveller already has vascular disease, then they are at a higher risk of blood clots forming or developing an embolism, which can be reduced by ensuring they are adequately hydrated when flying and avoiding foods which are high in salt and saturated fat.

Knowing what to choose in airport catering establishments and retail outlets is vital to successfully achieve a healthier business travel existence. So, we've done some searching for you and found healthier lighter meals for you to try. To further help you, we have also listed several approaches to choosing healthier, lower energy-dense foods. First, let's explain what health professionals really mean by a healthier meal option.

What constitutes a healthier meal option

Consuming a healthier, lighter meal will not only make you feel more comfortable during your journey, but it will also make your long-term goals for better health and enhanced well-being easier to achieve.

Unfortunately, airports are notorious for providing mainly unhealthy meal options. Equally, when restaurants and cafes do promote healthier choices, they are often far from what they claim. Moreover, it can be difficult to ascertain sufficient information to check what you are buying is indeed what they are asserting.

There is also a lot of misinformation as to what a healthier meal option should be. It's important to seek the right information from the outset of your business travel life, which is why you should only rely on evidence-based recommendations and follow a Registered Nutritionist or Dietitian and government-backed advice. To escort you through the maze of misinformation, we have put together a practical guide on what exactly constitutes a healthy option. It will support you in making healthier choices when passing through the airport and beyond.

We've also reviewed the restaurants and café's menus and done a lot of the research and scrutiny for you. As a result, we have listed suitable meal items available in Gatwick Airport's North Terminal later in this chapter. They are all based on the recommended dietary principles as described below.

A healthy balance of energy

Ideally, if you are eating regularly, inclusive of snacks, then your meal at lunch or dinner should provide no more than 30% of your total daily energy intake. If you are trying to maintain your weight, then this would represent, based on an average energy balance, no more than 600 calories per meal for women and 750 calories for men. If you are attempting to lose weight, then aiming for 350 to 450 calories at lunch or dinner for women and 450 to 600 calories per meal for men, would be a reasonable target.

Many airport meals have twice the quantity of calories that you need to maintain your weight. Nutritional information which we obtained indicated a whopping 1400 calories for one main meal, incorporating 65 grams of fat (enough for the entire day!). Not only is this excessive but it could also make an unpleasant flight if sitting cramped on a plane for several hours.

Your plate should be balanced too

Healthier lower energy dense meals are those which contain a good source of protein and fibre rich carbohydrates, but low in fat and calories. Healthier meals may incorporate legumes (beans, peas and lentils), potatoes, brown rice or whole grains, along with fish, skinless white meat, lean meats, low-fat dairy products or eggs.

For a balanced meal, you should aim for a meal with a moderate amount of lean protein and carbohydrates, adding a substantial portion of vegetables. **Ideally, your plate will have one-quarter protein, one-quarter carbohydrate foods and one-half from the vegetable food group**. You might add a dairy product as a sauce, drink or dessert, along with a little fat.

The protein and fibre help to slow down digestion to deliver a steady release of energy, so you are less likely to feel fatigued when you arrive at your destination. Protein takes some time to break down into smaller units so that it can cross the gastrointestinal lining, while fibre slows the absorption of small units (of protein, carbohydrate and fat) by inhibiting the access to the gastrointestinal wall.

If you choose a moderate to high-fat protein, then limit the inclusion of other moderate to high-fat items in your diet to no more than three times per week, and preferably not when you are going to board the plane. High-fat proteins include lamb, duck, oily fish, sausages and bacon. Look for cooking methods on the menus which are not flash or deep fried. For example, choose items which are grilled, barbequed, poached and baked.

Always aim to have whole grains if having bread, rice or pasta with a meal, and whole foods if having potatoes, e.g. baked potato or new potatoes steamed. Whole carbohydrate foods provide more nutrients and are a greater source of fibre. You should aim for approximately 30 g of fibre per day, which equates to 9 g per meal, which is equivalent to two to three portions of vegetables and a whole grain carbohydrate.

Combination foods

As mentioned, a balanced meal should include several of the basic food groups: protein, carbohydrates, vegetables, dairy products and a little fat. Combination foods incorporate a mixture of these various food groups into one item. Examples include lasagne, pizza, shepherd's pie, casseroles, baguettes or sandwiches.

You may need to scan the ingredients listed to see how many food groups have been included to ascertain whether it is a balanced meal, along with the cooking methods and the number of high-fat ingredients it contains. For example, a duck taco with avocado and sour cream has four food groups. However, three are high in fat. So, it may appear well balanced, but it is likely to be energy-dense.

Meals can be healthy if made with low-fat ingredients and include plenty of vegetables. Choose a pizza with a low-fat or little cheese topping and plenty of vegetables on top. If you wish to have a meat topping as well, then choose a low-fat protein such as chicken, seafood or ham, rather than chorizo or salami. If you have a baguette or sandwich for lunch, then select a low-fat protein and check to see if some vegetable or salad is included.

In comparison, some combination meals, such as shepherd's pie, are typically low in fat and if it contains vegetables and not solely meat with gravy, then it can also be low to moderate in calories. The same can be said for fish pie and casseroles with baked potatoes, but of course not for pastry pies, quiches or lattices.

Reducing saturated fat and total fat

Fats are a concentrated source of energy, and a high fat intake can lead to being overweight which increase the risk of joint problems, coronary heart disease, some cancers and type 2 diabetes. Diseases which frequent business travellers appear to be more susceptible.

Meals which are high in fat shouldn't be regularly included in a travellers' diet as they leave you feeling overfull, bloated and uncomfortable during the flight. They can also keep you from falling asleep. In contrast, a meal which combines protein and carbohydrate may help to induce sleep, which is useful if you're travelling long haul and catching an evening flight to arrive at your destination during the day. Also, fat has a lower satiety effect than protein and high fibre foods, leaving you feeling slightly less satisfied.

When travelling frequently, you should aim to have meals which are low to moderate in fat. Low-fat ingredients are less than 3 g of fat per 100g. Protein sources which are low in fat include white fish, crustaceans, skinless chicken, rabbit, venison and lean pork. When you combine low-fat protein sources with whole grain carbohydrates and vegetables, you can reasonably anticipate your meal will be low in fat, subject to cooking method and added fats or sauces.

To put this into perspective, a meal of 600 calories shouldn't provide more than 20 g of fat in total. For women attempting to lose weight, this would equate to no more than 15 g per 450 calorie meal and for a man or very active woman eating a 750-calorie meal, this would be no more than 25 g per meal.

While all fats are high energy-dense ingredients, some fats are much healthier than others. The two main types of fat are saturated and unsaturated. A meal comparatively high in saturated fat to unsaturated fat will increase the cholesterol circulating in your arteries. Over time a diet high in saturated fat may narrow your arteries by increasing fatty deposits. Thus, increasing your risk of heart disease, pulmonary embolisms, strokes and other cardiovascular diseases.

As a general rule of thumb, a man shouldn't eat more than a total of 30 g of saturated fat a day which is less than 10 g for a meal and a woman shouldn't eat more than a total of 20 g of saturated fat a day which is less than 7 g per meal.

Choose fats which are better for you

While too much-saturated fat in your diet may be bad for you, polyunsaturated and monounsaturated fats have the opposite effect regarding cholesterol, i.e., they help remove the cholesterol and transport it back to your liver.

So, choose foods which contain polyunsaturated or monounsaturated fats. These include olive oil, rapeseed, avocados, nuts, oily fish such as mackerel, kippers, herring, trout, sardines, salmon and tuna. Adding these to your diet will also increase other vital nutrients in your diet, such as fat-soluble vitamins A, D and E, along with providing some essential fats which our bodies can't produce.

However, fats which are healthier for you are still fats, so don't overeat these in the mistaken belief they will do you more good, as the opposite may be true if you overcompensate and start to gain weight.

Reducing salt

Foods with high salt contents are best avoided when flying. If you are a frequent business traveller, then meals with a high sodium content will contribute to high blood pressure and fluid retention, make you feel bloated and uncomfortable when flying. Cutting down on salt in the long-term will help to reduce high blood pressure and lessen the risk of heart disease, along with DVT and cancer.

You should aim for no more than 6 grams of salt per day which mean no more than 2.0 grams per meal. Airport food can be extremely high in salt, such as soups which are typically over 2.5 grams per serving and many Asian based dishes which use soy sauce. We have not included any meals which we know are excessively high in salt in any of our healthier meals options listed below or those listed under the Chapters 12, 14 and 15 on breakfasts, 5-a-day and snacks.

Obviously, this is subject to nutritional information being available. Where nutritional information is not available at the time of review, we have relied on the ingredients listed and deselected those which may contain high salt ingredients, such as soy sauce, seaweed, stocks and sauces. In some instances, where the rest of the nutritional content is fine, we have suggested how to alter the salt content, such as holding the soy sauce on a portion of sushi.

Airline food can also be heavily seasoned to counter the lack of taste at high altitudes. If you have high blood pressure, then it might be worthwhile considering either obtaining the lower sodium foods items available in the airport for you to take on board with you, packing food items from home and bringing them with you, or order a low-sodium meal option in advance when you book your ticket.

Sugar

A low sugar option should only contain 5 grams or less per 100 g. Foods with very high sugar contents contain over 22.5 grams of sugar per 100 g. Examples of these include muesli or cereal and protein bars, flavoured coffee drinks, bottled smoothies, sweetened breakfast cereals and soft drinks. Sugar doesn't provide any additional nutrients other than calories. If you're thinking honey, brown sugar, agave syrups or concentrated juice is healthier, then you've been misled. These ingredients are not healthier, as they still only provide energy without any significant contribution of vitamins and minerals to your diet. Also, a high fructose content may lead to long-term health problems.

Most meals are savoury based and low in sugar, except those which contain hidden sugars, such as soups, sauces, and salad dressings, and the more obvious accompaniments to a main meal such as preserves, drinks, baked goods and desserts. Avoiding high in sugar additions to your main meal will reduce its total sugar content.

If you have filled up sufficiently from your starter and main, you probably won't feel the need for a dessert. However, if there is still room, then a good rule of thumb to reduce the amount of added sugar while enhancing the nutritional quality of your diet is to choose either dairy or fruit-based desserts. The sugar naturally present in milk and whole fruit is not classified as a free (added) sugar.

Should you decide to deviate from either milk based or fruit to something more tempting, then try to choose something which will be low to moderate in sugar and fat. Remember to watch out for sugar alternatives such as honey or syrups, as these still count as added sugar.

Examples of lower sugar and fat desserts may include a low-fat frozen yoghurt such as on the Comptoir Libanais with varieties including Pomegranate & Orange Blossom and Halva & Roasted Pistachio. Other examples of desserts with low to moderate sugar contents are Yo! Sushi's chocolate mochi.

Plenty of vegetables

Your plate should comprise one-half of vegetables. Most vegetables are very low in calories as they have a high water and fibre content. Consequently, this makes them of a high volume or weight and low in energy density type food. They are also an excellent source of vitamins and minerals, many of which are not usually present in the protein, dairy or carbohydrate foods.

Choose menus which offer a selection of vegetable-based starters and sides. If you can't see these listed on the menu, then look at the mains which are salads and request a small portion to accompany without the additional protein and dressing. You can also add vegetables to your airport meal by requesting additional toppings such as peppers, tomato or onions.

We have listed menu items which are served with vegetables in the following section. We have also added suggestions from the starter and side sections on the menu.

How to reduce the energy density of meals when dining in an airport restaurant.

Reducing the energy density of your pre-flight meal is integral to making your meals healthier and lighter while keeping you feeling satisfied. It will ultimately help you achieve and maintain an appropriate weight in the long term, without making you feel hungry or uncomfortable during a flight.

Granted it can be a challenge to decipher how much energy a meal comprises when only faced with a short menu description. You'll be lucky to find any nutritional information on the menu or readily accessible in a separate document as few restaurants supply such. Most restaurants can provide ingredient information separately for allergy suffers, which is all they need to do by law. Regardless, diners are usually at the mercy of the chef as to how energy-dense a meal may be.

There are some simple steps you can take to reduce the energy density of your meal. Here are five ways to ensure your meal has a lower energy density.

Choose low energy dense foods as a starter

Choose salads, vegetable or broth-based soup options to start with rather than dishes with ingredients that are high in fat. Research shows we tend to eat the same weight of food each day, although the energy content can vary considerably. By selecting lower energy-dense foods for a starter, as your stomach expands your body will tell your brain a lot sooner you are full. It usually takes about 20 minutes to register, which is approximately the time your main meal will take to be served, leaving you less likely to overeat on the main. Some studies have shown that those who choose a salad (without dressing) before their main dish will on average consume 100 calories less per sitting.

For example, at Armadillo there is a Street Snack starter, and at Comptoir Libanais there is a selection of mezze style starters. While at the Red Lion you could choose a side salad to start.

Swap the high energy dense vegetables for a lower energy dense option

Many airport restaurants appear rather prescriptive with their inclusion of a carbohydrate vegetable, such as the traditional serving of chips on most of the dishes on the menu. However, the chef is usually quite happy to swap the fries for another carbohydrate item such as rice, steamed new or baked potatoes, especially if it is already served with other menu items. Lower energy dense foods which provide a similar weight of food will help you feel fuller on fewer calories.

For example, at the Red Lion, you can order the classic beef, classic chicken or vegetarian burger without chips and add a side salad. You already have the bun, so do you need the chips as a carbohydrate as well?

Similarly, other vegetables can be laden with fat through deep-frying or additions of butter, cream, sugar and honey. For example, at the Nicholas Culpeper you can request to have no honey added to the roasted carrots, and at Garfunkel's restaurant, you could ask for no butter on the Garden Vegetables.

Round your meals out with additional options

Some airport restaurants do not include vegetables with the main menu item, or if they do, the portion might be minuscule, leaving you with sufficient room for a sweet afterwards. As mentioned above, we should be aiming for half of our plate containing vegetables. When dining at these restaurants, it's better to order additional vegetables to have with the main meal, rather than settle for a dessert later. Choose side dishes which add bulk, such as beans, cabbage or salad, and avoid items which are fried or have added fat, such as onion rings or garlic bread to accompany.

Opt for the lower fat proteins

Lamb and beef naturally have a high marbled fat content compared to other meats such as chicken, venison and pork which have a much lower fat content. Similarly, low-fat cream cheese, fromage frais and yoghurts are lower in fat than traditional cheeses and cream. So, when you choose from a menu, select items which have a lower fat protein as their main ingredient.

For example, At Nicholas Culpeper, the grilled herby chicken served with brown rice, spinach and fresh lemon is a lean protein served with higher fibre rice, and vegetables. At Comptoir Libanais, the Chicken and Green Olive Tagine is a lower fat protein than the Lamb Kofta Tagine

Watch out for high energy-dense 'healthy' ingredients

Ingredients which contain 'healthy fats' such as avocado, nuts and olive oil, are still fats. Any menu items which has 'healthy fats' as a dominant ingredient will most likely be energy-dense. Similarly, desserts which advertise ingredients such as honey, maple syrup, agave syrup or fruit juice as a sweetener may also be high in sugar and packed with calories.

For example, the Armadillos' BBQ Confit Duck Tacos mentioned above, contains avocado making it appear healthier in balance, yet contributing to the total high-fat content. For a lighter taco, reduce or deselect the sour cream or smashed avocado and replace them with more salsa and beetroot.

Healthier, lighter meals at Gatwick Airport

Preparation and planning are essential for successful business travel, regardless of whether it is a long or short haul. Once you have your basic travel itinerary, meetings organised and work planned; it's the time to ensure you can choose healthier options en route. While at the date of booking your flight you can pre-order your in-flight meals to suit your needs, it is harder to know what is on offer in the terminal until you arrive at the airport.

Gatwick Airport's North Terminal offers an eclectic selection of cuisines for travellers to pick from as part of their journey through the airport. Passengers can choose from 'grab and go' items to casual or private dining options. However, as we have discovered during our review, many menu items are extremely high in calories, fat, saturated fat, salt and sugar.

As with most busy executives, you probably won't get the chance to search through each menu and find, if there is any, nutritional information before travelling, so we've done the exploration and assessment for you. All you need to do is to select from the lists of options below.

All of the items listed match the robust criteria for healthier choices as outlined above. We've scrutinised every menu to find the healthier options for you. Where nutritional analysis was not available at the time of review, we examined the description carefully and based inclusion on dietetic guidelines.

We've also included a selection of sides along with any suitable starters for inclusion as a low-energy-dense starter. For main meals, we have indicated where a simple modification might be necessary to reduce the added fat or sugar.

Here are the items we've looked at during our last review and have found they met the criteria outlined above.

Grab and go outlets

Arrivals, Ground Floor

If you have just landed and wish to grab something to eat while continuing with your journey, then there are a couple of stores surrounding the arrivals exit where you can pick up some items. If you're passing through security for departures, then don't forget you can take solids through, but not liquids or gels over 100 ml. Examples of foodstuff over 100 ml which you can't take through security include yoghurt, jelly and marmite.

M&S Simply Food

M&S Simply Food provides convenient shopping for business travellers who have either just arrived or are about to depart. In addition to sandwiches and wraps, M&S Simply Food offers several ready meals, including salads and prepared plates of foods, along with fresh fruit, yoghurts and snack foods for longer journeys.

For a main meal item, there is also the new Nourish range, which offers dishes that provide several of your five a day count, high in vitamins and minerals while contributing a high fibre content. If you wish to reduce the fat and calorific content further on any of the dishes below, then the simple solution for most of these items would be to not to use all the additional dressing supplied.

Open: 24 hours
Location: Opposite the Bureau de Change and next to Boots the Chemist

Wraps

Mexican Three Bean Wrap Three bean and tomato salsa, roasted sweet potato with cheese, soured cream and spinach in a tomato and chilli tortilla wrap. The wrap provides 440 kcal (1851 kJ)

Moroccan Style Chicken Wrap Carrot and coriander slaw with marinated roast British chicken, yoghurt and mint dressing and spinach in a pumpkin and wheat flour tortilla wrap. The wrap provides 403 kcal (1692 kJ)

Beetroot & Feta Wrap Beetroot, feta cheese and salad cheese with a pea, edamame soybeans and beetroot and wheat flour tortilla wrap. The wrap provides 410 kcal (1717 kJ)

Ready meals and food bowls

Chilli & Lime Chicken & Rice Salad Chilli and lime marinated chicken breast and rice salad with sesame, soy and ginger dressing. One portion provides 322 kcal (1357 kJ)

King Prawn Tomato & Basil Pasta Salad Pasta with king prawns in a tomato and basil dressing. One portion provides 510 kcal (2142 kJ)

Super Wholefood Salad Edamame (soy) beans, quinoa and spelt with a creamy lemon & mint dressing. One portion provides 371 kcal (1546 kJ)

Beetroot, Goat's Cheese & Lentil Salad Beetroot, lentils and aubergine salad served with a beetroot & mint dip and topped with goat's cheese. One pack provides 342 kcal (1431 kJ)

Hot Smoked Lochmuir Salmon and Potato Salad With a lemon vinaigrette. One portion provides 275 kcal (1153 kJ).

Nutty Super Wholefood Salad Cooked quinoa, cooked spelt-wheat, beans and soy and ginger dressing with a cannellini bean and sesame tahini dip. Leave the dressing off if you wish to reduce the fat content. One portion provides 385 kcal (1605 kJ)

Crayfish, Mango and Rice Salad Mixed rice, crayfish, mango and pea shoot salad with coconut and chilli dressing. You can reduce the fat content by not adding all the dressing. One portion provides 446 kcal (1879 kJ)

Nourish Bowl Sweet Potato Sweet potato bites, harissa spiced chickpeas, butternut noodles, red pepper & walnut dip. Leave the dressing off if you wish to reduce the fat content. One portion is 393 kcal (1642 kJ)

Nourish Bowl Avocado & Egg Sorghum with hard-boiled free-range egg with avocado, pickled red cabbage, cooked quinoa and kale with a cashew nut and sesame dip. Leave the dressing off if you wish to reduce the fat content. One portion is 333 kcal (1385 kJ)

Nourish Bowl Edamame & Black Rice Cooked black rice with roasted chickpeas, edamame beans and ginger bites, pickled beetroot and carrots, kale and sesame seeds with a soy sauce and chilli cashew dip. Leave the dressing off if you wish to reduce the fat content. One portion is 395 kcals (1649 kJ)

Desserts

Watermelon & Lime Jelly Watermelon and lime jelly watermelon and blueberries. This pot provides 95 kcal (397 kJ)

Banana, Almond and Honey Granola Fat-free Greek yoghurt, banana and an almond and honey granola. A pot provides 220 kcal (925 kJ)

Boots the Chemist

Conveniently located in the Arrivals Hall and the Departure Lounge, business travellers can shop in here for refrigerated meal options. There is plenty of fresh fruit, prepared salads, sandwiches and flatbreads.

There are several Boots the Chemist at Gatwick's North Terminal, including one before security (in the Arrivals Hall) and two within the Departure Lounge. You can pre-order online and collect either from Boots the Chemist within the North Terminal Departure Lounge or before security at Unit 2 near M&S Simply Food, opposite Costa Coffee on the ground floor, post-exit from Customs and Excise.

The larger of the two Boots the Chemist, at the far end of the Departure Lounge, has a broader selection of food items. It even has a sushi and salad island near the front of the Boots entrance for you to choose freshly sliced and healthier convenient food from.

Locations: Arrivals next to M&S. After security, on the right in the lower level of the Departure Lounge, next to The Bookshop by WHSmith, and at the far end of the Departure Lounge next to WHSmith.

Opening in Arrivals: 24 hours
Opening in Departure Lounge: 4.00 am to 8.300 pm
Telephone: 01293 569606
Website: www.boots.com

Sandwiches

Chicken & Avocado Roast chicken, avocado and chilli crush mayonnaise and lemon zest mayonnaise with tomato and spinach on malted bread. This packet provides 317 kcal (1563 kJ)

Cheese & Apple Slaw on Wholemeal Bread Reduced fat cheese with apple coleslaw, cucumber and lettuce on wholemeal bread. This packet provides 400 kcal (1677 kJ)

Houmous & Falafel on Wheat Flatbread Moroccan style houmous with carrot and coriander falafel, cucumber and mint yoghurt topped with spinach in a plain white flatbread. This packet provides 368 kcal (1548 kJ)

Katsu Style Chicken Cooked chicken breast with katsu style curry sauce, red pepper, spinach and cucumber with carrot, mooli and ginger mix, spring onion, mayonnaise, carrot and coriander on malted bread. This packet provides 315 kcal (1331 kJ)

Raspberry Jelly A raspberry flavour jelly with raspberries. This pot provides 25 kcal (105 kJ)

Public Dining

Arrivals, Ground Floor

Costa Coffee

Costa Coffee boasts to offers over 600 varieties of your favourite beverage, with a range of food items to accompany. While it may not be your first port of call for a healthy light meal, it is open 24 hours, so when you hop off the plane you can be guaranteed there is somewhere you can have a hot beverage and a quick bite to eat. If it is a healthier sandwich, salad or a wrap you prefer, then we've checked the nutritional analysis for you and have listed the options for you to try below.

Open: 24 hours
Location: At the far end of the hall, right opposite the exit from international arrivals. A small unit is at Check-in on level one.

Smoked Salmon & Cream Cheese Sandwich This sandwich provides 388 kcal (1627 kJ)
Roast Chicken Sandwich This sandwich provides 352 kcal (1482 kJ)
Chicken, Honey and Mustard Pasta This pasta provides 475 kcal (1997 kJ)
Chipotle Bean & Butternut Squash Wrap This wrap provides 264 kcal (1112 kJ)
Tuna Melt Panini This panini provides 470 kcal (1976 kJ)
Goats Cheese & Sweet Chilli Chutney Panini This Panini provides 447 kcal (1883 kJ)
Chicken Chorizo & Roasted Pepper Rice Box This box provides 327 kcal (1374 kJ)
Free Range Egg Sandwich This sandwich provides 342 kcal (1435 kJ)

Desserts
Fruit Pot This pot provides 45 kcal (190 kJ)
Portuguese Custard Tart This tart provides 169 kcal (707 kJ)

Check-in, Level One
Hampton by Hilton
Hampton by Hilton offers a bar menu for travellers who wish to dine without the chaos surrounding the other Check-in dining outlets. It's quiet and only two minutes from the main check-in for Easy Jet. Unfortunately, there was no nutritional analysis at the time of our review, so we've selected a couple of items for you to try based on their menu descriptions.

Open: A limited menu is available 24 hours a day. An additional bar menu operates daily from 4.00 pm to 10.00 pm daily.
Location: The entrance to this hotel is right near the Easy Jet Check-in on level one. Just follow the signs to the right of the check-in desk. You will see a sign above the entrance to the corridor for the Hampton by Hilton.

Items include:
Side Salad

Tomato and mozzarella salad Fresh Italian mozzarella and tomatoes with balsamic dressing and basil.

Salmon Salad Salmon fillet with lemon and French dressing.

Chicken Tikka Tender chicken served with basmati rice, naan bread and mango chutney.

Jacket Potato with Cheese and Beans Served with salad and coleslaw. Ask for no added butter.

Jacket Potato with Tuna Mayo. Served with salad and coleslaw. Ask for no added butter.

Check-in, Level Two

Jamie's Coffee Lounge

Jamie's Coffee Lounge is one of the many catering outlets owned by the world-renowned Chef Jamie Oliver. Backed by a team of qualified, Registered Nutritionists and Dietitians, Jamie Oliver is a leader in offering healthier options to customers.

This coffee lounge is one of the few places in Gatwick North's terminal which is open all hours to provide nutritious, great tasting food for those travelling on business.

The food items are made fresh each day, and while they provide guidance at a glance for allergens, this wasn't the same for nutritional information. We've listed some options for you based on their list of ingredients. There are some great tasting salad pots for you to try, along with some dessert pots. Both ideal as grab and go items.

Opening: 24 hours

Location: Directly between the escalator from Level One and the glass window frontage.

Items include:

Herby Chicken Salad Pot Free range chicken, bulgar wheat, lemon yoghurt, croutons, lettuce, dill, olives, tomatoes, cucumber, parsley, lemon, black sesame, pasteurised feta, chilli mint, salt and pepper.

Pastrami Salad Pot Barley, pastrami, beetroot, lemon, yoghurt, lemon horseradish, watercress, spinach, tomatoes, tarragon, walnuts, balsamic vinegar, extra virgin oil, thyme and salt.

Superfood Salad Couscous, lemon, yoghurt, chickpeas, pasteurised feta, pomegranate, lettuce, carrot, cucumber, orange, parsley, mint, sesame seeds, olive oil, chilli, salt and pepper.

Superfood Blueberry Pot Blueberries, banana, almond yoghurt, chia seeds, almonds and vanilla essence.

Strawberry Yoghurt Pot Strawberries, banana, almond yoghurt, chia seeds, almonds and vanilla essence.

Nicholas Culpepper

The Nicholas Culpeper offers homemade food for those wishing to dine in. As it's named after a famous English Herbalist and Physician, it should come as no surprise their dishes are made from scratch using the freshest of ingredients. Although no nutritional information was available at the time of review, we have carefully selected several items which appear to meet our stringent criteria. We've included a couple of sides and desserts which you can use as a low energy dense option for a starter or afters.

Open: 4.00 am to 8.30 pm
Location: In the front of large windows on the left-hand side as you travel up on the escalator from Check-in level one.

Starters, sides and desserts

Mixed Leaf Salad with Panzanella Dressing.

Honey Roasted Carrots & Seasonal Greens (request no additions, e.g., honey or butter).

Fresh Fruit Salad Served with fresh mango, pineapple, strawberries, pomegranate & Mascarpone cream.

Main meals

Grilled Herby Chicken served with brown rice, spinach & fresh lemon.

Naked Foxham Farm Beef Burger Comes served without bun or chips! Just with a mixed leaf salad and a chilli slaw.

Goats' Cheese & Roasted Beets Salad served with mixed salad leaves, freshly sliced apple, spinach & chopped hazelnuts.

King Prawn & Mixed Grains Salad Mixed salad leaves, carrot ribbons, goji berries & Panzanella dressing.

Orange Glazed Salmon Served with an Asian inspired fresh salad of wok-fried chilli, pak choi, fresh carrot & pea shoots.

Smashed Avocado on Toast with fresh mango, chilli, lime & coriander served with toasted bloomer bread.

Roasted Vegetable Cobbler Hearty roasted vegetable pie topped with creamy parsnip mash, served with honey roasted carrots and seasonal greens. (Ask for no honey on carrots if you wish to reduce the sugar content).

Departure Lounge, Lower Level

The lower floor of the Departure Lounge is mostly retail shops. You will find Caviar House and Prunier in the middle of the hall and The Red Lion at the far right-hand side just before the stairs to the upper level. There are also a couple of 'grab and go' retail outlets which we have already covered above, and near the far end of the Departure Lounge, there are several private lounges which offer more private dining (listed under private dining at the end of this chapter).

Caviar House & Prunier

Caviar House & Prunier pride themselves on offering the highest quality seafood for travellers who want a touch of luxury dining before departure. They provide a selection of the finest Prunier caviar, and Balik smoked salmon, along with crustacean platters and salads.

There are definite nutritional highlights when choosing crustacean for the main meal. It is low in fat and calories. However, it is also naturally high in sodium. So, if you are hypertensive without medication, you might find this comparatively high in sodium compared to other restaurant cuisines.

Open: 4.00 am to 8.30 pm
Location: Middle of Departure Lounge opposite Lacoste and World Duty Free

Main meals
Smoked Salmon and Shrimps Balk smoked salmon accompanied by marinated shrimps.
Crab Salad with fresh white crab meat.
King Crab & Caviar King crab legs accompanied by a spoon of Prunier Cavier.
Lobster & Caviar Lobster served with 20 g Prunier Cavier.
Scottish Smoked Salmon Finest Salmon from the pure waters of Scotland.
Lobster Salad Lobster served out of the shell, on a bed of mixed leaves, fresh mango and avocado.
Seafood Platter A combination of Balik Smoked Salmon, Balik Gravlax, Balik Tartar, shrimps, king prawn, an oyster and accompanied by Prunier caviar and new potato salad.

King Seafood Platter Four rock oysters, king crab, half lobster, prawns, shrimps, fresh white crab meat and 20 g caviar.

Tuna Tartar Tuna tartar on a bed of avocado, crispy onions served with a lemon-flavoured soy sauce. Hold the sauce if you wish to reduce the salt content.

Extras to accompany

Mixed Green Salad
Tomato & Onion Salad
Bread Selection

The Red Lion

The Red Lion is named after John of Gaunt's coat of arms, who was one of the most powerful men in English during the 14th century. It is a friendly, relaxed pub and serves traditional English food. Owned by the JD Wetherspoon chain, it provides calorific information on the menu for all its dishes and further nutritional information upon request. While many of the English favourites are high in calories, fat and salt, there are a couple of menu items which meet our set criteria. We have listed these below.

Open: 3.00 am to 8.30 pm
Location: At the end of the Departure Lounge on the right as you enter from security.

Starters, sides and desserts

Side Salad A serving is 82 kcals (343 kJ)
Quinoa Side Salad A serving is 252 kcal (1054 kJ)

Main meals

Fish Pie Hot-Kilm-smoked salmon, king prawns, Atlantic cod and haddock, in a mature Cheddar, spinach & British cream sauce, with a crunchy mash topping, vegetables. This dish provides 665 kcal (2782 kJ)

Quinoa Salad Quinoa, rice, avocado, adzuki beans, grilled red and yellow pepper, red cabbage, chia seeds, kale, buttermilk ranch dressing. This salad provides 498 kcal (2084 kJ)

Vegetable Burger Puy lentils, carrot, Davidstow Cheddar cheese, sweetcorn and mushrooms. This burger provides 575 kcal (575 kJ)

Departure Lounge, Upper Level
Armadillo

The Armadillo offers travellers a South Western style cuisine. Although they may not serve armadillo, they do serve several nutritious meals which appear low in energy density. Unfortunately, choosing such is hindered by the lack of nutritional information, so we've selected what we consider are the best options based on their menu description. In general, it would be wise to deselect the fries and choose green rice if you wish to reduce the fat and energy content.

Open: 4.00 am to 8.30 pm
Location: In the middle of the upper level of the Departure Lounge, overlooking the lower level below.

Starters, sides and desserts

Street Snack Salad. Mango, mouli & cucumber crudites with chilli salt & lime wedges, herby yoghurt dip (request no salt)
Green Rice
Little House Salad
Healthy Slaw
Fresh Fruit Bowl
Grilled Corn on the Cobb Hold the cayenne aioli.

Big Bowl Salads

Quinoa Green Green quinoa, crushed pecans, sugar snaps, apple, goat's cheese, market leaves, fresh herbs, avocado, green herby yoghurt dressing. Can add chicken or spicy prawns.
Spicy Prawns, Chicken & Mango Salad Baby gem lettuce, cucumber, radish, jalapeno and fresh herbs. Hold the honey mustard dressing.
Chopped Chef Salad Chopped chicken, hard-boiled free-range egg, blue cheese, radish, tomato, cucumber, tortilla strips, charred corn, fresh herbs, cumin and sweet onion vinaigrette. Hold the vinaigrette.

Main meals

Pan Roast Salmon Fillet. Served with pickled beetroot, mouli, pico de gallo salsa, charred corn, and the green rice option.
Grilled Citrus Chicken Breast Served with pico de gallo salsa, fresh herbs, chilli salt and healthy slaw with the green rice option.

Quinoa & Butternut Squash Quesadilla Filled and grilled soft tortilla, green quinoa, butternut squash caramelised onion, goat's cheese and mushrooms. Served with street snack salad and healthy slaw.

Veggie Chilli Burrito Filled and grilled soft tortilla, green rice, roasted rainbow veggies, smashed avocado, fresh coriander, toasted pumpkin seeds, sour cream and healthy slaw.

Black Bean Veggie Chili & Quinoa Bowl with toasted pumpkin seeds, guacamole, sour cream and fresh herbs.

Comptoir Libanais

Comptoir Libanais serves Middle East cuisine in a casual dining environment. You can either enjoy eating in or use their takeaway option for their wraps and salad. Unfortunately, no nutritional information was available at the time of review, so we've picked a selection for you based on the menu's description indicating it may be a lower fat, salt and sugar option.

Open: 4.00 am to 8.30 pm
Location: First restaurant on the upper level, next to the stairs and directly opposite the security entrance.

Starters and sides

Hommous Smooth, rich chickpea puree with tahini and lemon juice.

Baba Ghanuj Smoked aubergine, tahini and lemon juice with pomegranate seeds.

Muhammara Spiced mixed roasted nuts, roasted red pepper, cumin and olive oil.

Natural Labne Natural strained yoghurt with fresh mint, spring onion, olive oil & Nigella seeds.

Fattoush Baby gem lettuce, cherry tomatoes, mint and parsley, with toasted pita bread, fresh pomegranate and a sumac dressing.

Tabbouleh Chopped parsley, cracked wheat, tomatoes, mint and onions, with a lemon and olive oil dressing.

Freekeh Smoked green wheat, wild rocket, vine tomato, spring onion, apple vinegar and mint dressing.

Vermicelli Rice Pilaf rice mixed with vermicelli pasta.

Couscous A Middle Eastern side dish made from wheat durum granules.

Quinoa Vegan and gluten-free grains with olive oil and thyme.

Salads

Chicken Sirine Salad Chargrilled Lebanese spiced chicken breast, feta cheese, romaine lettuce, spring onion, mint, vine tomatoes, topped with pomegranate and pumpkin seed.

Quinoa & Feta Cheese Salad Quinoa, chickpeas, vine tomato, fresh mint, spring onion, topped with zaatar feta cheese, apple vinaigrette & pomegranate dressing.

Main meals

Chicken Shish Taouk Grilled marinated chicken breast with garlic, apple vinegar & fresh thyme, served with vermicelli rice.

Chicken Kofta Grilled minced chicken, herbs, onions and spices, served with vermicelli rice.

Spiced Lamb Kofta Grilled minced lamb, herbs, onions and spices, served with vermicelli rice.

Pan Roasted Salmon Pan roasted salmon fillet served with vermicelli rice, harissa sauce, pickles, fattoush salad and garnished with pomegranate seeds.

Chicken Taouk Wrap Sliced marinated chicken, pickled cucumber, tomato & garlic sauce, served with salad.

Lamb Kofta Wrap Spiced minced lamb, hommos, pickles, cucumber and tomato, served with salad.

Aubergine Tagines. Baked baby aubergine in a rich tomato & chickpea sauce. Garnished with mint yoghurt.

Desserts

Low-fat Frozen Yoghurt Choose from the following flavours;
Plain
Fresh Pomegranate seeds & orange blossom water
Halva & roasted pistachio

EAT

EAT offers a range of fresh food items which you can either eat in or take away. Their menu changes with the season so to use fresh seasonal produce and to provide variety all year round. Each item is made from scratch every day, and they donate as many leftover sandwiches and salads as possible to the Crisis charity for the homeless.

Open: 4.00 am to 20.30 pm
Location: Halfway along the upper level, just opposite Shake-A-Hula.

Soups

Italian Meatball A rustic soup of meatballs and cannellini beans in a chunky tomato sauce with chilli, basil and oregano, topped with Italian cheese. Regular size provides 304 kcal (1300 kJ)

Beef Ragu A tomato soup, with herbs, red peppers, mushrooms, minced beef and macaroni pasta. Regular size provides 283 kcal (1184 kJ)

Hot Pots

Texan Chilli Chilli con Carne with wild rice and crème Fraiche. Regular serving provides 386 kcal (1595 kJ)

Large salads & fit boxes

Houmous & Falafel Mezze Salad Mixed leaves with tabbouleh; a fresh herby mix of bulgar wheat, cucumber chunks, chopped fresh herbs and lemon juice. Topped with chunky houmous, carrot and coriander falafels, harissa spiced chickpeas and a crunchy Mezza slaw, with a vinaigrette dressing. Serving with dressing provides 493 kcal (2063 kJ)

Mexican Guacamole & Quinoa Mixed salad leaves served with quinoa, black bean, giant corn mix topped with guacamole, roasted sweet potato, chargrilled sweetcorn salsa and chargrilled red pepper. This dish provides 323 kcal (1351 kJ)

Sicilian Orzo & Roasted Vegetables An orzo based topped with sun-dried peppers, slow roast tomatoes, chargrilled courgette and capers. Served with toasted omega seeds spinach and an oregano vinaigrette. This dish provides 514 kcal (2151 kJ)

Spicy Chicken Noodle Salad Egg noodles mixed with crunchy vegetables and a hot and spicy chilli peanut relish, topped with sliced of chilli chicken, red chilli, sesame seeds and a wedge of lime. Serving provides 401 kcal (1678 kJ)

Spicy Crayfish Noodle Salad Egg noodles with crayfish tails and a chilli pepper relish. Topped with carrot, pak choi, Chinese cabbage, spring onion served with chopped red chilli and fresh coriander. Regular size provides 352 kcal (1473 kJ)

Super Nutty Fit Box Cashew and pistachio nuts served on a bed of quinoa, black rice and pickled beetroot, served with a side of houmous and chargrilled broccoli with chilli and garlic. Serving provides 343 kcal (1435 kJ)

Grills

Butternut, Chickpea & Harissa Flatbread A vegan Moroccan wrap with roasted butternut squash, harissa houmous, spiced chickpea, spinach, fresh herbs and pumpkin seeds in a khobez wrap. This flatbread provides 506 kcal (2117 kJ)

Firecracker Chicken Flatbread Spicy chicken breast with red and yellow peppers, chopped jalapenos and red pepper and crème Fraiche tapenade on a khobez wrap. This flatbread provides 436 kcal (1824 kJ)

Sandwiches, Baguettes & Wraps

Avocado Banh Mi Baguette A fresh Vietnamese-style vegan baguette with creamy avocado, pickled veg and fresh coriander. This baguette provides 384 kcal (1607 kJ)

Chicken Salad Sandwich Freshly baked malted break filled with chicken mayonnaise, crisp lettuce and juicy tomatoes. This sandwich provides 319 kcal (1335 kJ)

Smoked Salmon & Soft Cheese Sandwich Malted bread frilled with peppered soft cheese and Scottish smoked salmon. This sandwich provides 367 kcal 1535 kJ)

Turkey and Cranberry Sandwich Malted bread filled with cranberry sauce, sliced turkey breast, fresh rocket and mayonnaise. This sandwich provides 396 kcal (1657 kJ)

Chicken Salad Wrap Chicken breast with herbs, tomato, cucumber and mixed leaf salad wrapped in a kibbled rye tortilla wrap. This wrap provides 452 kcal (1891 kJ)

Chunky Houmous Wrap Chunky houmous & onion mix with fresh cucumber and spinach wrapped in a kibbled rye tortilla wrap. This wrap provides 377 kcal (1577 kJ)

Falafel & Houmous Wrap Falafel mixed with harissa houmous, chickpeas and spinach wrapped in a kibbled rye tortilla wrap. This wrap provides 477 kcal (1996 kJ)

Garfunkel's

Garfunkel's proudly promotes 'there is something for everyone' with its menu reflecting a multi-cultural world that includes British favourites as well as European, Asian and American popular dishes. Unfortunately, no nutritional information was available at the time of review, so we have chosen a selection of healthier options based on their description from the menu. For some menu items, you may need to request a slight modification e.g. swap the chips for new potatoes. We've highlighted the items which are easy to modify so to increase the number of options available.

Open: 4.00 am to 8.30 pm
Location: At the back on the upper level, opposite the Armadillo restaurant.

Starters and sides

Bruschetta Grilled flatbread topped with a cherry tomato and coriander salsa, fresh avocado, spring onion and drizzled with lime and olive oil.

Avocado on Toast Smashed avocado, mango, coriander & lime with a hint of fresh red chilli, served on toasted bread.

Mixed Salad green leaves, cucumber and tomatoes with a French dressing.

Garden Vegetables Carrots, tender stem broccoli and French beans (request no butter)

Main meals

Grill Chicken Breast served with a choice of marinades (Cajun spices or lemon & herb) and mixed salad.   Ask an alternative to chips, ask for herby grains and watercress on the side.

Cottage Pie Warming beef mince and peas, topped with mashed potatoes and served with buttered carrots, tender stem broccoli and French beans. (Request no butter on the vegetables)

Meadow Salad Goat's cheese, roasted baby potatoes, mixed grains and roasted pepper, tossed with a fennel and rocket salad with basil dressing.

Omelettes A selection of omelettes to choose from (plain, single or double fillings), all made with three eggs. Choose the mixed salad.

Frittata Packed with onions, potatoes, sliced mushrooms and roasted peppers.

Penne Arrabbiata Penne pasta tossed in a Neapolitan, with slow roasted tomato and goat's cheese topped with rocket and chilli flakes. Optional extra to add Spicy Chicken.

Grilled Chicken Burger A grilled chicken breast with lettuce, tomato, red onion and mayonnaise. Reduce the fat by swapping the chips for a side salad and asking for no mayonnaise.

Veggie Stack Burger A stack of grilled goats cheese, roasted peppers and a flat mushroom served with watercress and pesto mayonnaise. Reduce the fat by swapping the chips for a side salad and asking for no mayonnaise.

Jamie's Italian and the Union Jack Bar

Jamie Oliver and Gennaro Contaldo (Jamie's Italian Mentor) are the co-founders of Jamie's Italian which they started in 2008. They now have over 60 restaurants worldwide and continue to offer fresh, authentic Italian dishes, including pasta and antipasti.   The restaurant also has a big focus on nutrition, promoting health alongside taste, and employs a team of Registered Nutritionists and Dietitians to support all new recipe creations. They were operating a summer 2018 menu at the time of review. You can order your meal in the Union Jack Bar or the Italian Restaurant opposite.

Open: 4.30 am to 10.00 pm

Location: At the far corner of the upper level on the right-hand side as you pass through the security exit.

Starters and sides

Tomato Bruschetta Slow-roasted cherry tomatoes, with garlic & oregano, torn buffalo mozzarella, extra virgin olive oil & basil. Serving is 188 kcal (787 kJ)

Rocket & Radicchio with aged balsamic. A serving is 70 kcal (293 kJ)

Charred Broccoli With extra virgin olive oil, chilli and garlic. A serving is 128 kcal (536 kJ)

Mains

Prawn Linguine Garlicky prawns, tomatoes, shaved fennel, saffron, chilli & rocket. Small portion 353 kcal (1477 kJ) Large portion 708 kcal (2962)

Tagliatelle Bolognese Rich port, beef & red wine Ragu with Parmesan. Small portion 314 kcal (1314 kJ)

Veggie Tagliatelle Bolognese Tomato, lentil & porcini Ragu with garlic and veggie Parmesan. Small portion 322 kcal (1347 kJ)

Tagliatelle Pomodoro Small portion provides 297 kcal (1242 kJ) Large portion 593 kcal (2481)

Casarecce Puttanesca Fiery tomato & garlic sauce with black olives, capers, extra virgin olive oil & veggie Parmesan. Small portion provides 341 kcal (1427 kJ) Large portion provides 661 kcal (2766 kJ)

Casarecce Arrabbiata Fiery tomato and basil sauce with Parmesan & extra virgin olive oil. Small portion provide 294 kcal (1230 kJ) Large portion 582 kcal (2435 kJ)

Pret A Manger

Opened in 1986, Pret now has over 350 cafes worldwide and operates in many UK airport terminals. Everything is made fresh daily, and all unsold food is given to charities at the end of the day. Pret has a real focus on healthier options as well as treats. We've chosen a selection of lunch and dinner items which match our stringent criteria below for you.

Open: 3.00 am to 8.30 pm

Location: Far left-hand corner on the upper level, overlooking the World Duty Free and main departure board.

Salads

Sweet Potato Falafel & Smashed Beets Veggie Box Turmeric & sweet potato falafel, smashed beetroot hummus, avocado and long-stem broccoli on a bed of brown & black rice. Hold the dressing to reduce the fat content. Per serving 407 kcal (1695 kJ)

Tuna Nicoise Salad (without dressing) Pole & line caught tuna and sliced free-range egg, with sweet baby plum tomatoes, kalamata olives, served with freshly sliced cucumber, red onion, salad leaves and a wedge of lemon. Hold the dressing. Per serving 176 kcal (738 kJ)

Sesame Salmon & Black Rice Roasted salmon coated with sesame seed paired with black rice. Served with long-stem broccoli, pickled cabbage, carrot salad and edamame beans. Hot the dressing to reduce the fat content. Per serving 369 kcal (1541 kJ)

Sandwiches

Chicken & Cucumber Sandwich Chicken sandwich with cucumber on granary bread. Sandwich provides 389 kcal (1628 kJ)

Chicken Avocado Sandwich British Chicken breast with avocado, salad leaves and a yoghurt mayonnaise. Sandwich provides 484 kcal (2017 kJ)

Cracking Egg Salad Sandwich Chunky egg mayo with slices of tomato, on the fresh wild rocket. Sandwich provides 375 kcal (1575 kJ)

Crayfish & Avocado Sandwich Crayfish from the Yangtze River, combined with sliced avocado, mixed salad leaves, yoghurt dressing and a squeeze of lemon juice. Sandwich provides 383 kcal (1600 kJ)

Curried Chickpeas & Mango Chutney Sandwich Lightly-spiced curried chickpeas combined with spring onion, raisins, red peppers and our sweet mango chutney. Finished with a handful of spinach leaves and fresh coriander. Sandwich provides 476 kcal (2003 kJ)

Free Range Egg Mayo Sandwich Free range eggs with mustard and cress. Sandwich provides 367 kcal (1541 kJ)

Baguettes

Chipotle Mozzarella Hot Baguette A hot stone baked baguette with melted mozzarella, chipotle ketchup, fresh red peppers, roasted tomatoes and our delicious Italian matured cheese. A baguette provides 422 kcal (1756 kJ)

Wraps

Avocado and Chipotle Chickpeas Salad Wrap A vegan salad wrap filled with creamy avocado covered with chipotle chickpeas, charred corn and black bean salsa, topped with fresh coriander and mixed salad leaves. A serving provides 444 kcal (1855 kJ)

Humous and Crunchy Veg Salad Wrap Generous amount of humous onto a kibbled rye wrap, pickled onions and a pile of fresh, aromatic coriander, topped with slices of fresh red peppers, crunchy cucumber sticks and a handful of spinach. A serving provides 392 kcal (1638 kJ)

Soups

Chicken, Broccoli & Brown Rice Soup Chunky British chicken broth simmered with vegetables, baby broccoli florets and brown rice. A 370 g serving provides 137 kcal (576 kJ)

Smokey Chorizo Chicken Soup Chunks of smoky chorizo simmered with chicken, tomatoes, cannellini beans, celery, peppers and carrot. Finished with smoked paprika and a mix of herbs. A 370 g serving provides 223 kcal (931 kJ)

Souper Tomato Chopped, super-ripe plum tomatoes simmered with crushed tomatoes, diced tomatoes, onion, celery, carrots and rich tomato puree. A 370g serving provides 199 kcal (831 kJ)

Veggie Chilli Soup Black turtle beans, red kidney beans and black-eyed beans, peppers, sweetcorn, brown rice and quinoa with ancho chilli, cocoa, jalapeno chilli and a hint of lime. A 370 g serving provides 216 kcal (909 kJ)

Vegetable Tagine Soup Roasted courgettes and peppers cooked in vegetable stock with cumin, turmeric red chilli and cinnamon. Served with tomatoes, chickpeas, buckwheat and red lentils. A 370 g serving provides 188 kcal (788 kJ)

Desserts

Diary-Free Chocolate Chia Pot A rich and creamy vegan chia pot, combining soaked chia seeds, dairy-free coconut yoghurt alternative and a dark chocolate sauce topped with fresh blueberries and pomegranate. A pot provides 161 kcal (632 kJ)

Mango & Lime Chunks of mango and a squeeze of lime. A pot provides 92 kcal (384 kJ)

Pret's Fruit Salad Pineapple, melon, mango, apple, kiwifruit and blueberries. A pot provides 113 kcal (473 kJ)

Superfruit Salad Chunks of mango, kiwi fruit, pomegranate seeds and blueberries. A pot provides106 kcal (450 kJ)

Watermelon & Lime Watermelon with a wedge of lime. A pot provides 48 kcal (204 kJ)

Nectarine & Raspberries Perfectly ripe nectarines served with tangy raspberries. A pot provides 56 kcal (238 kJ)

Starbucks

Starbucks has over 17,000 stores worldwide, and you'll find it in many airport terminals. Starbucks pride themselves on the quality of their coffee, ethical sourcing and providing an excellent environment for the business traveller to relax, chat and work. You can grab several healthier options here to either eat in or take away.

Open: 24 hours
Location: Halfway along, at the back of the upper level between Jamie's Italian and EAT restaurants.

Items selected include:

Smoked Salmon Bagel One portion is 472 kcal (1985 kJ)
Vegan Wrap with Falafel & Slaw Wrap provides is 261 kcal (1096 kJ)
Californian Chicken Sandwich Sandwich provides 393 kcal (1653 kJ)

Desserts

Whole Bananas provides 108 kcal (448 kJ)
Mango and Lime Fruit Pot One pot provides 87 kcal (367 kJ)
Fruit Mix Pot One pot provides 72 kcal (301kJ)
Berry Crunch Pot One pot provides 250 kcal (1051 kJ)

Yo! Sushi

Visit Yo! Sushi for great Japanese street food and sushi. Yo! Sushi offers casual dining with over 80 items on their menu to choose from either as you dine in or to take away. While many Asian cuisines have a high fat and salt content, Yo! Sushi has plenty of items which when combined meet the criteria for a healthier light meal.

Open: 6.00 am to 8.30 pm
Location: Overlooking the lower level at the far end of the balcony.

Salads

Edamame Pods sprinkled with salt flakes and spring onion. One serving is 135 kcal (565 kJ)
Spicy Chicken Salad Kimchi grilled chicken thigh and crunchy salad in a sesame soy dressing. One serving is 206 kcal (862 kJ)

Rolls

Spicy Tuna Rolls Chopped yellowfin tuna, spicy sriracha and rayu chilli oil with shichimi powder. One serving is 119 kcal (498 kJ)
Ebi Roll Prawn katsu and avocado with mayo and dried purple shiso yukari. One serving is 135 kcal (565 kJ)
Avocado Maki 6 pieces. A serving is 212 kcal (887 kJ)
Cucumber Maki 6 pieces. A serving is 149 kcal (623 kJ)
Salmon Maki 4 pieces. A serving is 125 kcal (523 kJ)
Tuna Maki 4 pieces. A serving is 119 kcal (498 kJ)

Nigiri (rice blocks with a topping)

Tamago Sweet and light egg omelette and nori. One serving 262 kcal (1096 kJ)
Salmon Nigiri Fresh cut salmon and a touch of wasabi. One serving is 99 kcal (414 kJ)
Ebi Sushi Poached butterflied prawns with a washbi kick. One serving is 137 kcal (573kJ)
Beef Nigiri Seared beef with nori and seven chilli shichimi powder. One serving is 102 kcal (427 kJ)
Assorted Nigiri & Maki Salmon, tuna and Ebi Nigiri, avocado and cucumber maki. 218 kcal (912 kJ)

Sashimi (premium slices of fish or meat)

Salmon Fresh cuts of thick-sliced salmon with mooli and lemon A serving is 140 kcal (586 kJ)
Tuna Thick cut slices of yellowfin tuna, with mooli and lime. A serving is 106 kcal (444 kJ)
Beef Taraki Pepper seared rare beef and tangy coriander pesto. A serving is 97 kcal (406 kJ)

Salmon Selection Two slices of sashimi and two pieces of maki and nigiri all on one plate. A serving is 220 kcal (920 kJ)

Temaki (hand rolls)
Salmon & Avocado Fresh salmon, avocado, mayo and toasted sesame seed in a nori rice cone. A serving is 163 kcal (682 kJ)
Yasai Cucumber, inari and tamago with mayo, wrapped in a nori rice cone. A serving is 230 kcal (962 kJ)

Yakisoda (stir fried noodles)
Plain Yakisoda A serving is 78 kcal (326 kJ)

Ramen (soup, noodles and broth)
Pork Ramen. A serving is 478 kcal (2000 kJ)

Desserts
Fresh Fruit A palate cleanser of fresh and healthy fruits. A serving is 46 kcal (192 kJ)
Chocolate Mochi Sweet Rice balls with a rich chocolate ganache centre. A serving is 236 kcal (987 kJ)

Private Dining

Dining in one of the many lounges at Gatwick's North Terminal offers the privacy to conduct meetings or to work on your laptop while having a meal. Here's the rundown on what the private lounges offer the hunger business traveller for lunch and dinner.

No. 1 Lounge

No. 1 Lounge has a dine-in bistro as well as a self-service buffet for snacks, salads and desserts. Hot dishes in the bistro dining area are made to order. When we reviewed this lounge, it offered a soup of the day, salads, fish finger sandwiches and a small bowl of lamb hotpot. On another occasion, it offered Lemon Chicken Tagine, Spinach & Ricotta Pasta Shells as the hot dishes. All the dishes we tried were delicious. The bowl sizes are not very large, so you definitely won't be going overfilled onto your flight!

Open: 4.00 am to 10.00 pm

Location: On the lower level of the Departure Lounge, after security, near gates 101 - 113.

Directions: Head towards gate 101 – 113, as you pass London News Company turn right into the corridor, you will see another hallway on your right.   Enter the hallway and walk through the double glass doors. No.1 Lounge is directly ahead.

Aspire Lounge

The buffet option in the middle of the Aspire Lounge is of mixed fare. The options are more for a snack or a light meal and often include a variety of pasta dishes (self-serve) or soup of the day. If it is a light meal or snack you are after, then there are several healthy options to consider.

Open: 4.00 am to 10.00 pm, with a slight seasonal variation.
Location: First floor of the Departure Lounge.
Directions: Head towards gate 101 – 113, as you pass London News Company, you will see a corridor on your right. Go through the double glass doors and take the lift to the first floor. The lounge is located on the right-hand side.

My Lounge

Although more informal than the No. 1 Lounge or Aspire Lounge, there is also a buffet where you can help yourself to snacks or a hot item which usually comprises a vegetarian option such as vegetable curry or vegetarian chilli. Although you can visit the hot food as often as you like, it remains of a limited range for a main meal. Nevertheless, our travel health consultant enjoyed the both vegetable curry and vegetarian chilli during her reviews.

Open: 6.00 am to 8.00 pm.
Location: Departure Lounge, lower level.
Directions: Head towards gate 101 – 113, as you pass London News Company, you will see a corridor on your right. Turn right and proceed through the double glass doors. The lounge is located on the left-hand side just before the lifts.

Chapter 14: Five-a-day is beneficial for busy travellers

Most of us fail to eat adequate amounts of fruit and vegetables when we are at home or in the office. If truth be told, only 15% of adults meet the recommended target of five portions a day, with the majority of us eating less than three portions a day. Research has also found that travelling is cited as a primary reason for not reaching the recommended consumption.

There are many possibilities as to why this might be the case. When you're travelling on business, your daily routine is disrupted making it less feasible to stick to the fruits and vegetables you usually enjoy. Moreover, the availability of fruit and vegetables can be rather hit and miss when in transit. There's also the hustle and bustle of getting somewhere which unpredictably leaves little time to source fresh fruit or vegetables. The combination of multiple barriers means business travellers find it more challenging to consume adequate fruit and vegetables. The outcome tends to be to leave it until arrival or wait until you are back on familiar ground.

We know frequent business travellers are more likely to suffer from cancer, cardiovascular disease and diabetes than non-frequent business travellers. While we don't fully understand the underlying reasons as to why business travellers are more at risk, we recognise regular business travellers are more likely to be, on average, heavier in weight, have higher blood pressure, blood lipids, cholesterol and sugar levels. All of which can be related to dietary causes. In contrast, those who consume a minimum of 400 grams of fruit and vegetables a day, usually as five portions of different items, tend to have a lower risk of severe health problems, including heart disease, stroke and some cancers.

The World Health Organisation (WHO) analysed a large number of research studies, and it is the totality of this research which validates people who consume above-average amounts of fruit and vegetables have below-average rates of heart disease, stroke and cancer. From this evidence base, the WHO estimated that 2.7 million deaths globally each year are due to low fruit and vegetable consumption. It has also been acknowledged diet contributes to the development of one-third of cancer, and eating more fruit and vegetables is the second most important action to be taken to prevent cancer after not smoking.

It's not just about quantity either. While the advice is to eat at least 400 g of fruit and vegetables a day, it is recommended that this should be in five portions as a mix and match approach is more effective if consumption is from a selection of fruit and vegetables. Each fruit or vegetable offers different nutrients which support a range of biological functions and help prevent an array of diseases. This is why the WHO recommendation of at least five portions a day has been used around the world as a vital health campaign to help reduce diet-related disease. For this reason, business travellers are advised to consume a 'rainbow' each day. Hence the minimum 400 grams of fruit and vegetables should be broken into at least five portions, spread throughout the day, and from an assortment of colourful fruit and vegetables.

How business travellers benefit from a variety

The benefits of consuming a rainbow selection of fruit and vegetables each day serve to counteract many of the ailments pertinent to business travellers' health and wellbeing. Here's how those travelling regularly on business can benefit.

Lower business traveller's cancer likelihood

While some research indicates frequent flyers, particularly crew, may be exposed to greater cosmic radiation, Cancer Research UK advise the amount of exposure by itself may not affect the risk of cancer. However, if you have a lack of fruit and vegetables in your diet, this will increase the possibility of cancer, irrespective of how often you fly. Fruit and vegetables contain many nutrients which lessen cancer likelihood. They are an excellent source of dietary fibre as well as numerous vitamins, minerals and other substances, including antioxidants. Vitamins and minerals are crucial for preventing disease as well as being used in metabolism.

In addition to their metabolic roles, vitamins such as vitamin A, E and C also act as antioxidants and protect the body from harmful free radicals (negatively charged atoms or molecules) that may cause cancer. Vitamin A is found in orange and yellow fruits, along with orange, red and green vegetables, such as carrots and peppers, whereas Vitamin E is found in nuts, avocado and berries, along with cereals. Vitamin C is found in all fruit and vegetables and is exceptionally high in peppers, oranges and kiwi fruit.

For this reason, alone, it is essential to choose a 'rainbow' selection of fruit and vegetables, and not just the green variety to accompany your snacks and meals each day.

Reduce fatigue

In metabolism, B vitamins aid the release of energy from carbohydrates, along with the breakdown of fat, metabolism of amino acids and formation of red blood cells. There are many B vitamins, each used in several different biochemical pathways. Business travellers who feel fatigued not only need to select a range of fruit and vegetables but also should include legumes, nuts and cereals into their diet to provide the majority of B vitamins.

Good sources of B vitamins, such as riboflavin, pantothenic acid, pyridoxine and folate, are found in a variety of fruits and vegetables, including bananas, dried fruits, avocado, green leafy vegetables, leeks, mushrooms, nuts, seeds and legumes. While other B vitamins, such as thiamine, biotin and niacin, which also aid the release of energy from food, include cereals, oatmeal and soya. The WHO recommendation of at least 400 grams of fruit and vegetables is currently divided into five 80 g portions a day from an assortment of fruit and vegetables, with nuts, legumes and cereals on top of this to safeguard good health and wellbeing.

Maintain good circulation

Minerals are also found in fruits, green leafy vegetables, dried fruits and nuts. Again, variety plays a vital role in preventing dietary related diseases and enhancing traveller wellbeing. Potassium, found in dried fruits, bananas, beetroot, spinach and avocado, helps to maintain fluid balance, regulate blood pressure and is essential for heart function, whereas iron plays a crucial role in carrying oxygen around the body, and is also found in green leafy vegetables, peas, dried apricots and nuts. Calcium is not just essential for bones, but also for muscular contractions. It is found in green leafy vegetables, dried figs, sesame seeds and tofu. All these minerals are especially relevant for the frequent business traveller who may suffer more from fatigue and circulatory problems.

Lessen the risk of blood clots

Meanwhile, other nutrients found in fruit and vegetables, such as flavonoids may also be cardioprotective as they also function as antioxidants and may decrease the risk of blood clotting. Flavonoids are easy food sources to identify as they are usually responsible for the vivid colour pigments in fruit and vegetables, such as red, blue and yellow. Another reason why the consumption of a 'rainbow selection' of fruit and vegetables is essential in the diet.

Enhance hydration

Fruits and vegetables also contribute fluid to our daily diets, as they typically have a high water content. On average, food supplies one litre of water to our diet. If you consume the minimum recommended 400 grams of fruit and vegetables a day, comprising at least three-quarters of water, then your consumption will contribute 300 ml of water on top of any beverages you may drink. Fruits with the highest water content (over 85%) include melons, berries and citrus fruits, and vegetables with the highest water content (over 90%) include salad vegetables, green leafy vegetables and squash.

Enhances overall wellbeing

Fruit and vegetables are also a good source of fibre. Fibre helps to keep our blood sugar at healthy levels, reduces blood cholesterol, the incidence of stroke, coronary heart disease and aids in the prevention of bowel cancer. In fact, vegetable fibre is particularly noted for supporting the reduction of cardiovascular disease and reducing the incidence of coronary heart disease, while fibre within cereals has shown to be effective in lowering blood pressure (oat fibre in particular), total cholesterol, LDL cholesterol, blood lipids and type 2 diabetes.

Ease discomfort from constipation

Fibre also helps to maintain a healthy gut and prevent constipation, something that majority of business travellers find a challenge. In particular, fibre from fruit and vegetables, such as carrots, potatoes, prunes and citrus fruit, have been found to aid the movement of waste through the intestine. The fibre from legumes, wheat, rye, barley, maize and rice bran are good at absorbing fluids which may also aid movement. If you are prone to traveller's constipation and suffer from tiredness, then including at least a couple of fruits, three portions of vegetables a day as well as eating whole grains, will help when travelling on business. Research has also shown eating a banana is particularly good if you suffer from diarrhoea as well as constipation.

Lessen risk of travel Infections

As well as helping prevent chronic diseases, such as cardiovascular diseases, diabetes and some cancers, adequate fruit and vegetable intake also helps increase resistance to infectious disease. Something that many business travellers wish to avoid while travelling on business. So, aim for, at the very least, five portions of fruits and vegetables per day, from a variety, when travelling on business. These can include dried as well as fresh items.

Five fun approaches to increasing your fruit and vegetable intake when travelling

There are many ways you can incorporate fruit and vegetables into your travelling regime. Here are the five best approaches.

1. Building up your breakfasts

Breakfast is a great place to start if you want to raise the number of portions of fruit and vegetables you consume each day. You may find it easier to begin increasing your consumption at home first. Once you have found an approach which suits your taste and lifestyle, then it will become easier when you're away on business. The good news is that retail shops, cafes and restaurants in airports are increasingly offering breakfast menu items which either have fruit or vegetable ingredients or menu items which you can easily add to with a side dish.

Here are our top tips on how to maximise fruit and vegetable intake at breakfast time.

Just one fruit at a time

Get effortlessly underway by endeavouring to add just **one** fruit at this meal time to begin. Simple additions can include choosing a fruit juice first when you reach for your usual morning cuppa, packing a banana or apple in your hand luggage when you leave in the morning or picking up a container of fruit salad en route from one the retail outlets at the airport. You can increase your portions on future trips once you've succeeded with an easy addition first.

Sweet toppings

Alternatively, you might prefer to adapt your usual breakfast by adding a little fruit as a topping.

Before leaving home or hotel: If you have time to spare and wish to eat breakfast before setting out, try to add fruit to your porridge or cereal instead of adding sugar, honey or syrup. You could add mashed or sliced banana, fresh or thawed frozen berries, fruit compote, canned peaches or dried fruits. These all add sweetness in addition to many other nutrients.

On the go: If you arrive at the airport with little time to spare, then head straight for one of the retail shops, such as London News Company, Boots the Chemist or one of the many cafes which offer yoghurt or porridge to go options. You will also find packets of dried fruit near the counter and sliced fresh fruit or salad in the chilled section. Simply add the dried or fresh fruit to the top of your yoghurt or porridge.

In a restaurant: Several restaurants offer a healthy option on the menu, e.g. porridge with fruit. For example, at the Armadillo restaurant, there is porridge with strawberries, blueberries and pumpkins seeds and at the Red Lion, you can order MOMA porridge with banana.

If you prefer to treat yourself to a pancake for breakfast, then you can also add fruit instead of syrup. For example, at Garfunkel's, you can order Buttermilk pancakes with summer berries and Greek-style yoghurt.

Adding a little veg

Adding a little vegetable to your cooked breakfast also works wonders. Here are a couple of easy yet practical options.

Before leaving home or hotel: The simple omelette can also be made with additional vegetables. You could add almost any vegetable you like, including onions, tomatoes, diced peppers, mushrooms, broccoli, spinach, spring onions and chives. Herbs are exceptionally high in some vitamins and minerals, even in small amounts they can add taste and contribute a little to the overall diet. Hotel kitchens are often happy to cater for impromptu requests, so don't hang back when the waiting staff take your order.

At the airport: There is the obvious baked beans, tomatoes or mushrooms which you can add to toast or substitute in an English breakfast. At some airport restaurants, they have already done the combinations for you. For example, the Comptoir Libanais restaurant offers Feta, avocado, cherry tomato and olives on toast.

Omelettes are also readily available usually in a variety of options. At Gatwick airport, some of the restaurants have come up with innovative combinations. For example, at Garfunkel's, there are several omelettes, including an Egg White Omelette made with spinach, red onion and served with smashed avocado with mango, coriander, chilli & lime, a grilled tomato and pea shoots. While at Wagamama, there is a vegetarian Japanese inspired omelette (Yasai Okonomiyaki) made with shiitake mushrooms, red cabbage and leeks.

Even scrambled eggs are getting more innovative, for example at the Armadillo restaurant; you could choose Avocado Southwest from the menu, made from scrambled eggs, smashed fresh avocado, red chilli, watercress and salsa on a muffin.

2. Sort out your snacking

Snacking between meals is a perfect opportunity to get to your target of five-a-day. Try to include a fruit or vegetable with each snack. Here are some quick and easy ways of adding more fruit and vegetables at snack time.

Grab and go bags

Before leaving home: If you are travelling and time is limited before you set off in the morning, then prepare some grab and go bags the night before. Cut up carrots, celery, cucumber and peppers into a plastic bag and add some cherry or mini vine tomatoes, olives or even some cocktail onions or pickled gherkins with a couple of cocktail sticks. Alternatively, make it a fruit grab and go, with orange segments, grapes, chopped pineapple and melon.

At the airport: You may even find some grab and go options at the airport. Some of the small retail outlets, such as Boots and London News Company offer small containers of pepper slices with cheese, carrots sticks with hummus, apple and grape bags or sliced fresh fruit. Cafes, such as Pret Manger, Costa Coffee, Jamie's Coffee Bar and Starbucks offer grab and go fruit or vegetable snacks.

Pick of the pantry

While fresh fruit and vegetables may supply more of some nutrients than preserved, it isn't always possible to take quickly perishable items with you. It may be preferential if you select less fragile items from the stores of the pantry.

Whole dried fruits, such as raisins, apricots, prunes, cranberries, blueberries and cherries all count towards your five a day. A portion size is 30 g which is equivalent to 1 heaped tablespoon. Take care when incorporating dried fruit as a snack as they are a concentrated calorie and sugar source and it's easy to consume a lot before stopping. Dried fruit is better when combined with other foods or eaten after a meal as residue can to stick between the teeth and cause damage.

Before leaving home: Boxes or small packets of dried fruits can be easily stored and retrieved from the pantry when in a hurry. They are nicer and more satisfying when combined with other snack items such as seeds, nuts, apples, mini cheeses and vegetable sticks. Don't neglect to think of items such as olives, gherkins, cocktail onions and pickled garlic as a combination to include.

At the airport: Dried fruit in packets can be purchased now in most of the cafes, such as Pret A Manger, Starbucks and Costa coffee at Gatwick Airport, as well as at some of the retail stores such as Boots the Chemist, London News Company and Marks and Spencer. We've listed where you can find these below and in Chapter 15 on snacks.

Add seasonal variety with vegetables

Vegetables are typically less expensive when they are in season, and they also taste better.

Before leaving home: Bite-sized cubes of cooked vegetables like potato, pumpkin, sweet potato, swede and turnip, steam or roasted can also make excellent snack packs. When combined with segments of cheese or cubes of cured meats, such as prosciutto, pancetta or even smoked chicken, they can make a tasty snack alternative.

On route: Cafes and retail shops are now supplying nibbles in the form of vegetable bites or sticks. For example, Boots the Chemist stock packets of wasabi peas and Edamame beans, while at Marks and Spencer's Simply Food minimarket you can pick up a small bowl of fresh ready to eat vegetables.

3. Manage your main meals

Try to incorporate fruit and vegetables into every meal time. Aim to cover half your plate with vegetables or salad. Here are some suggestions on how to make a difference to your main meals.

Spruce up your lunch sandwiches

Before leaving home: Add fresh seasonal vegetables to your sandwiches, rolls and wraps. If sliced tomato, cucumber or lettuce is not available, then opt for grated carrot, radishes, cooked beetroot or shredded cabbage as an alternative.

At the airport: Purchase items which include salad vegetables, such as salad-based sandwiches, vegetarian wraps and roasted vegetable baguettes.

Alternatively, select a meal deal which offers a side salad or fruit as the second item.

Pre-dinner nibbles

Vegetable nibbles can assist to ward off hunger and subsequently help to prevent you from overeating or fill up on dessert after dinner. There are plenty of pre-dinner vegetable-based nibbles to choose from when you know where to look.

On route: Retail outlets and cafes now sell packaged takeaway items which can be purchased for nibbling. Examples include a container of edamame beans in their pods, red pepper sticks and cheese carrots batons and hummus, or a crunchy raw rainbow super bowl.

At the airport: Some restaurants provide various forms of starters; anything from speciality salads to sharing bowls of olives and pickles. For example, Armadillo Restaurant offers a street snack salad comprising mango, mouli, and cucumber crudites. While Wagamama offers side dishes such as edamame beans, wok-fried greens or a raw salad).

Sidesaddle with a salad

Starting your meal with a salad can be refreshing. Alternatively, if your main course doesn't come with many vegetables, then supplement with a side salad or selection of meze items. For example, the Comptoir Libanais offers meze menu items, such as Fattoush (tomatoes, cucumber, radish, mint and parsley salad), tabbouleh (parsley, cracked wheat, tomatoes and mint) or **Freekeh** (smoked green wheat, wild rocket, vine tomato, spring onion, apple vinegar and mint dressing). All of which you could choose either before or at the same time as your main course.

Eat a rainbow!

Variety really is the spice of life. Different coloured vegetables contain a complementary blend of vitamins and minerals. So, make sure you select a vegetable from each colour group. Choose at least two vegetables from orange, green, yellow and red vegetables, including the less popular colours such as white (turnip, onions and garlic) or purple (aubergine or broccoli spears) per meal.

4. D-Day for desserts

Desserts can add a nutritious element to your diet, especially if you opt for a dessert which is fruit or dairy based. Unfortunately, many of the desserts available are either high fat or sugar (or both), so you need to search for the healthier options when you're travelling. Try these options to increase your fruit intake.

On route: Takeaway yoghurts with fruit is now readily available from most small cafes or retail outlets, such as Boots, WHSmith or M&S Simply Food stores. Some are stretching their selection to include more innovative tastes and choices. For example, EAT offers Bio-Live yoghurt with berries.

At the airport: Restaurants tend to offer the basic menu items for healthier fruity desserts. Fruit salads and apple crumble with custard remain firm favourites. More restaurants are beginning to offers smoothies which can double up as a dessert on the menu. Wagamama's offers smoothies made from fruit and frozen yoghurt, making an excellent dessert option.

5. Drink it up

Smoothies, juices, soups are all ways in which you can increase your fruit and vegetable intakes. 150 ml smoothie or a glass of unsweetened 100% fruit or vegetable juice is equivalent to one of your five a day. However, only one portion counts per day.

Take from home: You can purchase either cans or containers of tomato juice or vegetable juice from the supermarket to add to your non-perishable travelling stock items in your pantry. Tomato juice is an excellent taste stimulator and can be consumed on the aeroplane to enhance the flavor of your airline food.

On route: Grab a small takeaway bottle of fruit juice or a smoothie from one of the retail outlets at the airport. There is now a wider selection of fruit juice and smoothies available.

At the airport: It's becoming more common for airports to have a dedicated smoothie/juice bar which offers freshly squeezed juice or smoothies. Care needs to be taken when choosing smoothies at airports as they can be enormous and contain more calories than a meal! At the moment, Gatwick Airport doesn't have a juice/smoothie bar, but you can obtain freshly squeezed juices and smoothies at a variety of restaurants and cafes. See the list below for more details.

Where to find-five-a-day

Given travelling is one of the primary reasons cited for eating insufficient fruit and vegetables, it goes without saying that information on where to find healthy fruit and vegetable options at Gatwick Airport's North Terminal might be useful. So, we've sent a Registered Nutritionist to research where to find whole fresh fruit and take away vegetable items. Availability and choice will naturally depend on whether you want to take food with you on your flight or you've just landed and want something for the remainder of your journey.

Whole fruit is available in some retail outlets, most lounges and a few restaurant counters. While fresh whole fruit is best, dried fruit and fruit salads will offer variable nutrients and fibre as well.   So, we've also found outlets which offer dried fruit along with some restaurants and cafes which provide mixed fruit salads, fruit-based desserts and smoothies to take away.

Vegetables in the form of prepared packs and salads are also available in certain retail stores. Some restaurants also offer a takeaway service where you can also purchase a selection of fresh 'buffet' salads, large salad portions or vegetarian main dishes, starters and freshly made smoothies to take on board. These are also listed below.

Buyer beware:

While many prepared salads and vegetable-based dishes, including side dishes and soups, also contribute to your five a day we found many of those available in Gatwick Airport North Terminal's cafes and restaurants had excessively high salt contents. Some were also too high in fat.

Although the advice is to increase the consumption of fruit and vegetables to help your wellbeing and combat fatigue, we don't recommend increasing the salt and fat content unduly at the same time. A side portion of vegetables which contributes only 60 kcals needn't provide one-sixth of the maximum daily intake of salt.

Nor is it appropriate for a salad which is only 300 kcals to supply half of the maximum daily salt intake of 3 g. And we certainly wouldn't recommend soups as part of your 5-a-day, particularly when flying, that contain a full teaspoon of salt (just under the maximum daily salt intake) in one portion while only contributing one-quarter of your total energy intake. Likewise, we wouldn't recommend stir-fries which contain the equivalent to a full day's fat content.

Consequently, salads or vegetable-based dishes with excessively high salt or fat contents have not been listed in the suggestions below. What we have listed is where you can obtain fresh fruit, salads and vegetable dishes with minimal salt or fat added.

Retail shops which offer fruit and vegetables

M&S Simply Food

M&S Simply Food is the only onsite mini supermarket and is open all day. It offers a wide selection of fresh fruit and vegetables, prepared salad options and snacks. You can take whole foods through security, provided they are not a liquid or gel exceeding over 100 mls.

Open: 24 hours
Location: Opposite the Bureau de Change and next to Boots the Chemist.

Fresh fruit

You can get a variety of whole fruit at M&S Simply Food. Either purchase as a single item, fruit salad or as a package.

Portion size fruit salads

Banana and Berries 160 g portion provides 96 kcal (405 kJ)
Pineapple, Melon and Grape 120 g portion provides 52 kcal (218 kJ)
Purely Pineapple 190 g portion provides 87 kcal (367 kJ)
Melon and Grape 210 g portion provides 90 kcal (380 kJ)

Dried fruit and vegetables

Raisins 50 g portion pack. Partially rehydrated jumbo raisins. A 50 g pack provides 145 kcal (615 kJ)
Dried Apricots 80 g portion pack. Dried soft apricots. An 80 g pack provides 147 kcal (615 kJ)
Wasabi Peas 50g portion pack or £1.50 for a 200g pack. Roasted green peas with a flavoured wasabi coating. A 50 g pack provides 214 kcal (1403 kJ)

Fruit Mix 70g pack. A selection of raisins, sultanas, sweetened dried cherries, sweetened dried cranberries and dried apricots. A 70 g pack provides 230 kcal (976 kJ)

Packaged additions

Reduced Fat Houmous with Crunchy Carrot Sticks (130g) Comprises carrots and reduced fat houmous. Good source of fibre. Consume this snack within a few hours of purchase. 130 g portion provides 157 kcal (651 kJ)

Mini salads

Sweet and Crunchy Side Salad Salad with sweetcorn, cabbage, carrots and red peppers. Salad provides 48 kcal (202 kJ)

Beetroot & Santini Tomato Side Salad Beetroot, Santini tomato and cucumber leafy salad with a creamy lemon dressing. Salad provides 117 kcal (491 kJ)

Edamame & Sesame Side Salad Cabbage and Edamame soybean salad with shredded broccoli, vinegar infused cucumber, mooli, coriander, sesame seeds and a soy and lime dressing. Salad provides 118 kcal (488kJ)

Nutty Super Wholefood Salad Cooked quinoa, cooked spelt-wheat, beans and soy and ginger dressing with a cannellini bean and sesame tahini dip. A salad provides 385 kcal (1605 kJ)

Super Wholefood Salad Edamame (soy) beans, quinoa and spelt with a creamy lemon & mint dressing. Salad provides 371 kcal (1546 kJ)

Freekeh Couscous & Cauliflower in a tahini & lemon dressing. Pack provides 238 kcal (992 kJ)

Courgettes, Beans, Wheatberries & Toasted Fregola with a lemon & parsley dressing. Pack provides 130 kcal (546 kJ).

Glorious Greens & Seeds Veggie Pot Edamame soybeans, sugar snap peas, spinach and lemon roasted seeds with a pea dip with mint infused sunflower oil. The pot provides 159 kcal (660 kJ)

Boots the Chemist

If you didn't manage to take advantage of the excellent range of fruit and vegetables at M&S Simply Food before moving through security, then head straight down to the larger of the two Boots the Chemist stores in the Departure Lounge where there is a fruit and vegetable island. Here there are plenty of pre-made fresh fruit salads and mixes to choose from. Although both Boots the Chemist stores offer fresh fruit and vegetables in pots, there is less variety at the smaller of the two stores, and the fruit & vegetable island is well worth a visit.

Unfortunately, we were unable to find whole fruit at either store when we visited, but there were plenty of pre-made pots to choose from.

Locations: Arrivals. After security, next to the security exit and at the far end of the Departure Lounge.
Open: 4.00 am to 8.30 pm

Fresh fruit and vegetables

Grape, Apple and Strawberries Packet provides 53kcal (225 kJ)
Apple and Grape Bag Packet provides 48 kcal (205 kJ)
Apple Pieces Packet provides 46 kcal (205 kJ)
Pineapple, Grape & Carrot Pack provides 123 kcal (520 kJ)
Melon & Grapes 110 g Pack provides 44 kcal (189kJ)
Carrot Sticks and Hummus Pack provides 110 kcal (457kJ)
Red Pepper Sticks and Cheese Pack provides 160 kcal (669 kJ)
Olives 70 g Pack provides 113 kcal (465 kJ)
Carrots Sticks 80 g Pack provides 27 kcal (115 kJ)

Salads and Sushi

Shapers Veggie Sushi Snacks Edamame, carrot and red cabbage California roll with beetroot rice, two cucumber Hosomaki and two red pepper Hosomaki. Low salt soya sauce is provided separately. Sushi provides 93 kcal (395 KJ)

Moroccan Style Veggie Couscous Salad Seasoned couscous with roasted butternut squash and aubergines, cos lettuce and a Moroccan style dressing. Salad provides 161 kcal (676 kJ)

Kimachi & Edamame Salad with Brown Rice Kimchi, edamame and mango on a mixed vegetable and seasoned rice bed, topped with coriander and served with a bottle of gluten-free low salt soya sauce. Salad provides 184 kcal (777 kJ)

Dried fruit and vegetables

Another option, especially if you are in a hurry, is to opt for the dried fruit and vegetables available at their counter. Here is a quick list of some items you can grab when queuing for the check-out.

Edamame Beans 50 g Per pack 210 kcal (882 kJ)
Wasabi Peas 50 g Per pack 201 kcal (847 kJ)
Apricots 35 g packet Per portion 92 kcal (390 kJ)
Apple & Cinnamon Clusters 20 g Per portion: 68 kcal (288 kJ)

WHSmith & London News

WHSmith has a selection of fruit and vegetable items. If you're in a hurry, the service here is usually quick, and you can grab either whole fruit from their stand near the food counter, or a vegetable snack or salad from the refrigerator. Some items count as part of their meal deal offer. There are also plenty of dried fruits and nuts in large and small packets to choose.

WHSmith opening hours: Before security; 24 hours, and post-security; 3.00 am to 10.00 pm
WHS Locations: Between The Bookshop and Fat Face; and Gates 101 – 113.
London News Company opening hours: Before and after security 4.00 am to 9.00 pm.
London News Company Locations: Opposite M&S Simply Food in the Arrival Hal; opposite Excess Baggage in the main entrance of Check-in, level one; upstairs of Check-in, level two just opposite Moneycorp Bureau de Change.

Fresh Fruit and Fruit Salad
Apples
Bananas
Oranges
Apples and Grapes This pack provides 90 kcal (384 kJ)
Apple, Grape & Cheese Apple slices, whole grapes and mild cheddar cheese chunks. This pack provides 147 kcal (620 kJ)
Del Monte Rainbow Fruit Salad 160 g pot Watermelon, cantaloupe melon, kiwi, mango and pomegranate. One pot provides 40 kcal (166 kJ)
Del Monte Fruit Salad 160 g Orange, pineapple, apples and grapes. One pot provides 46 kcal (197 kJ)

Fresh Vegetables and Salad
Edamame Beans and Houmous Houmous with Edamame beans, sugar snap peas and pumpkin seeds. One pot contains 178 kcal (747 kJ)
Carrots and Houmous Carrot batons with houmous. This pack provides 110 kcal (460 kJ)
BolFood Mediterranean Salad Jar Chickpeas, carrot, courgette, butternut squash and feta with lemon and sun-dried tomato. This jar provides 323 kcal (1347 kJ)
BolFood Japanese Salad Jar Cooked black rice, raw slaw, edamame beans, black beans, tender stem broccoli with a soy and ginger dressing. This jar provides 275 kcal (1150kJ)
BolFood Mexican Salad Jar Cooked white quinoa, chargrilled sweetcorn, black beans, cooked black barley and Provola Cheese with a jalapeno & lime dressing. This jar provides 316 kcal (1320 kJ)
BolFood Moroccan Salad Jar Grilled aubergine, creamy feta cheese and fresh spinach on a bed of beetroot with whole wheat couscous and crunchy pumpkin seeds, served with a lightly spiced orange and Harissa dressing. This jar provides 298 kcal (1250 kJ)

Supergreen Salad Jar Chargrilled broccoli & sprouts, feta cheese, quinoa, peas & a lemon, mint & spirulina dressing. This pot provides 275 kcal (1150 kJ)

Dried Fruits and Nuts

Urban Magnificent Mango 100 g or 35 g snack pack. Not only is it a good source of fibre but mango is also known for their vitamin C content, modest amounts of other vitamins (folate, E and K) and phytonutrients. 35 g portion provides 104 kcal (434 kJ)

Urban Cheeky Cherries. 100 g or 35 g snack pack. Just the cherries, which are gently baked. Good source of fibre and melatonin, along with vitamin C. Studies on tart cherries offer many nutritional properties. Some claim to decrease inflammation and reduce the risk of heart disease. A 35 g snack pack provides 93 kcal (391 kJ)

Urban Perfect Pineapple 100g or 35 g snack pack. Excellent source of fibre and vitamin B Folate. A 35 g snack pack provides 100 kcal (420 kJ)

Urban Ravishing Raspberry 100 g or 35 g snack pack. Good source of anthocyanin, vitamins E and K. A 35 g snack pack provides 104 kcal (434 kJ)

Urban Smashing Strawberry 100 g or 35 g Just strawberries and a bit of apple juice. Good source of fibre, vitamin C, manganese, folate and potassium. A 35 g pack provides 103 kcal (431 kJ)

Munch Raisin Shots 25 g packet Flame raisins, golden raisins and sultanas. This packet provides 84 kcal (352 kJ)

Lounges which offer fruit and vegetables

If you are fortunate to gain entry to one of the lounges you will find complimentary fruit and vegetable options in each lounge. They range in variety, so here is a quick summary;

No. 1 lounge

No. 1 Lounge had the best selection of salads. We counted five when we visited on several occasions. They also offered a different selection of the 'usual' whole fruit compared to the other lounges, which included plums and pears as well as apples and bananas.

Open: 4.00 am to 10.00 pm
Location: On the lower level of the Departure Lounge, after security, near gates 101 - 113.
Directions: Head towards gate 101 – 113, as you pass London News Company, turn right into the corridor, you will see another hallway on your right. Enter the hall and walk through the double glass doors. No.1 Lounge is directly ahead.

Aspire Lounge

On the self-service counter, you will find fresh fruit and dried fruit snack items. We found a choice of three fruits, including apples (red and green) and oranges in large fruit bowls. There were also dried fruits and olives in other snack bowls.

Open: Open hours are from 4.00 am to 10.00 pm, with a slight seasonal variation.
Location: First floor of the Departure Lounge.
Directions: Head towards gate 101 – 113, as you pass London News Company, you will see a corridor on your right. Go through the double glass doors and take the lift to the first floor. The lounge is located on the right-hand side.

My Lounge

Hot vegetable chilli or vegetarian curry is available in the self-service area, along with a selection of finger vegetables, such as carrot sticks and mange tout. There are large bowls of fruit, namely apples and oranges, in the middle of the large table situated in the centre of the room. Just help yourself!

Open: 6.00 am to 8.00 pm
Location: Departure Lounge, lower level.
Directions: Head towards gate 101 – 113, as you pass London News Company, you will see a corridor on your right. Turn right and proceed through the double glass doors. The lounge is located on the left-hand side just before the lifts.

Restaurants which offer takeaway fruit and vegetables

Arrivals, Ground Floor

Costa

Costa Coffee offers a whole fruit selection along with some prepacked grab and go items, including dried fruits at the counter and freshly prepared salads in the fridges.

Locations: Arrivals Hall, right next to the International Arrivals exit, and Check-in Level 1.
Opening in Arrivals: 24 hours

Opening in Check-in: 4.00 am and 8.00 pm

Fresh fruits7
Apple

Banana

Dried fruits
Fruit and nut mix Comprises of raisin, cashew nuts, almonds & walnuts. Per pack 204 kcals (847 kJ)

Dried Mango Per Pack 204 kcals (847 kJ)

Fresh fruits
Apple

Banana

Dried fruits
Fruit and Nut Mix Comprises of raisin, cashew nuts, almonds & walnuts. Per pack 204 kcals (847 kJ)

Dried Mango Per Pack 204 kcals (847 kJ)

Tropical Fruit Mix. A mix of dried pineapple, mango, physalis & raisins. Per pack 135 kcal (571 kJ)

Wraps and Salads
Chipotle Bean & Butternut Squash Wrap Per wrap 264 kcal (1112kJ)

Fruit Pot 160 g One pot is 45 kcal (190kJ)

Departure Lounge, Lower Level
Caviar House & Prunier
Caviar House & Prunier Seafood Bar offer a couple of side and seafood salads which you can take on board your flight with you. Unfortunately, there was no nutritional information available when we reviewed their items, so here are a couple of suggestions based on their menu descriptions.

Open: 4.00 am to 8.30 pm

Location: Middle of Departure lounge opposite Lacoste and World Duty Free

Main salads
Crab Salad with fresh white crab meat.

Lobster Salad Lobster served out of the shell, on a bed of mixed leaves, fresh mango and avocado.

Extras
Mixed Green Salad
Tomato & Onion Salad
New Potato Salad

The Red Lion

The Red Lion is part of the Weatherspoon's chain which supplies calorific information on their menu to aid choice. You can request a main meal as a takeaway with a side salad to accompany or a large salad as a main.

Open: 3.00 am to 8.30 pm
Location: At the end of the Departure Lounge on the right as you enter from security.

Quinoa salad. Quinoa, rice, avocado, adzuki beans, grilled red and yellow pepper, red cabbage, chia seeds and kale with a buttermilk ranch dressing. Per portion: 498 kcal (2084 kJ)
Quinoa side salad Per portion 252 kcal (1054 kJ)
Side Salad Per Portion: 201 kcal (841 kJ)

Departure Lounge, Upper Level
Comptoir Libanais

Comptoir Libanais pride themselves on offering fresh, healthy food. They operate a takeaway service so you can take salads (and wraps) with you on your flight. The salads can be viewed in the counter refrigerator. Beware if you have any food allergies or intolerances as sometimes cross-contamination can occur when foods are served from buffet style environment. Unfortunately, no nutritional information was available at the time of review, so we are unable to verify the nutrition content. Here are a couple of suggestions to help increase your fruit and vegetable intake based on their menu description.

Open: 4.00 am to 8.30 pm
Location: First restaurant on the upper level, next to the stairs and directly opposite the security entrance.

Fresh fruit
Apple & Oranges are available on the counter.

Mezze salads

Tabbouleh. Chopped parsley, cracked wheat, tomatoes, mint, spring onions, lemon and olive dressing.

Fattoush Baby Gem lettuce, cherry tomatoes, mint & parsley with toasted pitta bread, fresh pomegranate and a sumac dressing.

Freekeh Smoked green wheat, wild rocket, vine tomato, spring onion, apple vinegar & mint dressing.

Baba Ghanuj Smoked aubergine, tahini and lemon juice with pomegranate seeds.

Lebanese Hommos Smooth, rich chickpea puree with tahini and lemon juice.

Muhammara Spiced mixed roasted nuts, roasted red pepper, cumin & olive oil.

Large Salads

Falafel & Fattoush Salad Falafel served with romaine lettuce, cucumber, radish, vine tomato, flatbread croutons, mint and parsley with sumac dressing.

Quinoa & Feta Cheese Salad Quinoa, chickpeas, vine tomato, fresh mint, spring onion topped with zaatar feta cheese, apple vinaigrette & pomegranate dressing.

Sides

Batata Harra Spiced cubed potatoes with red pepper, fresh coriander, garlic and chilli.

Baba Ghanuj Smoked aubergine, tahini and lemon juice with pomegranate seeds.

EAT

In addition to sandwiches and meat-based dishes, EAT offers a variety of fruit and vegetable items. It is one of the few places in the Departure Lounge where you can easily purchase fresh whole fruit. You'll find whole fruit in their baskets between the refrigerator and service counter, dried fruit at the counter, along with packets of whole grapes and fruit salads in the refrigerator. They also stock prepared salads and soups.

Open: 4.00 am to 20.30 pm
Location: Halfway along the upper level, just opposite Shake-A-Hula.

You can choose from;
Whole fruits

Grapes, whole in a punnet or bag

Banana, whole
Apple, whole
Pear, whole
Seasonal fruit, e.g. nectarines or clementines

Fruit salads

Rainbow Fruit Salad. Mango, kiwi fruit, blueberry and pomegranate. Per pot 66 kcal (276 kJ)

Mango & Lime slices Per pot 85 kcal (356 kJ)

Big Fruit Salad Per serving 120 kcal (502 kJ)

Summer Berries Per serving 40 kcal (167 kJ)

Dried fruit

Fava Beans, Chickpeas & Roasted Pumpkin Seeds Per packet 156 kcal (653 kJ)

Natural Nuts A mix of almonds, pistachios, hazelnuts and cashews. Per packet 222 kcal (929 kJ)

Vegetable soups

The options listed below are based on a small portion of soup. Larger portions have an increased salt content, often higher than recommended by health professionals.

Creamy Slow Roasted Tomato A rich soup with intense flavours from the slow-roasting. Per small soup 240 kcals (993 kJ)

Small Crudite Pots

Houmous & Crudite Pot Creamy houmous salad with crunchy carrot batons and sweet sugar snap peas. Per serving 246 kcal (1029 kJ)

Large salads served as a main

Super Nutty Fit Box Cashew and pistachio nuts served on a bed of quinoa, black rice and pickled beetroot, served with a side of houmous and chargrilled broccoli with chilli and garlic. Per portion with dressing; 343 kcal (1436 kJ)

Houmous & Falafel Mezze Salad Mixed leaves with tabbouleh, a fresh herby mix of bulgur wheat, cucumber chunks, chopped fresh herbs and lemon juice. Topped with chunky houmous, carrot and coriander, falafels, harissa spiced chickpeas and a crunch mezze slaw. Per portion with dressing; 493 kcal (2063 kJ)

Mexican Guacamole & Quinoa Mixed salad leaves served with quinoa, black bean, giant corn mix topped with guacamole, roasted sweet potato, chargrilled sweetcorn salsa and chargrilled red pepper. Served with a lime wedge. Per serving 323 kcal (1351 kJ)

Middle Eastern Tabbouleh Middle Eastern tabbouleh, combining mixed salad leaves with roasted butternut squash, pomegranate and dukkah seeds and crumbled feta.

328

Served with roasted carrot houmous and harissa chickpeas. Hold the dressing to reduce the fat content. Per serving 367 kcal (1536 kJ)

Sicilian Orzo & Roasted Vegetables A orzo base topped with sun-dried peppers, slow roast tomatoes, chargrilled courgette and capers. Served with toasted omega seeds spinach and oregano vinaigrette. Per serving 514 kcal (2150 kJ)

Garfunkel's

Garfunkel's offers the option of ordering a takeaway meal for your flight. If you choose to purchase a main item to take with you, then don't forget to order some side dishes. Or better still try the large salad as an alternative to the main. No nutritional information was available at the time of our review, so we've based suggestions on the menu descriptions.

Open: 4.00 am to 8.30 pm
Location: At the back on the upper level, opposite the Armadillo restaurant.

Main salads

Meadow Salad Goat's cheese, roasted baby potatoes, mixed grains and roasted red pepper, tossed with a fennel and rocket salad with basil dressing.

Side vegetables.

Garden Vegetables Carrots, tender stem broccoli and French beans.
Mixed Salad Green leaves, cucumber and tomatoes in French dressing.

Jamie's Bakery

Jamie's Bakery has several fresh salads at the deli counter which you can pick and choose according to your taste and lifestyle. You can order either a small or a large carton to take out a salad, which they will fill up for you. When we visited, there were six salads to choose. Naturally, we chose all of them to try. The cost for a large box with all six salads was £6.50, and a small box was £4.50.

Beware if you have any food allergies or intolerances as sometimes cross-contamination can occur when foods are served from buffet style environment. Unfortunately, we were unable to access any nutritional information at the time of review.

Open: 4.00 am to 8.30 pm
Location: Next to Jamie's Italian Restaurant and just opposite Yo! Sushi.

Whole fruit is available in a bowl on the counter.
Takeaway boxes of salad are available, freshly made on the day.

Pret A Manger

There are several fresh vegetable pots and soups made daily as part of Pret A Manger takeaway items, along with fresh and dried fruit. Many of these contribute to your five a day, without excessive fat, salt or sugar. Pret A Manger also offers a variety of salads, suitable either as a side, starter, snack or main.

Open: 3.00 am to 8.30 pm
Location: Far left-hand corner on the upper level, overlooking the World Duty Free and main departure board.

Whole fruit

Apple Chopped apple. The variety depends on the season. 85 kcal (358 kJ)
Bananas from Costa Rica by the Rainforest Alliance certification. 62 kcal (258 kJ)
Nectarines 53 kcal (227 kJ)

Dried fruits and seeds

Pret A Mango Chopped dried and into bags. Per bag 119 kcal (506 kJ)
Tamari Pumpkin Seeds A little bag full of tamari-coated pumpkin seeds. A bag provides 189 kcal (784 kJ)

Fruit Pots

Mango and Lime Shipped in from tropical regions when they are at their seasonal best. A pot provides 92 kcal (384 kJ)
Pret's Fruit Salad A selection of freshly prepared chunks of pineapple, orange flesh melon, mango, pink apples, kiwifruit and whole blueberries. This salad provides 113 kcal (473 kJ)
Superfruit Salad Chunks of mango, kiwifruit, pomegranate seeds and blueberries. This salad provides 106 kcal (450 kJ)
Watermelon and Lime Watermelon with a wedge of lime. The pot provides 48 kcal (204 kJ)
Nectarine and Raspberries This pot provides 56 kcal (238 kJ)

Vegetable Pots

Avocado & Super-Green Veggie Pot Avocado, peas, edamame and coriander with a sprinkling of sesame seeds and served with a pot of zingy green dressing. Per pot 170 kcal (706 kJ) Hold the dressing to reduce the fat content.

Soups

Souper Tomato 370 g Chopped, diced and simmered super ripe plum tomatoes, tomato puree, vegetables and herbs. A 370 g serving provides 199 kcal (831 kJ)

Souper Tomato Side Soup 220 g Chopped, diced and simmered super ripe plum tomatoes, tomato puree, vegetables and herbs. A 220 g serving provides 119 kcal (495 kJ)

Vegetable Tagine Side Soup 220 g Roasted courgettes and peppers cooked in vegetable stock with cumin, turmeric, red chilli and cinnamon. Served with tomatoes, chickpeas, buckwheat and red lentils. A 220 g portion provides 112 kcal (469 kJ)

Vegetable Chilli Side Soup 220 g Vegan chilli combines three beans (black turtle beans, red kidney beans and black-eyed beans), peppers, sweetcorn, brown rice and quinoa. A 220 g serving provides 130 kcal (541 kJ)

Salads and salad boxes

Sweet Potato Falafel & Smashed Beets Veggie Box Turmeric and sweet potato falafel, smashed beetroot hummus, avocado, broccoli on a bed of black and brown rice, and red quinoa served with a pot of zingy green dressing. A box provides 407 kcal (1695 kJ)

Starbucks

Starbucks has several items which can quickly contribute to your fruit and vegetable intake, including fresh whole fruit, dried fruit snack bags, salads and fruit pots.

Open: 24 hours
Location: Halfway along, at the back of the upper level between Jamie's Italian and EAT restaurants

Whole fruit

Bananas Sweet, ripe fairtrade banana. 108 kcal (448 kJ)

Fruit Mix A mix of pineapple, melon, mango, kiwi and blueberry. A pot provides 82 kcals (301 kJ)

Mango with Lime Fruit Pot Mango chunks with a slice of lime. A pot provides 87 kcals (367 kJ)

Dried fruit

Almonds, cashews, cranberries & raisins. Unsalted nuts and dried berries. A packet provides 233 kcal (975 kJ)

Wraps

Vegan Wrap with Falafel & Slaw Sweet potato falafel with mixed peppers, rainbow slaw and a tomato salsa dressing. A wrap provides 261 kcal (1096 kJ)

Smoothies

Smoothies and juices can also be consumed as an approach to increasing your fruit and vegetable intake. One glass (150 ml) smoothie or a glass of unsweetened 100% fruit or vegetable juice is equivalent to one of your five a day. But it only accounts for one portion per day.

The nutritional content of a smoothie depends on the mix of ingredients. While they are promoted as a convenient alternative to eating whole fruit and fresh vegetables, there is a downside to smoothies. The natural sugar content can be extremely high, due to the number of fruits and vegetables being juiced for one drink. What's more, as the fruit is no longer whole, the sugar has been released from fruit's cells during processing turning it into a 'free' sugar. This allows it to interact more efficiently with your teeth, increasing the risk of decay. Health professionals advise that the sugars freed from the whole fruits and vegetables during the juicing process can cause damage to your teeth especially if you have more than one portion a day and between meals.

In addition, the fibre content has been altered mechanically during the process, which enables a quicker release of energy into one's bloodstream, and you won't feel as full as you would have if you had eaten several whole fruits, vegetables or salad. So if it's to accompany a meal or sandwich, it can provide a valuable addition to your diet, but if you are hungry and want something for satiety (a full sensation), then this feeling won't last for long when consumed by itself. For this reason, smoothies and fruit juices are best served with or just after a meal in place of a dessert.

Watch out for some smoothies as they can also be extremely high in their calorific value. Some restaurants, cafes, etc. add protein powder to their smoothies to increase the nutritional value, which also means the calorific value has been increased as well. In fact, smoothies with protein powder added are often over 400 kcals per serving. While this may make it an ideal approach for gaining weight, it may not be precisely the outcome you desire.

As a rule, smoothies can have a high calorific content simply because they contain several fruits and vegetables in one drink. So choose your smoothie or fruit juice wisely. Aim for 150 ml serving (not the 500 ml often served in fresh smoothie bars), and choose one which suits the calorific value you wish to add to your diet, preferably to accompany your main meal.

Where to find fresh smoothies to take with you

There are only a couple of restaurants and cafes which sell freshly made smoothies and fruit juices which you can take with you. Failing this, you can obtain a smoothie or juice from one of the retail stores such as Boots the Chemist, WHSmith or London News Company.

Comptoir Libanais

Comptoir Libanais blend all their juices fresh to order. They offer some great combinations. All combinations cost £3.95.

Open: 4.00 am to 8.30 pm
Location: First restaurant on the upper level, next to the stairs and directly opposite the security entrance.

Smoothies/Juices include:

Apple
Apple, Cucumber & Orange
Carrot
Carrot & Orange
Carrot & Ginger
Mixed Juice

EAT

EAT is one of the few places in the Departure Lounge where you can easily purchase smoothies to take away. Their creatively interesting smoothies, listed below, provide a good source of nutrients. For example, the Cherry Berry Almond Smoothie is a natural source of melatonin which may aid sleep, antioxidants which may help to lower inflammation, mono-unsaturated fats from the almonds and fibre from the oats to aid the reduction of cholesterol. Whereas, the Berry Beet juice is a good source of potassium and nitrate which may help to reduce blood pressure, along with anthocyanins which may lower insulin resistance and improve blood sugar control.

Open: 4.00 am to 20.30 pm
Location: Halfway along the upper level, just opposite Shake-A-Hula.

BD Eat Smoothie Mango & Passionfruit

Berry Beets Juice A zingy cold-pressed blend of apples, strawberries, raspberries and beetroot. 115 kcal (481 kJ)

Cherry Berry Almond Smoothie Cherries, blueberries and oats blended with almond milk. 162 kcal (678 kJ)

Cool Carrot Juice A cold-pressed blend of apples, carrots, pineapple, lemon and cooling mint. 90 kcal (376 kJ)

Drama Green Juice A refreshing blend of cold-pressed apples, cucumber, celery, basil and lemon. 105 kcal (439 kJ)

Pret A Manger

Pret A Manger offers a variety of smoothies, freshly made each day. This is probably one of the best places to get a smoothie at Gatwick's North Terminal, simply due to the range on offer. While just like cafes' smoothies they offer a range of nutrients, make sure you take care to choose wisely based on the calorific value they provide. Whatever possible benefit they might provide would be short-term, if consumed on a regular basis with other meal items and you end up gaining weight! Although saying this, they could be used as an alternative to a dessert.

Open: 3.00 am to 8.30 pm

Location: Far left-hand corner on the upper level, overlooking the World Duty Free and main departure board.

Smoothies include:

Avo Smoothie Apple, pear, cucumber and spinach blended with creamy avocado. 400 g serving provides 272 kcal (1140 kJ)

Berry Blast A mix of raspberries, chopped mango, apple juice and blackberries. 410 g serving provides 239 kcal (1004 kJ)

Cranberry & Raspberry Pure Pret Still Red grape juice, cranberry juice, raspberry juice, fruit and vegetable concentrates. 500 g serving provides 175 kcal (740 kJ)

Daily Greens Cold pressed pear, apple, cucumber, romaine lettuce, spinach and celery, with lime and yuzu. 400 g serving provides 124 kcal (520 kJ)

Ginger Beets Cold pressed beetroot, fruity apples and fiery ginger. 110 g serving provides 28 kcal (116 kJ)

Mango Smoothie Made with squished mangoes, bananas and passion fruit. 250 g serving provides 143 kcal (603 kJ)

Strawberry and Banana Smoothie. Frozen strawberries, banana, apple and lemon. 400 g serving provides 211 kcals (886 kJ)

Super Greens Apple juice, cucumber, avocado, baby spinach and shredded ginger. 379 g serving provides 265 kcal (1100 kJ)

Vitamin Volcano Forest fruits, including blackberry, boysenberry, raspberry and strawberry blended with banana and apple juice. 250 g serving provides 130 kcal (548 kJ)

Pure Juices

Apple Juice 400 ml serving provides 120 kcal (505 kJ)
Large Orange Juice, 400 ml serving, provides 168 kcal (708 kJ)

Starbucks

They have recently launched a few new smoothie drinks without added sugar. Some stores will have several choices. We tried the Green Smoothie, having found the raw ingredients in a pot in the refrigerator, which they blend upon purchase.

Open: 24 hours
Location: Halfway along, at the back of the upper level between Jamie's Italian and EAT restaurants.

Smoothies include:

Teavana tea and ice. Mini: 132 kcal (562kJ), Tall (156 kcal (665 kJ), Grande 190kcal (808 kJ)
Mini Raspberry Blackcurrant Frappuccino Blended raspberry and blackcurrant juice with brewed Teavana tea and ice. Mini 133 kcal (565 kJ), Tall 157 kcal (668 kJ), Grande 191 kcal (812 kJ)

Wagamama

Wagamama offers two sizes for their smoothies; regular and large. Unfortunately, no nutritional information was available on the smoothies at the time of our review, so we can't verify the nutritional content of these. However, there was nutritional content available on the juices, so we've included the nutritional content for those. Freshly made on the premises to order; we enjoyed testing them out.

Open: 4.00 am to 8.30 pm
Location: At the far end of the Upper Level, to the right, just opposite Jamie's Italian Restaurant and Yo! Sushi.

Smoothies include:

Banana Banana, apple and passion fruit juice blended with plain frozen yoghurt.
Mango & Chilli Mango blended with plain frozen yoghurt and a touch of chilli
Pineapple & Coconut Pineapple blended with coconut reika.

Juices include:

Repair Juice Kale, apple, lime and pear. 188 kcal (785 kJ)
Raw Juice Carrot, cucumber, tomato, orange and apple. 97 kcal, (406 kJ)
Fruit Juice Apple, orange and passionfruit. 146 kcal (611 kJ)
Orange Juice Orange juice, pure and simple. 110 kcal (460 kJ)
Carrot Juice Carrot with a dash of fresh ginger. 72 kcal (302 kJ)
Super Green Juice Apple, mint, celery and lime. 128 kcal (534 kJ)
Clean Green Juice Kiwi, avocado and apple. 174 kcal (728 kJ)
Tropical Juice Mango, apple and orange. 167 kcal (697 kJ)
Blueberry Spice Juice Blueberry, apple and carrot with a taste of ginger. 193 kcal (808 kJ)

Mixed juices:

Positive Juice Pineapple, lime, spinach, cucumber and apple. 159 kcal (667 kJ)
Power Juice Spinach, apple and ginger. 160 kcal (669 kJ)

Chapter 15: Smart Snacking

While there has been an increase in business trips over the last 50 years, there has also been a change in our snacking patterns. Unlike 50 years ago, we now snack more regularly, and subsequently eating between meals during a business trip has become a typical part of our daily routine. Today, 95% of us snack at least once a day and about half of us snack two to three times per day. In effect, at least 25% of our daily energy intake now reportedly comes from snacks. This is more than health professionals advise for a healthy diet.

One of the main influences on the change in our eating patterns is to do with multi-national food companies who have invested heavily in research to explore food acceptability. They found, around 50 years ago, that while restrictive rules appear to apply to meals, they do not apply to snacks. Although meals will remain a structured food event with set times, various courses, made up of particular food groups and usually eaten in the company of others, snacks have never followed the same set of standards. We tend to eat snacks in any order, combination, by ourselves and at any time.

Given the routine changes when travelling on business, along with the adaptation to different time zones, availability of food in airports, and provision of snacks on the flight at a collective time; it is hardly surprising travellers are more likely to snack at 'unscheduled' times. What's more, many of us will snack when stressed or bored. For business travellers who experience a higher number of stressors and are more likely to suffer from weight-related illnesses, this makes snacking a lifestyle change many of us need to consider.

Despite the shift in consumption patterns and the rise of related diseases, health professionals advocate snacking can contribute to a healthy diet but only when structured into our overall daily intake. It is because they acknowledge snacking can have many nutritional benefits. Choosing a healthy snack can contribute vital nutrients which we may not achieve in a sufficient amount from three meals alone. Indeed, there are specific nutrients which many of us are not consuming to meet a recommended daily intake, and some of these missing nutrients are especially pertinent to business travellers.

Also, there are benefits associated with maintaining a healthy weight and controlling blood glucose levels. Snacks high in complex carbohydrates, such as whole-grain bread and cereals, not only provide B vitamins which are essential for energy production, but are also good sources of fibre which is beneficial for lowering cholesterol, controlling energy uptake and keeping blood glucose levels stable. When protein is added, a greater variety of nutrients become available, it supports stabilising blood glucose levels, and satiety increases resulting in better control of our appetite.

While in the past, many of the snacks commercially available have been high in fat, salt and sugar, the good news is that food manufacturers have realised there is a growing consumer demand for healthier food, including snacks. Market surveys are now reporting a rise in the availability of healthier snacks to meet consumer pressure. Subsequently, we are beginning to see more variety on offer in airports, with a shift away from only providing crisps, chocolate and fatty fast food.

However, not all snacks promoted as healthy are any healthier for you than their traditional counterparts or better than their fresh food group components. In many instances, we have found some snacks are still too high in sugar, salt and fat to be considered healthy on their own or even as a contribution to a healthy diet.

The trick for the business traveller is to know not only where to find foods suitable for healthy snacking in the airport but also how to make what is on offer healthier while fitting the snack into their daily requirements. This chapter is aimed at guiding you towards what constitutes a healthier snack, where to find snacks at Gatwick Airport's North Terminal and how to fit the items found in your personal eating pattern and travel schedule.

Benefits of healthy snacking

Contrary to common belief, snacking can be incorporated into a healthy diet, especially into a nutritious business traveller's diet. Here are the benefits you can gain when you incorporate healthy snacking into your travelling regime.

Complements insufficient dietary intakes

We briefly mentioned above that snacking can contribute to a healthy diet by providing nutrients that you may not get in sufficient amounts from your main meals. In particular, some nutrient intakes are harder to meet when there is a change in our diet due to travelling. For example, foods which are good sources of calcium are often missed out at meal times. Calcium is vital for healthy bones, teeth and contributes to muscle function. Many of us struggle to meet the recommended daily amounts of calcium. This is when snacking can help. When you choose a snack, reflect on whether you are likely to have two to three portions of dairy or dairy alternatives that day. If it is unlikely, then you might consider including milk, yoghurt, low-fat cheese or other calcium-rich sources as part of your snack.

Another instance where healthy snacking can make a difference is with vitamin D. Many of us fail to meet the recommended levels of vitamin D, particularly over the winter months. If you're not getting sufficient sunlight during the day due to travelling arrangements, then consider opting for snack foods which are a good source of vitamin D, such as boiled eggs or smoked salmon. You will find a list of food items available at the airport in Chapter 10, and we've listed some snacks with good sources of vitamin D below. You might also consider choosing a dairy alternative such as soy milk which states it is fortified with Vitamin D as well as calcium.

If you suffer from mild anaemia, then consider complementing your meals with snack foods which are a good source of iron, such as dried apricots, pumpkin seeds, quinoa, hummus or meat. When you fly at 35,000 feet or above, the cabin is pressurised to 6,000 to 8.000 feet, which is comparable to climbing at a high attitude. While there might be a drop in the level of oxygen, a reduced level shouldn't pose a threat to those in good health. Travellers with certain conditions, including severe anaemia, may experience hypoxia (insufficient oxygen circulating in the body) and will require a doctor's advice before flying. If you are mildly anaemic, you may feel more fatigued than normal. We've included snacks which are good sources of iron below.

Reduces the symptoms of fatigue

Healthy snacking not only reduces the risk of poor health but also helps to keep you from getting fatigued when travelling. Eating at regular times is an excellent way to ensure your blood sugar is steady for longer periods, which helps to prevent the onset of fatigue and tiredness.

Snacking is often considered a 'bridge' between two meal times. Consuming an early breakfast at the crack of dawn before commencing your journey packed day, then waiting for lunch in the afternoon, might just be a road too far. Consider having a snack to connect that hunger gap.

If it has been more than three to four hours since your last meal, then your body may start to produce glucose to keep a constant amount of energy circulating to your brain and other vital organs. As soon as your blood glucose drops below a certain level, your body will need to start producing its own. Having a snack which is high in fibre, complex carbohydrate and protein will keep your blood glucose more constant until the next meal time.

Take care not to opt for high sugar foods and low in complex carbohydrate and fibre, as this will raise your blood sugar quickly, causing insulin to bring it back down to a more desirable level, and making you soon feel hungry again. If you choose, however, to base your snacks on high fibre, starchy carbohydrate foods you will be providing your body with a constant supply of energy throughout the day, along with B vitamins which aid energy metabolism.

Helps to maintain weight

Making sure your blood sugar levels are constant throughout the day, avoiding peaks and troughs from large meals and significant gaps in between, not only helps to kerb fatigue between meals but can stop you from becoming over-hungry and subsequently overeating at the next meal time. Managing your appetite more efficiently will help you to maintain your weight.

The trick is to choose foods which keep us satisfied. This is why eating whole foods which are high in fibre, and slow-burning carbohydrates are essential. The longer it takes to break down and absorb your food, the greater the satiety value (sensation of fullness). Fibre helps to slow down the uptake of digested food across the gut wall. A perfect example of this is the comparison between eating whole fruit and drinking a juice drink. The slower consumption and the fibre being left intact mean the whole fruit is digested more slowly and leaves you feeling fuller for a greater time.

What's more, if you add some protein to your carbohydrate snack base it can also help to increase satiety and facilitate weight-loss. Protein takes longer to break down, and research has found that in doing so it leaves you more satisfied for longer.

Aids your body clock synchronisation

Eating at regular times and sticking to your usual snacking routine in line with your destination's new awake hours can help to synchronise your body clock when you fly over several time zones.

When you eat at regular intervals, you are communicating with your metabolic processes the time of day, and your body knows from routine when your next meal should be coming, which in turn helps to control the feelings of hunger and sustain your energy levels. In fact, food availability is known as a 'time-giver', providing information to your peripheral body clocks as to the time of day and acts as a feedback mechanism to your master body clock.

The digestive process helps to regulate your awake/sleep cycle. While the master clock will instantly start to communicate to the various parts of your body its new time zone, it can take days for your body to readjust and your organs may synchronise at a different rate. The difference is due to the master body clock being alerted to time zone changes as soon as daylight hits your retina, which in turn signals your organs through the nervous system, hormonal and metabolic changes that there has been a phase shift. These activities can take some time, which may explain some of the symptoms of jet-lag, such as indigestion and disruption to bowel function. Your organs will continue to secrete digestive enzymes at your usual feeding times until they are aware of a time shift.

The peripheral clocks, however, in some of our organs are also influenced by food availability and routine which triggers a feedback mechanism to our master body clock. By eating at regular times throughout your destination's awake time, your body will begin to synchronise by prompting metabolic and hormonal changes. What's more by the regulation of food intake, physical activity and metabolic processes, both the brain and peripheral body clocks help to maintain a precise energy balance which contributes to long-term weight stability.

So, if you are travelling long-haul, adjusting your snacking times to match your destination time may help reduce the effects of jet-lag and shorten the time of adjustment, along with contributing to control appetite and maintain your weight.

What constitutes a healthy snack for business travellers?

The key to achieving healthy snacking is to choose foods which render us feeling satisfied and provides some energy between meals, as well as contributing to a variety of nutrients over the course of the day. We previously mentioned that foods which provide a good satiety value are those which take longer to break down during digestion, therefore releasing energy more slowly.

Starchy foods, such as rice, bread and pasta, comprise long–chain carbohydrates (often termed complex) take longer to digest and absorb than simple carbohydrates (including honey, sugar and syrups). Complex carbohydrates need to be broken down into the smaller units for absorption to occur. Whole grains which incorporate fibre (brown rice and wholegrain bread) are slower to digest than refined starchy foods (such as croissants and cake) as fibre further inhibits the absorption of smaller particles. Consequently, our blood sugar levels remain more even rather than incurring peaks and troughs throughout the day.

The rise in blood sugar is often referred to as in a glycaemic index value (GI). You may notice some snack items state a GI value on the packet. This value is derived by measuring how quickly 50 g of carbohydrate within a food item will take to digest and be absorbed into our blood. The higher the GI value, the higher the peak in the blood sugar. It means your body will need to drop your blood sugar back down to a safe level quickly, which may leave you feeling fatigued, as well as empty and hungry again very soon. In contrast, carbohydrates high in fibre, such as whole grains, have a lower glycaemic index than their counterparts and as they remain longer in your stomach, they provide a prolonged sensation, as well as releasing energy into our bloodstream more slowly.

However, snacks generally contain much less than 50 g of pure carbohydrate per portion, and more importantly, snacks should be a mix of carbohydrate, protein, fat and fibre. It is the combination of nutrients, along with the type of carbohydrate and the portion of food consumed which will influence the rate of digestion and the subsequent rise in blood sugar.

When accounting for the presence of other nutrients, health professionals prefer to use a glycemic load value (GL), which also accounts for the composition and amount of food. This is why rice crackers topped with cream cheese or peanut butter may have a lower GL value than if the rice cracker was eaten by itself (GI value). It is also one of the reasons it is better to select a combination of food groups, high in fibre as well as supplying some energy in the form of carbohydrate.

It is also why health professionals recommend incorporating protein into your snack to help maintain even blood sugar and to provide other essential nutrients. Protein offers a high satiety value, as it takes some time to break the bonds between the protein units (amino acids) so they can be transported across the gut wall. In doing so, they also make us feel fuller for longer. Research also indicates that the value of protein is more complicated than previously thought.

To this end, a healthy snack would comprise more than one food group and often include foods which we generally don't get sufficient of at our meal times. For example, most of us do not eat adequate fruit and vegetables to reach at least five a day, nor do we tend to achieve enough insoluble fibre in our diet. Consequently, the basis of a good snack might start with a complex carbohydrate, e.g., whole wheat cracker, and a dairy (e.g., cream cheese) and vegetable toppings such as tomato, cucumber or avocado.

Ideally, your snacking should provide no more than 20% of your total daily energy intake. That's one-fifth less than most of us are currently consuming from snacking. If you are trying to maintain your current weight, then this would leave approximately 400 calories for breakfast, 600 calories for both lunch and dinner, when on a 2000 calorie intake. Active business professionals and most men may require a higher energy intake of at least 2500 calories.

To be more precise; a snack for an inactive business professional could contribute around 200 calories twice a day and similarly 200 – 300 calories for an active business professional, twice a day. Don't forget if you are attempting to lose weight, you may prefer snacks with a lower energy content but will still help prevent overeating at meal times.

Some health professionals suggest aiming for snacks which provide at least 5 g fibre and 10 g protein to keep feeling full for longer. Examples of these include some of the items we've listed below, such as an Egg and Avocado Protein Pot (M&S Simply Food), or Muki beans with Humous and Pumpkin Seed (Boots the Chemist). Combining dried fruit with nuts or dairy products is another approach to increase satiety. For example; a portion of cheese with rye crackers and dried apricots, or low-fat Greek yoghurt with nuts and dried fruit.

What healthy snacks are not, are those snacks which are high in fat, sugar or salt. It would be convenient to suggest these are the traditional commercial snacks such as chocolate or crisps. However, there are plenty of new snacks on the market which would also deliver a similar unhealthy profile, such as some muesli, cereal or protein bars.

To summarise; a healthy snack comprises a variety of food, usually from more than one food group, a good composition embracing complex carbohydrates containing

fibre, and some protein, supplying around 10% of your total calorie intake, fitting into your overall diet without adding excess energy, fat, salt or sugar.

We have listed several snacks below this section which we have found at Gatwick Airport's North Terminal, that match the criteria outlined above. These include both fresh and non-perishable snacks options, available before and post-security.

When to snack

Not everyone needs to snack and too much snacking or snacking on foods which are high in fat, sugar and salt will lead to serious health problems, including high blood pressure, weight gain, type 2 diabetes and cardiovascular disease.

So, when should you snack?

Missed meal opportunity

If you know your next meal will be on a delayed flight or your boarding time is at your regular meal time, then you might like to consider a small nutritious snack to tide yourself over. After all, your body becomes accustomed to eating at a regular time and may start the digestive process in anticipation of food. A stitch in time saves nine, so a small snack may equally save consuming a more substantial portion later.

Bridge between meals

If the last time you ate is more than three or four hours, and it will be several hours before your next meal, then it might be worthwhile considering a healthy snack. Snacking between meals which are six to eight hours apart will help to prevent you from overeating at the next meal time or to become desperate for something just before a meal and reaching for the first item to satisfy the desire to refuel your body. Planning can make the duration between meals easier to bear and could help you control your appetite and weight.

When you are hungry

Many of us snack not because we are hungry, but because we are fatigued, stressed with travel arrangements or just bored between transfers and waiting to embark. Hunger usually occurs when you haven't eaten for several hours, resulting in a feeling of weakness, headache or a rumbling stomach. If your last meal was in the past few hours, you might like to ask yourself why you're reaching for food.

Craving versus hunger

Are you truly hungry or simply craving a specific food? Hunger isn't usually associated with one particular food. Researchers have recently suggested there are different types of hunger and how we respond to them is essential to prevent eating more than we need.

Physical (homeostatic) hunger is when we are eating to satisfy a need for energy, while hedonic hunger is just wanting to eat highly palatable food. The latter hunger has more to do with the wide variety of delicious food now available and seeking pleasure rather than just needing the energy to maintain energy balance (homoeostasis). Research suggests it is the way you respond to these feelings of hunger which determine whether a craving develops.

Cravings for particular food items are influenced more by mood than when you last ate. Negative emotions such as travel fatigue, lack of sleep, flight anxiety or boredom when waiting to board are more powerful when triggered by environmental clues, such as the smell and visibility of food. It's important to know how to respond to the development of cravings to prevent yourself from overeating en route.

Foremost ask yourself, if you didn't have the particular food you're craving, would you want something else instead? If the answer is no, then it's more likely to be hedonic hunger cravings than physical hunger. There are many ways to reduce the impact of cravings, such as distracting yourself to block the intrusive thoughts of specific foods or being mindful of how you feel. Consider the time of your next meal and decide which approach might work best for you.

Snacking mindfully

Munching while working on your laptop is one way not to notice what you are consuming, never mind how much. Research shows that those who eat without distractions feel more satisfied and eat less over the entire day. It's worthwhile taking a break to refuel and make the most of the moment. It will also give your cognitive thinking some downtime, placing your mind in default mode so that your creative thoughts and problem-solving ideas have a chance to surface.

How to snack healthy when travelling

Snacks can be a healthy part of your day if you choose wisely. It can also play a significant role in reducing fatigue, maintaining your weight and health when travelling on a business trip. So here are our top tips on how to snack healthily.

Have a brilliant breakfast

No doubt you put fuel in your car before setting out on a long journey. It's no different when you're travelling on business. You've been fasting all night, but the engine has still been running. Breakfast is the time to break the fast and refuel to prevent it running to empty and stalling.

Having breakfast not only provides your body with immediate fuel but also with essential nutrients to help the body run more efficiently. If you miss breakfast, you increase the likelihood of becoming run down from missing vital nutrients as well as overeating later. In fact, evidence shows people who eat breakfast are generally slimmer than those who skip it, and they also eat more healthily throughout the day.

Don't miss meals

Missing a meal, such as lunch or dinner, is also a sure-fire way to feel fatigued and hungry for the rest of the day. If you're travelling, it's the last thing you need as it leaves you more open to constant grazing, grabbing unhealthy snacks and feeling more jet-lagged. It also makes it harder to reach all your recommended nutrient intakes leaving you more susceptible to being irritable, dehydrated and unproductive.

Drink first!

It's not unusual to mistake thirst for hunger. After all, it is the same part of your brain which is responsible for interpreting thirst which also interprets hunger signals. If you have eaten in the last three or four hours, then it might be thirst more than hungry. It's important to know the difference between thirst and hunger, particularly when travelling.

Being thirsty might indicate you are already slightly dehydrated. So, before you have a snack, consider having a drink first. Wait ten minutes and then check if you still feel hungry. Otherwise, you could be consuming more calories than you need by snacking more often than you need to.

Have a two-snack maximum

Having a more structured approach to snacking will support a healthier travel regime. Health professionals recommend limiting your snacks to a maximum of two a day as a good rule of thumb unless you are very active. If you are travelling with an early morning start and arriving at your destination late in the evening, then that's two bridges you can cross en route.

Start with your first 'danger' time of the day, let's say mid-morning when the gap between an early breakfast and lunch is longer than usual or before you pass through security as snack options post security might be less healthy. Then you can have a second snack option later in the day before hunger strikes again.

Go for whole grains

Make the basis of your snack a whole grain. Whole grains, whether it be wheat, rice, maize, oats, barley, rye and millet, have all parts of the grain left intact by minimal processing necessary to make it palatable. Having not been refined through further processing to remove various components, they contain, in addition to complex carbohydrates, more vitamins, minerals and more fibre, and subsequently take longer to digest.

As a result, whole grains offer a slower release of energy compared to refined grains, along with greater satiety. Science also shows people consuming whole grains have a lower risk of type 2 diabetes and heart disease.

The combo snack

Think about what you may miss out during the day. If your last meal lacked one of the basic four food groups (vegetables & fruit, protein, carbohydrate and dairy products) then consider adding these foods to your snack regime. For example, if your breakfast is mainly carbohydrate, such as toast, then consider adding dairy, fruit and protein to your mid-morning snack. Combinations, such as fruit and nuts sprinkled on plain yoghurt, or hummus, pine nuts and carrot sticks, are great ways to increase your calcium, protein and soluble fibre which your breakfast may have been lacking in.

Food Swaps

If you recognise your hunger is more hedonic (craving pleasurable foods) than needing to supply more energy to the body, then consider food swaps. Try to 'kerb' your desire to eat something sweet (chocolate) or crunchy (crisps) with something less 'damaging'. So instead of reaching for a biscuit with your coffee, tempt yourself with banana, or rather than grabbing a packet of crisps in a hurry, try replacing it with carrots and hummus. If you lack the conviction to swap, then ask yourself: are you really hungry or just craving a particular food or taste sensation?

Incorporate one of your five a day

At least five portions of fruit and vegetables each day are recommended by health professionals to supply sufficient nutrients and fibre for your daily diet. Yet, two-thirds of us do not consume the minimum five portions a day, and most of us do not consume sufficient fibre. Travelling on business can make the challenge to meet this requirement even more problematic. You never know what is available or on offer until you start your journey.

For this reason, you may prefer to take your own fruit or vegetable items with you. Many fruit and vegetables are perfectly packaged for snacking on the go. Apples, bananas, satsumas, dried fruit mixes, mini bags of carrots, cucumber sticks or cherry tomatoes can make a great addition to your trip regime.

We've also done some exploring for you. Snacks which incorporate fresh fruit and vegetables found at Gatwick's North Terminal are listed below this section. In addition, we have listed where to find fresh fruit, salads, soups and vegetable portions in Chapter 14.

Mix and match

Combining commercial snack packets can reduce the amount of fat, salt and sugar per portion. If you combine half a portion of a savoury snack, such as walnuts or roasted corn with half a portion of a sweet snack such as dried apricots, then you will get half the proportion of sugar, fat and salt in a whole portion.

We've listed all the packets of dried fruit, nuts and seeds we found at Gatwick's North Terminal below.

Ready snacks to go

Planning in advance is a great way to make sure your snacks are healthy, satisfying and to your taste. Not only does it eliminate the supermarket sweep at the last minute in the airport café, where most items are unsuitable, but it is also less expensive. Keep a pantry of non-perishable items which you can quickly throw in your hand luggage. Items could include small packets of raisins, UHT rice pudding, a small packet of olives or gherkins, oat biscuits, high fibre crackers, cereal, beef jerky, larger packets of baked corn, popcorn, nuts and seeds.

Remember, the last thing you want is travellers' tummy, so take care with perishable items which need refrigeration. These are best either left at home or purchased post-security and eaten within two hours. There is also the option of taking a 25 ml or 50 ml freezer block through security. For more information, go to our website review at http://www.extravitality.co/which-ice-packs-are-best-when-travelling/

Make your own trail mix

Making your trail mix enables you to control the taste as well as the nutritional content. If you have a fondness for certain nuts, seeds and dried fruit, or a specific dietary requirement, you can bring these with you rather than relying on what you can gather at Gatwick Airport's North Terminal.

Where to find great snacks to take with you

Catering establishments are beginning to realise their customers want healthier options and are starting to supply items which may be suitable. So, we've explored Gatwick Airport's North Terminal for you to find a selection of healthier snack options for you to choose from. Some are packaged, enabling the items to travel with you, and others are freshly served, making them better suited to immediate consumption while relaxing.

We've listed items which match the criteria we have outlined above. Sole food items or items from one food group will never supply a perfect nutrient profile, so sometimes it is better to mix and match pieces to provide a healthier option, such as an apple with cheese or dried fruit with nuts. Items high in added fat, sugar or salt have been excluded from this selection. Milk-based or fruit options where they contain intrinsic sugars (those naturally present in a whole food) have been included, but snacks with excess added sugar, honey or syrup have also been excluded.

Sometimes snacks come with optional items to add, such as soy sauce or dressing. Where this may add excessive salt or fat, we have included the snack but suggested without the addition of the option provided. Sometimes a food item might provide a set of nutrients which are often missing from diets, but they might be high in fat, such as cheese, avocado or eggs. In this instance, we've assessed the merit of the food as a contribution to the diet as a whole, although we may also suggest moderation.

Beware of dried fruit as a regular snack as it can cause tooth decay by becoming stuck between your teeth. Dried fruit is best eaten after dinner in exchange for a dessert or with another food, for example, raisins to complement nuts or a dairy product such as apricots with cream cheese on crackers or dried berries to top yoghurt.

Alongside each suggestion, we have stated any calorific information supplied by the catering establishment and food manufacturers. We rely solely on the provision of information supplied as being accurate and in accord with EU regulations. Where they haven't provided any nutritional information, we have only listed foods that are either from a single food group, e.g. salad, yoghurt, cheese, fruit or combination items which match recommended dietary guidelines.

Snacking to take with you

The snack options listed in this section are those which you can eat while you travel or are suitable to take on board the plane. They are all in sealed packages and are ready for transport.

We would add, that if you are taking nuts on a plane to ask the air staff if there is anyone with nut allergies on board first. In particular, we would urge you to consult those sitting around you before opening a nut-filled snack packet.

Boots the Chemist

Boots the Chemist is located on the lower level of the Departure Lounge and in the Arrivals Hall, next to M&S Simply Food. There are two Boots shops in the Departure Lounge. The nearest one to the security exit is the smaller. They stock a limited range of food items, both fresh and dried. The second, the larger of the two, is at the far end of the lower level, where they stock a much broader range of snack items. There is also a fruit and vegetable bar where you can buy fresh packets of freshly sliced fruit and fruit pots.

Although the selection isn't as vast as M&S Simply Food pre-security, you won't have any problems with security and can stock up on other options as well, including yoghurts, jellies, smoothies and water.

Opening in Arrivals: 24 hours
Opening in Departure Lounge: 4.00 am to 8.30 pm

Items to consider include:

Dried snacks

Apricots 35 g packet Dried apricots are a good source of fibre and iron. They also offer some vitamin C and vitamin E, along with some antioxidants. When combined with another snack such as walnuts, it can provide an excellent combination of nutrients for a busy traveller. This packet provides 92 kcal (390 kJ)

Walnuts 40 g packet. Walnuts are high in fat, mainly derived from unsaturated fat, and high in vitamin E. They are also a good source of other vitamins and minerals, along with melatonin, which helps reduce the time for the onset of sleep. However, if it's only an afternoon snack you desire, then consider combining half the packet with other snacks, such as the apricots mentioned above, to reduce the calorie content while boosting the nutritional content. This packet provides 287 kcal (1186 kJ)

Edamame Beans 50 g These are very high in protein and fibre, and low in salt, making them a great alternative to other dried snack foods. This packet provides 210 kcal (882 kJ)

Wasabi Peas 50 g Although a high source of protein and fibre, these peas are dried, and salt has been added. This packet provides 201 kcal (847 kJ)

Mixed Nuts This packet provides 177 kcal (741 kJ)

Urban Magnificent Mango 100 g or 35 g snack pack. Not only is it a good source of fibre but mango is also known for their vitamin C content, modest amounts of other vitamins (folate, E and K) and phytonutrients. 35 g portion provides 104 kcal (434 kJ)

Urban Perfect Pineapple 100g or 35 g snack pack. Excellent source of fibre and vitamin B Folate. A 35 g snack pack provides 100 kcal (420 kJ)

Fresh food snacks

Carrot Sticks and Hummus Pack provides 110 kcal (457kJ)

Spinach and Egg One free-range hard-boiled egg and fresh spinach. Consider adding a source of whole grain, such as one of the other dishes or some rye crackers to complement this dish further. Portion provides 106 kcal (442 kJ)

Cheddar Cheese and Red Pepper 70 g Comprises cheddar cheese, red pepper and a smoky barbeque dip. Cheese is a good source of protein, calcium, vitamin A and riboflavin (a B vitamin). Red peppers complement the taste and the nutritional value by adding fibre, vitamin C and vitamin A. Packet provides160 kcal (665 kJ)

Apple and Cheddar Apple wedges with Cheddar Cheese. This pack provides 93 kcal (388 kJ)

Avocado Houmous with Veggies Carrot and cucumber batons with avocado houmous. This packet provides 76 kcal (313 kJ)

Beetroot Houmous with Breadsticks Miniature breadsticks with beetroot houmous. This packet provides 136 kcal (569 kJ)

Muki beans with Humous and Pumpkin Seed 105 g Make bean (soya) and humous with pumpkin seeds and chilli. The soya beans, pumpkin seeds and chickpeas both supply protein, along with fibre and iron. There is a little carbohydrate, so if you're hungry, you might want to combine this with another option such as vegetable sticks or whole grain flatbreads. Portion provides 190 kcal (789 kJ)

Smoked Salmon Sushi Snack One smoked salmon in sweet chilli California roll with black sesame seed coating, two cucumber hosomaki, two smoked salmon hosomaki, one bottle of gluten free, low salt soya sauce. Boots have used a low salt soya sauce, so if you want to reduce the salt content further, do not add the sauce to the sushi. The pack provides 103 kcal (437 kJ)

Prawn & Salmon Sushi Prawn mayonnaise and red pepper California rolls with black sesame seed coating. Surimi and Edamame bean California roll with a black sesame seed coating. Smoked salmon nigiri. King prawn nigiri. Smoked mackerel mayonnaise hosomaki. Wasabi sachet. One bottle of gluten free low salt soya sauce. Boots have used a low salt soya sauce, so if you want to reduce the salt content further, do not add the sauce to the sushi. The pack provides 204 kcal (861 kJ)

Veggie Sushi Snack Edamame, carrot and red cabbage California roll with beetroot rice, cucumber Hosomaki, red pepper Hosomaki. This packet provides 93 kcal (395 kJ)

Veggie Quinoa Sushi. A selection of Californian and Nigiri vegetable sushi. The packet provides 172 kcal (727 kJ)

Pulled Pork Rice Burger Pulled pork, Yuzu sauce and pickled cucumber sushi burger with sesame seed topping, and an Edamame and Coriander Hosomaki. Bottle of gluten free low salt soya sauce. The packet provides 187 kcal (792 kJ)

Small Salads

Rainbow Salad Carrot, mixed grains, beetroot, butternut squash and broccoli with an orange and mustard dressing. This packet provides 154kcal (643kJ)

Moroccan Style Veggie Couscous Salad Seasoned couscous with roasted butternut squash and aubergines, cos lettuce and a Moroccan style dressing. Salad provides 161 kcal (676 kJ)

Kimchi & Edamame Salad with Brown Rice Kimchi, edamame and mango on a mixed vegetable and seasoned rice bed, topped with coriander and served with a bottle of gluten-free, low salt soya sauce. Salad provides 184 kcal (777 kJ)

Costa Coffee

Many of the options available at Costa Coffee are over 200 calories. As a result, our list is currently limited in choice for a snack. We hope to see a wider range over the next year or so. For now, the fruit and nut options are a suitable quick grab option to take on board.

Locations: Arrivals Hall, right next to the International Arrivals exit, and Check-in Level 1.
Opening in Arrivals: 24 hours
Opening in Check-in: 4.00 am and 8.00 pm

Items to consider include:

Dried Mango Simply dried mango. Naturally, high in sugar, this snack is a great topper to yoghurt or mixed with additional nuts and seeds. The packet provides 120 kcal (511 kJ)

Fruit & Nut Mix Comprises of raisin, cashew nuts, almonds and walnuts. The packet provides 204 kcal (847 kJ)

Fresh Fruit Pot The pot provides 45 kcal (190 kJ)

Free Range Eggs Hard boiled eggs with spinach leaf. The pot provides 116 kcal (483 kJ)

Bananas are found next to the cash register.

Mixed Berry Compote 38 kcal (161 kJ)

Tuna Nicoise Salad Salad provides 219 kcal (914 kJ)

Roast Chicken Salad Salad provides 223 kcal (929 kJ)

Organic 0% Fat Greek Style Yoghurt This pot provides 67 kcal (286 kJ).
Sprinkle the yoghurt with:
Raspberry Coconut and Seed Sprinkle A sprinkle provides 87 kcal (361 kJ)
Maple Granola & Coconut Sprinkle A sprinkle provides 85 kcal (355 kJ)

London News Company

London News has a limited selection of snacks which fitted our specific criteria for a healthier snack. Here are a couple which you might take with you on board.

Location: Arrivals and Departure Lounge.
Open: Arrivals 24 hours, Departure Lounge 4.00 am to 8.30 pm

London News Company Locations: In the far-left corner of the Check-in, level two, next to Moneycorpo. On the upper floor of Departures opposite BLOC hotel entrance, and just before World Duty Free on the left-hand side on the lower level of the Departure Lounge, post-security.
Opening hours: Before security 24 hours and post security 4.00 am to 9.00 pm

Proper Corn - Lightly sea salted popcorn 20 g Low in fat, sugar and protein per portion, mainly complex carbohydrates and some fibre. While this is a low energy option, satisfying the need for some crunch, it may not fill you up for long. Portion provides 88 kcal (368 kJ)

Urban Magnificent Mango 100 g or 35 g snack pack. Not only is it a good source of fibre but mango is also known for their vitamin C content, modest amounts of other vitamins (folate, E and K) and phytonutrients. 35 g portion provides 104 kcal (434 kJ)

Urban Cheeky Cherries. 100 g or 35 g snack pack. Just the cherries, which are gently baked. Good source of fibre and melatonin, along with vitamin C. Studies on tart cherries offer many nutritional properties. Some claim to decrease inflammation and reduce the risk of heart disease. A 35 g snack pack provides 93 kcal (391 kJ)

Urban Perfect Pineapple 100g or 35 g snack pack. Excellent source of fibre and vitamin B Folate. A 35 g snack pack provides 100 kcal (420 kJ)

Urban Ravishing Raspberry 100 g or 35 g snack pack. Good source of anthocyanin, vitamins E and K. A 35 g snack pack provides 104 kcal (434 kJ)

Urban Smashing Strawberry 100 g or 35 g Just strawberries and a bit of apple juice. Good source of fibre, vitamin C, manganese, folate and potassium. A 35 g pack provides 103 kcal (431 kJ)

M&S Simply Food

M&S Simply Food at Gatwick North is a small supermarket offering packaged food items which you can take on board with you. Provided they are not liquid or a gel exceeding 100 ml they should make it through security. The store is open all day making it ideal if you have just arrived and need something to sustain you while you continue your journey.

Snack items range from packets of dried fruit and nuts to fresh protein pots, mixed salads and sushi. You can purchase the dried fruits and nuts either in a small individual portion or a large packet. The protein pots also make an excellent snack, supplying fibre and protein in decent amounts, packed full of nutrients, while at the same time restricted in fat, saturated fat, sugar and salt.

Fresh sushi is also available to take on board. If you choose a fresh item, then ensure you eat it soon after purchase to avoid any unwanted traveller's tummy. All items have a use by date and nutritional information on the package. Healthier items are sometimes on special offer and display an 'Eat well' logo.

There is also plenty of fresh fruit, yoghurts and other essential food commodities.

Open: 24 hours
Location: Arrivals Hall, just opposite the International Arrivals exit.

Items to consider include:

Packet dried food snacks

Wasabi Peas 50g portion pack or a 200g pack. Roasted green peas with a flavoured wasabi coating. – High in complex carbohydrate and a good source of fibre and protein. 50 g pack provides 214 kcal (903 kJ)

Raisins 50 g portion pack. Partially rehydrated jumbo raisins. 50 g pack provides 145 kcal (615 kJ)

Dried Apricots 80 g portion pack. Dried soft apricots. Dried apricots are a good source of iron, potassium and vitamin K. 80 g pack provides 147 kcal (615 kJ)

Seed & Nut Mix 70 g packet. Available also in a 200 g packet. Roasted sunflower seeds, pumpkin seeds, almonds and cashew nut halves with soy sauce. High in fat, derived mainly from unsaturated fats within the nuts and seeds. Excellent amount of protein, a good source of fibre and zinc. For a healthier snack of 200 calories, consume half of the packet. 70 g pack provides 427 kcal (1766 kJ)

Walnut Halves 85 g pack. Guidelines on this pack are for a 30 g portion. Walnuts are a good source of melatonin, the 'sleep' hormone. Walnuts are also a good source of fibre, vitamin E and high in fat, mainly unsaturated fat. Research suggests walnuts may help to reduce inflammation and LDL cholesterol. They are also linked to lower blood pressure and improved blood vessel function. Per 30 g portion 212 kcal (874 kJ)

Lightly Salted Giant Corn Snacks 140 g According to the packet information, this contains four portions of snacks. Corn offers a good source of fibre, complex carbohydrate and protein. Corn also contains several antioxidants. 30 g serving provides 134 kcal (565 kJ)

Jalapeno Giant Corn 140 g The packet information indicates a portion is 30 g or approximately five portions in this pack, which is quite small. You might find it easier to divide the pack into three (50 g) and follow the nutritional information for a third of the pack. A 30 g serving provides 135 kcal (566 kJ)

Superberry and Almond Mix 150 g Described as a mix of dried fruit, honey-coated almonds and roasted almonds. This pre-mixed packet contains raisins, goldenberries, sour cherries, blueberries, golden raisins and almonds. A portion is labelled as 25 g. 25 g portion provides 127 kcal (529 kJ)

Fresh food snacks

Anti Pasta Selection Pitted Halkidiki olives with mozzarella cheese and marinated semi-dried tomatoes. The packet provides 115 kcal (475 kJ)

Oak Smoked Salmon & Egg Protein Pot Boiled egg, smoked salmon and spinach. The pot provides 106 kcal (442 kJ)

355

Reduced Fat Houmous with Crunchy Carrot Sticks 130g Comprises carrots and reduced fat houmous. Good source of fibre. The pack provides 157 kcal (651 kJ)

Chicken & Avocado Protein Pot Cooked chicken breast, couscous, red quinoa and spinach with avocado dip. Pot provides 171 kcal (714 kJ)

Egg and Avocado Protein Pot 140 g This pot contains boiled free range eggs, quinoa and avocado with parsley and light soy sauce. Avocados are an excellent source of fibre and monounsaturated fat, which both help to lower cholesterol. Both eggs and avocado offer different B vitamins and complement each other. Where they may lack some minerals, the quinoa makes up for it, particularly with iron and fibre. You can reduce the salt content by not adding the soy sauce. Pot provides 185 kcal (776 kJ)

Free Range Egg & Spinach Protein Pot. 105 g. Two cooked free-range eggs and spinach. Eggs are an excellent source of protein containing all the indispensable amino acids we need for our nutritional requirements, as well as a good source of vitamin D. The pot provides 152 kcal (633 kJ)

Glorious Greens & Seeds Veggie Pot Edamame soybeans, sugar snap peas, spinach and lemon roasted seeds with a pea dip with mint infused sunflower oil. Pot provides 159 kcal (660 kJ)

Beautiful Beets & Feta Veggie Pot Cooked beetroot, feta cheese, rocket and toasted pumpkin seeds with a beetroot and mint dip. Per pot 182 kcal (676 kJ)

Turmeric Chicken Salad Bites in mooli ribbons with a chilli, lime and coriander sauce. The pack provides 66 kcal (276 kJ)

Tempting Taster Two soy and ginger chicken, and two pea puree and pickled carrot California rolls with soy sauce. The pack provides 164 kcal (689 kJ)

Sushi Snack One tuna and cucumber California roll, red pepper and a cucumber maki with soy sauce. To reduce the salt content, do not use the soy sauce. Snack pack provides 115 kcal (486 kJ)

Vegetable Sushi Comprises chargrilled yellow pepper nigiri, one asparagus and sugar snap pea, one mango and red pepper and one pea puree and pickled carrot California rolls; two pickled carrot maki with soy sauce, pickled ginger and wasabi with optional soy sauce. To reduce the salt content, do not add the soy sauce. Sushi provides 182 kcal (769 kJ)

Strawberry Quinoa Yoghurt Pot Strawberry compote, quinoa and fat-free Greek-style yoghurt topped with mixed seeds. Per pot: 171 kcal (718 kJ)

Small Salads

Sesame King Prawn & Rice Salad with a teriyaki dressing. Hold the dressing to reduce the salt content. Salad provides 242 kcal (1017 kJ)

Sesame Chilli Chicken & Red Rice Salad with a hot sriracha chilli dressing. Salad provides 229 kcal (964 kJ)

Honey Smoked Salmon & Lentil Salad with a creamy lemon dressing. Salad provides 253 kcal (1063 kJ)

Starbucks

Starbucks is located on the upper level of the Departure Lounge. It offers a selection of dried snack packets. There is also whole fruit and some fruit salads which you can add as a snack item before boarding.

Open: 24 hours
Location: Upper Level in the Departure Lounge, next to Jamie's Italian Restaurant.

Whole Fruit Bananas, apples, oranges
Fruit Mix One portion provides 82 kcal (350 kJ)
Starbucks Almonds, Cashews, Cranberries & Yellow Raisins. One packet provides 187 kcal (780 kJ)

Snacking while relaxing

Departure Lounge, Lower Level, Lounges

If you prefer to snack when taking a break or trying to relax before your flight, then the airport lounges are ideal if you are a member. They offer a variety of snacks. The snack items range from a small bowl of nibble style snacks to hot dishes on a buffet. While one lounge may offer a more informal setting with a restricted range compared to another lounge, they all have something for the business traveller who may want a quick healthier snack before their flight.

No. 1 Lounge

No. 1 Lounge has an extensive range of snacks and nibbles for the weary traveller, including salads, soup, baked goods, fruit and finger nibbles. As you walk into the lounge from the reception, head straight through the bar area, down a few steps, to the buffet selection which awaits you. Here, depending on the time of day, you will find a range of fresh food waiting for you. At the time of review, No. 1 Lounge had an impressive array of five salads in addition to other typical snacks.

Open: 4.00 am to 10.00 pm
Location: On the lower level of the Departure Lounge.
Directions: Head towards gate 101 – 113, as you pass London News Company, turn right into the corridor, you will see another hallway on your right. Enter the hallway and walk through the double glass doors. No.1 Lounge is directly ahead.

Aspire Lounge

The buffet options in the middle of the Aspire Lounge are of mixed fare. The snacks options include a hot penne pasta or soup, fruit, baked items and dried nibbles. If it is a light snack you are after then this is satisfactory.

Open: Open hours are from 4.00 am to 10.00 pm with a slight seasonal variation.
Location: First floor of the Departure Lounge.
Directions: Head towards gate 101 – 113, as you pass London News Company, you will see a corridor on your right. Go through the double glass doors and take the lift to the first floor. The lounge is located on the right-hand side.

My Lounge

Although more informal than the No. 1 Lounge and the Aspire Lounge, there is also a buffet of snacks. These include a hot vegetable dish which you can add accompaniments to and a selection of nibbles. What it does lack are the baked goods. However, this is a good thing, as those typically offered in other lounges usually comprise cakes, biscuits and pastries, and so this is no loss to the healthier selection available. In its place, it offers a fresh selection of vegetables and dried snacks.

Open: 6.00 am to 8.00 pm.
Location: Departure Lounge, lower level.
Directions: Head towards gate 101 – 113, as you pass London News Company, you will see a corridor on your right. Turn right and proceed through the double glass doors. The lounge is located on the left-hand side just before the lifts.

Departure Lounge, Upper Level

Many of the restaurants and cafes are located on the top level of the Departure Lounge. We have found an array of healthier snack options for you to choose. Wherever possible, we have listed the calorific content so that you can choose according to your individual requirements.

Where nutritional information has not been available, we have selected options which stand out as being a healthier option compared to their menu counterparts which would be higher in fat, salt and sugar.

Armadillo

Armadillo offers a South West cuisine. Nutritional information was not available for this restaurant, making it difficult to choose with accuracy which items could be regarded as healthier snacks. Therefore, we have selected a couple which should be suitable. These are all from the small plate selection.

Location: At the end nearest to the security exit, overlooking the balcony, opposite from Garfunkel's.
Open: 4.00 am to 8.30 pm

Healthier snacks options may include:

Street Snack Salad mango, mouli, cucumber crudites with chilli salt and lime wedge, additional herby yoghurt dip.
Homecooked Tortilla Chips and Dips Choose from green chilli tomatillo sauce, guacamole, pico de gallo salsa.
Little Kale Caesar Salad Smokey Caesar dressing, crushed chilli croutons, Grana Padano.
Grilled Corn on the Cob

EAT

Eat is a very busy café, with seating spread out over two areas. You can either snack in the café or take the items with you on board your flight. Snack item range includes half portion wraps, salad protein pots, fresh fruit and dried snacks packets. There's certainly more variety here than the other cafés pre-security.

Location: In the middle of the upper level, next to Garfunkel's and opposite Shake-A-Hula
Open: 4.00 am to 8.30 pm

Healthier snacks options may include:

Grape bag One small bag provides 90 kcal (377 kJ)
Mango & Lime One small packet provides 85 kcal (356 kJ)
Big Fruit Salad This salad provides 120 kcal (502 kJ)
Rainbow Fruit Salad Mango, kiwi, blueberries and pomegranate combined in a colourful rainbow fruit salad. One small pot is 66 kcal (276 kJ)
Summer Berries This mix provides 40 kcal (167 kJ)
Smokey Almond & Corn 30 g A mix of smoked flavoured roasted corn and almonds. A snack which contains corn with almonds essentially combines to form a good

quality source of protein, fibre, along with other vitamins and minerals. This packet provides 141 (590 kJ)

Fava Beans, Chickpeas & Roasted Pumpkin Seeds Roasted and salted fava beans, chickpeas and pumpkin seeds. This packet provides 156 kcal (653 kJ)

Natural Nuts A mix of almonds, pistachios, hazelnuts and cashews. This packet provides 222 kcal (929 kJ)

Smoky Almonds & Corn Almonds and corn with a hickory smoke flavour. This packet provides 141 (590 kJ)

Smoked Salmon & Egg Fit Box Smoked Salmon served with egg, chargrilled garlic and chilli broccoli, spinach and salsa verde dressing. This box provides 202 kcal (845 kJ)

Free-range Egg & Chilli Greens A whole free-range egg served with edamame beans, peas, spinach and chilli with a dash of lemon juice. This snack provides 116 kcal (485 kJ)

Houmous & Crudite Pot Creamy houmous served with crunch carrot batons and sweet sugar snap peas. This snack provides 246 kcal (1029 kJ)

Tuna & Cucumber Half Baguette Dolphin friendly skipjack tuna mayonnaise mix with cucumber on a freshly baked white baguette. This half baguette provides 263 kcal (1100 kJ)

Italian Meatballs Small Soup A rustic soup of meatballs and cannellini beans in a chunky tomato sauce with chilli, basil and oregano. A small portion provides 228 kcal (954 kJ)

Jamie's Italian

For a more luxury snack attack, you might like to consider Jamie's Italian Restaurant. It has several healthier items on the menu which would work well for an early morning to late afternoon snack. You can also pop to the bakery and choose a small salad selection (there are at least four) to take with you on board the plane if time is a little too tight. Alternatively, you could also choose the Union Jacks bar as the menu is the same as the main restaurant.

Location: Far end of the upper level, next to Wagamama and opposite Yo! Sushi.
Open: 3.30 am to 8.30 pm

Healthier snacks options may include:
Tomato Bruschetta Slow-roasted cherry tomatoes, buffalo ricotta, basil & extra virgin olive oil. Tomatoes are often a forgotten vegetable, yet they are high in lycopene, which reduces the risk of prostate cancer and supports cardiovascular health. Per portion 188 kcal (787 kJ)

Margherita Arancini Tomato & mozzarella-stuffed risotto balls with Pomodoro sauce. This dish provides 272 kcal (1138 kJ)

Bread Board Freshly baked focaccia, music bread, grissini & black olive tapenade. This breadboard provides 282 kcal (1180 kJ)

Super Food Salad Avocado, roasted beets, pulses & grains, broccoli, pomegranate, spicy seeds & harissa. A small portion provides 179 kcal (749 kJ)

Pret A Manger

Pret A Manger is a small café close to the escalator at the far end of the upper level. It offers takeaways as well as seating, inside the café and on the balcony overlooking the lower level. We've selected several snack options here for you to choose.

There is a good assortment of snacks here, including veggie pots, salad boxes, sandwiches and soups. Although many of the soups at Pret A Manger are under 200 calories, they are proportionally high in salt. We've chosen only two soups as they have the lowest salt content and are only one-sixth of the maximum daily amount health professionals recommend. Similarly, the open sandwiches are also moderately high in salt, mainly from the rye bread base. We've selected sandwiches which are low in calories making them more suitable for a snack, and a good source of other vital nutrients for you to try.

Location: On the left at the far end of the upper level, opposite the escalator.
Open: 3.00 am to 8.30 pm

Mango & Banana Sunshine Bowl Blended mango and banana, with a splash of coconut milk and dash of turmeric, topped with granola, blueberries and coconut chips. Per portion; 253 kcal (1042 kJ)

Avo & Super-Greens Veggie Pot 136 g serving. Avocado, peas, edamame and coriander with a sprinkling of sesame seeds and served with a pot of our zingy green dressing. This small vegetable pot is a good source of fibre, and a modest amount of protein derived mainly from the edamame beans. Naturally high in fat which is primarily unsaturated fat from the avocado. Avocados are also a good source of B vitamins and vitamins C, E, K, along with potassium and antioxidants. This vegetable pot provides 222 kcal (918 kJ)

Smoked Salmon & Egg Protein Pot Scottish smoked salmon and a free-range egg with baby spinach. Served with a lemon wedge and seasoning. Per portion 134 kcal (560 kJ)

Soups

Souper Tomato 370 g serving. Tomato soup with chopped, diced and simmered super-ripe plum tomatoes, tomato puree, vegetables and herbs. Good source of fibre, moderate fat content, and moderate salt content. 370 g serving provides 199 kcal (831 kJ)

Vegetable Tagine Side Soup 220 g serving Roasted courgettes and peppers cooked in vegetable stock with cumin, turmeric, red chilli and cinnamon. Served with tomatoes, chickpeas, buckwheat and red lentils. 220 g serving provides 112 kcal (469 kJ)

Smoky Chorizo Chicken Side Soup 220 g serving. Chunks of smoky chorizo simmered with chicken, tomatoes, cannellini beans, celery, peppers and carrot. Finished with smoked paprika and a mix of herbs. 220 g serving provides 132 kcal (554 kJ)

Veggie Chilli Side Soup 220 g serving. Black turtle beans, red kidney beans and black-eyed beans, peppers, sweetcorn, brown rice and quinoa with ancho chilli, cocoa, Jalapeno chilli and a hint of lime. 220 g serving provides 130 kcal (541 kJ)